Brief Dynamic Interpersonal Therapy

Brief Dynamic Interpersonal Therapy

A Clinician's Guide

SECOND EDITION ■

ALESSANDRA LEMMA
FELLOW, BRITISH PSYCHOANALYTIC SOCIETY
VISITING PROFESSOR, PSYCHOANALYSIS UNIT,
UNIVERSITY COLLEGE LONDON
CONSULTANT, ANNA FREUD CENTRE

**MARY HEPWORTH
(FORMERLY MARY TARGET)**
CHARTERED CLINICAL PSYCHOLOGIST;
FELLOW, BRITISH PSYCHOANALYTIC SOCIETY
PROFESSOR OF PSYCHOANALYSIS,
UNIVERSITY COLLEGE LONDON

PETER FONAGY
FELLOW, BRITISH PSYCHOANALYTIC SOCIETY
PROFESSOR OF CONTEMPORARY PSYCHOANALYSIS
AND DEVELOPMENTAL SCIENCE,
UNIVERSITY COLLEGE LONDON
CHIEF EXECUTIVE, ANNA FREUD CENTRE

DEBORAH ABRAHAMS
CLINICAL PSYCHOLOGIST AND PSYCHOANALYST,
BRITISH PSYCHOANALYTIC SOCIETY
PROGRAMME DIRECTOR OF DIT, ANNA FREUD CENTRE

PATRICK LUYTEN
PROFESSOR OF CLINICAL PSYCHOLOGY,
UNIVERSITY OF LEUVEN
PROFESSOR OF PSYCHODYNAMIC PSYCHOLOGY,
UNIVERSITY COLLEGE LONDON

OXFORD
UNIVERSITY PRESS

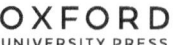

Great Clarendon Street, Oxford, OX2 6DP,
United Kingdom

Oxford University Press is a department of the University of Oxford.
It furthers the University's objective of excellence in research, scholarship,
and education by publishing worldwide. Oxford is a registered trade mark of
Oxford University Press in the UK and in certain other countries

© Oxford University Press 2024

The moral rights of the authors have been asserted

All rights reserved. No part of this publication may be reproduced, stored in
a retrieval system, or transmitted, in any form or by any means, without the
prior permission in writing of Oxford University Press, or as expressly permitted
by law, by licence or under terms agreed with the appropriate reprographics
rights organization. Enquiries concerning reproduction outside the scope of the
above should be sent to the Rights Department, Oxford University Press, at the
address above

You must not circulate this work in any other form
and you must impose this same condition on any acquirer

Published in the United States of America by Oxford University Press
198 Madison Avenue, New York, NY 10016, United States of America

British Library Cataloguing in Publication Data
Data available

Library of Congress Control Number is on file at the Library of Congress

ISBN 978–0–19–886747–0

DOI: 10.1093/med-psych/9780198867470.001.0001

Printed and bound by CPI Group (UK) Ltd,
Croydon, CR0 4YY

Oxford University Press makes no representation, express or implied, that the
drug dosages in this book are correct. Readers must therefore always check
the product information and clinical procedures with the most up-to-date
published product information and data sheets provided by the manufacturers
and the most recent codes of conduct and safety regulations. The authors and
the publishers do not accept responsibility or legal liability for any errors in the
text or for the misuse or misapplication of material in this work. Except where
otherwise stated, drug dosages and recommendations are for the non-pregnant
adult who is not breast-feeding

Links to third party websites are provided by Oxford in good faith and
for information only. Oxford disclaims any responsibility for the materials
contained in any third party website referenced in this work.

The manufacturer's authorised representative in the EU for
product safety is Oxford University Press España S.A. of el Parque
Empresarial San Fernando de Henares, Avenida de Castilla, 2 –
28830 Madrid (www.oup.es/en).

PREFACE TO SECOND EDITION

Dynamic interpersonal therapy (DIT) was developed in 2009. The first iteration of the DIT model was published by OUP in 2011. DIT was the product of a collaboration with colleagues committed to improving access to psychoanalytic interventions in the National Health Service (NHS) in the United Kingdom and beyond. We wanted to distil best practice and engage in a research programme to contribute to a more substantive body of evidence supporting psychoanalytic interventions for a range of clinical presentations. We want to thank the Tavistock and Portman NHS Trust and the Anna Freud Centre for supporting this work and, in particular, Matthew Patrick, Louise Lyon, and Ros Bidmead for facilitating a rich and productive collaboration across these two leading mental health organizations.

We first piloted DIT in a dynamic and thriving NHS primary care psychology service based in Tower Hamlets, London, which was at the time led by Mary Burd and her wonderful team. Without their vision and enthusiasm for trialling the model we would not have been able to carry out the first pilot study and write the first edition of this book. Several colleagues from this team have since become valued supervisors and trainers in DIT, and we are very grateful to them: Tamara Gelman, Jane Gibbon, Lucy Marks, and Anne McKay.

Over the past 13 years we have developed further specific applications of the model, and we describe these in this new edition. The twenty-six-session model of DIT for complex care (DITCC) was first piloted in an NHS secondary care service in Newham, London. We are deeply grateful to Amra Rao for her leadership and facilitation, along with her colleagues' commitment to implementing this model and refining it through their clinical experience. In particular, we would like to thank Gosia Fijak-Koch, Anne McKay, and Marta Sosnowska.

Jeremy Clarke has been a constant advocate of psychoanalytic approaches in the NHS and we are grateful to him for his support in establishing DIT provision within the NHS. We are also much indebted to Tamara Ventura Wurman for her operationalization and development of a measure of therapist competence for DIT.

The training and research developments over the past 13 years that have contributed to this second edition would not have been possible without the notable contributions of Deborah Abrahams and Patrick Luyten, who have joined us as co-authors. Patrick has led not only on the development of DIT for functional somatic disorders and internet-delivered DIT (i-DIT) but also in researching these new applications. Deborah is now the director of DIT training at the Anna Freud Centre and has been central in ensuring the continued development of all DIT trainings, making these accessible to more clinicians in the UK and internationally. We are deeply grateful to Deborah and Patrick for bringing renewed vigour and creativity to the development of DIT.

Last but by no means least, we want to extend our deep gratitude to all the colleagues who chose to train in DIT in the UK and internationally, and to all our patients. Their feedback has been central to refining the model.

Professor Alessandra Lemma
Professor Mary Hepworth (formerly Mary Target)
Professor Peter Fonagy

ACKNOWLEDGEMENTS

We would like to thank our editor at OUP, Martin Baum, for encouraging us to produce a second edition and for his patience.

We are indebted to all our colleagues who—as students, supervisors, and trainers—have contributed to the development of DIT over the past 13 years.

We are very grateful to Liz Allison and colleagues at the UCL Psychoanalysis Unit for their invaluable editorial help.

CONTENTS

List of figures xvii
List of tables xix
List of boxes xxi
List of abbreviations xxiii

1. Why Dynamic Interpersonal Therapy for Mood Disorders? 1
   The rationale of DIT 1
   Psychodynamic approaches and diagnostic classification 3
   Mood disorders: depression and anxiety 7
   Assessing suitability for DIT 12
      The patient's response to an exploratory approach 12
      The patient's interest in working with interpersonal and affective themes 14
      The patient's capacity to reflect on the therapeutic relationship 15
      The patient's curiosity about their role in their difficulties 15
      The external resources that could support the patient during the course of DIT 18
      The therapist's experience with the patient in the session 19
   This second edition 20

2. Key Analytic Models and Psychoanalytic Concepts Informing Dynamic Interpersonal Therapy 25
   The theoretical framework of DIT 25
      Object-relations theory 26
      Ego functioning and theories of attachment 30
      Interpersonal psychoanalysis: The contribution of Harry Stack Sullivan 33
      Mentalizing 36
   Key psychoanalytic technical concepts that inform DIT 37
      Ability to establish and manage the therapeutic frame and boundaries 38
      Ability to work with unconscious communication 40

    Ability to recognize and work with defences 42
    Attachment perspective on defences 45
    Ability to work in the transference 46
    Ability to work with countertransference 48
    Ability to make dynamic interpretations 49
  Conclusions 51

3. Core Features and Strategies 59
  Aims 59
  Trajectory of the therapy 60
    The initial phase (sessions 1–4) 61
    The middle phase (sessions 5–12) 62
    The ending phase (sessions 13–16) 63
  The DIT foci 64
    The interpersonal-affective focus 64
    Here-and-now focus 66
    Focus on the patient's mind 68
  Therapeutic stance 70

4. The Initial Phase 75
  Engagement 75
  Listening out for 'cautionary tales' 78
    Case examples of 'cautionary tales' 80
  What do we need to know in order to formulate a dynamic focus for intervention? 81
    History-taking versus history-making 82
    History of the presenting problem: the symptom/problem from the patient's point of view 84
    Family history 85
    Medical history and the patient's bodily self 86
    Mapping the interpersonal landscape 87
  How many relationships need to be explored before sharing a formulation with the patient? 97
  Negotiating the therapeutic content and goals for therapy 97
  How much information does the patient need about DIT in order to consent to it? 98
  Managing risk and self-harm 100
  Managing the frame and the setting 101
  The use of outcome monitoring and video/audio recording of sessions 102

5. The Interpersonal-Affective Focus 109
   What is a psychodynamic formulation? 109
   The interpersonal-affective focus: an overview 110
   The patient's experience of the IPAF 113
      Case example 115
   Constructing a formulation: a step-by-step guide 118
      Step 1: Describe the problem 118
      Step 2: Describe the cost of the problem 118
      Step 3: Contextualize the problem 118
      Step 4: Describe the recurring object relationship that is meaningfully connected to the onset and/or maintenance of symptoms and the affect that is linked with the activation of the pattern 120
      Step 5: Identify the defensive function of the recurring pattern 120
   The trial interpretation: working towards sharing the IPAF 121
   Using the patient's language and metaphors 122
      Case example 123
   Using the transference and countertransference to inform the formulation 125
      Case example 126
   How to select a focus 128
   Sharing the IPAF with the patient 129
      Case example 131

6. The Middle Phase 139
   Aims 139
   Sequence of movement in middle phase sessions 140
   Tracking the IPAF: eliciting interpersonal narratives to illustrate the activation of the IPAF 143
   Staying focused 145
      Case example 147
   Working in the transference 149
   Working with defences 150
   Supporting attempts at new behaviour in relationships 153

7. Techniques 157
   Listening with an analytic ear 157
   Emergence versus structure in the sessions 160
   Expressive/exploratory techniques 162

Confrontation 162
Clarification 164
Interpretation 166
Features of helpful interpretations 169
Focusing on affect 170
Supportive techniques 171
Mentalizing interventions 172
How to identify failures of mentalizing 172
How to use mentalizing interventions 175
Communication analysis 178
Directive interventions 178

8. Working in the Transference 183
Using the transference to explore the IPAF 183
Formulating a transference interpretation 186
Criteria for interpreting the transference in DIT 189
Case example 191
The bridge to change 195
Case example 195

9. The Ending Phase 199
The patient's response to endings 199
Preparing for ending 201
Interpreting the unconscious meaning of endings 203
Paranoid and manic phantasies 204
Neurotic phantasies 204
Premature and prolonged endings 205
The therapist's perspective on ending 206
The goodbye letter 207
The goodbye letter in practice 208
Examples of goodbye letters 211
Revisiting the attachment descriptors 216
Working with resistances in the ending phase 216
Therapeutic stance in the ending phase 217

10. When Things Go Wrong 219
Managing difficulties in the therapeutic relationship 219
Reflective practice: monitoring the countertransference 220
Therapeutic stance when managing misunderstandings and misattunements in the therapist–patient relationship 222
Case example 223

Forms of resistance 226
  Requests for information about DIT 227
  Personal questions about the therapist 228
  Requests for direction or advice 229
  Challenging the boundaries of the therapeutic relationship 230
  The IPAF as an intellectual defence against feeling 230
  The compliant patient 230
  Difficulty in being the patient 231
  Idealizing the therapist 231
  Sexualized behaviour 232
  The therapist's resistance to time-limited work 232
Working with resistance 233
When things go wrong for the DIT therapist when learning this model 236
  Initial phase difficulties 238
  Middle phase difficulties 240
  Ending phase difficulties 241
Summary 242

11. Frequently Asked Questions 245
    How does DIT differ from interpersonal psychotherapy? 245
    How does DIT differ from other brief psychodynamic therapies? 245
    Is DIT a supportive psychotherapy? 246
    Is DIT an adaptation of mentalization-based treatment for mood disorders? 246
    How central is working in the transference in DIT? 247
    What training do I need to practise DIT? 248
    Does the DIT therapist work with dreams and unconscious phantasies? 248
    Does the DIT therapist use the countertransference as the basis for intervening? 249
    Does DIT focus on the patient's past? 249
    What should I expect if I choose to train in DIT? 250

12. Research on Psychotherapy Outcomes, Fidelity and Mechanisms of Change in Dynamic Interpersonal Therapy 253
    The meta-analytic evidence base of psychodynamic therapy for depression 254

The evidence base for DIT 257
Research on fidelity to psychodynamic principles in DIT 262
　Fidelity as a predictor of outcome 263
　Developing a measure of competence 264
　Clinical implications 266
Working mechanisms of DIT 267
Conclusions 269

13. Dynamic Interpersonal Therapy for Complex Care (DITCC) 277
Who is DITCC for? 277
The complex case: the failure of mentalizing in depression 279
DITCC and DIT: commonalities and differences 283
DITCC in practice 284
　Structure of DITCC 287
　The model in detail 288
　Techniques in DITCC 293
Summary 300

14. Dynamic Interpersonal Therapy for Patients with Functional Somatic Disorders 303
The DIT approach to understanding patients with functional somatic disorders 304
　Introduction 304
　A contemporary psychodynamic approach to FSDs 306
DIT-FSD 313
　Background and basic principles of DIT-FSD 313
　The initial phase (sessions 1–4): engagement and case formulation 313
　The middle phase (sessions 5–12): fostering embodied mentalizing and working through 316
　The ending phase (sessions 13–16): empowerment and improvement 322
Conclusions 323

15. Internet-Delivered Dynamic Interpersonal Therapy (i-DIT) for Depression and Anxiety 327
The structure of blended i-DIT 329
Specific competences needed to deliver blended i-DIT 333
　Assessment of suitability 334

Motivating patients to engage in online work 337
   Recognizing and dealing with resistance to online work 338
   Formulation of the IPAF 340
   Balancing the content focus and the process focus 341
   Managing the ending phase 342
  Conclusions 344

16. Future Directions for Dynamic Interpersonal Therapy 347
   The broadening scope of DIT 348
   Training in DIT 350
   Conclusions 351

Appendix 1 Patient Information Leaflet: Dynamic Interpersonal Therapy (DIT) for Depression and Anxiety 353
Appendix 2 DIT Checklist 359
Appendix 3 DIT Competence Rating Scale 361
Appendix 4 DIT Patient Complexity Subscale 365
Appendix 5 Training and Supervision Model for DIT 367
Index 381

FIGURES

1.1 Dimensions to be explored when assessing suitability for DIT 13
4.1 The interpersonal map 87
4.2 Interpersonal contexts yielding information about key attachment patterns 90
5.1 The IPAF dimensions 111
5.2 Carol's IPAF 117
5.3 Criteria for selecting an IPAF 129
5.4 Marc's IPAF 136
6.1 Middle phase strategies 142
6.2 Sequence of movement in the middle phase sessions 142
6.3 Abstracting interpersonal-affective patterns from interpersonal narratives 144
6.4 Strategies for exploring defences 152
7.1 Levels of listening 161
10.1 Steps for interpreting resistance in the therapeutic relationship 235
14.1 Factors that predispose to, precipitate, and perpetuate functional somatic disorders 306
15.1 Structure of blended i-DIT 330

TABLES

- 3.1 Initial phase: sessions 1–4 61
- 3.2 Middle phase: sessions 5–12 62
- 3.3 Ending phase: sessions 13–16 63
- 4.1 Relationship questionnaire rating scale 92
- 14.1 Prototypical IPAFs as a function of attachment style in patients with functional somatic disorders 310
- 14.2 Basic principles for fostering embodied mentalizing 317
- 14.3 Somatic markers of inner mental states 318

BOXES

3.1 Core features of DIT 60
4.1 Assessment of the problem/symptoms 85
5.1 DIT formulation aide-mémoire 119
6.1 Staying focused on the IPAF 146
7.1 Characteristics of helpful questions 168
7.2 Characteristics of helpful interpretations 170
7.3 What does good mentalizing look like in relation to other people's thoughts and feelings? 173
7.4 Steps in making an intervention 176
8.1 Criteria for interpreting the transference in dynamic interpersonal therapy 190
9.1 Ending phase strategies 202
9.2 Preparing for ending 203
9.3 Guidelines for writing the goodbye letter 210

ABBREVIATIONS

ADM	antidepressant medication
BACP	British Association for Counselling and Psychotherapy
BPC	British Psychoanalytic Council
BPD	borderline personality disorder
CAT	cognitive analytic therapy
CPD	continuing professional development
DIT	dynamic interpersonal therapy
DITCC	DIT for complex care
FSD	functional somatic disorder
GAD	generalized anxiety disorder
GP	general practitioner
GST	general supportive therapy
HCPC	Health and Care Professions Council
IAPT	Improving Access to Psychological Therapies
ICC	intraclass correlation coefficient
i-DIT	internet-delivered DIT
IN	interpersonal narrative
IPAF	interpersonal-affective focus
IPT	interpersonal psychotherapy
IWM	internal working model
MBT	mentalization-based treatment
NHS	National Health Service
RCT	randomized controlled trial
REDIT	Randomized Evaluation of DIT
RIB	relationship-interfering behaviour
TCS	Therapist Competence Scale
UKCP	UK Council for Psychotherapy

1
Why Dynamic Interpersonal Therapy for Mood Disorders?

THE RATIONALE OF DIT

We are short of neither psychodynamic therapies nor acronyms. Inevitably, by developing dynamic interpersonal therapy (DIT) and publishing the first edition of this book in 2011, we added to an already long list. Why, then, did we do this? DIT's techniques and theoretical underpinnings are not novel and will be broadly familiar to psychodynamically trained practitioners. Rather than offering a new model of psychodynamic therapy, DIT was first developed in response to the erosion of provision of psychodynamic therapy within the public health care system, and the high demand for brief interventions in the private sector.

We wanted to develop a protocol that would be relatively easy to acquire and that could assist psychodynamically trained clinicians to *work to a specific focus* relevant to the difficulties commonly encountered by patients with depression and/or anxiety. DIT was thus developed primarily for pragmatic reasons so that clinicians who had undertaken psychodynamic psychotherapy or counselling training could readily acquire the specific priorities and competences associated with time-limited therapeutic work with depressed and/or anxious patients, and have a common name for it, especially within public health care. DIT provides a way of delineating a particular focus for intervention within a time limit, set at sixteen sessions in the original protocol and twenty-six sessions in its most recent adaptation for more complex cases (DIT for complex care (DITCC); see Chapter 13).

When we developed the original protocol, we set the number of sessions at sixteen because this was consistent with many other models of brief intervention, and with the framework of a national public mental health programme in the UK. We wanted to develop a protocol that would also allow us to test its effectiveness in outcome trials; hence, making the length of the treatment comparable to other brief models guided our decision about the number of sessions. Moreover, it is our clinical experience that much can be achieved with the patient in sixteen sessions, and it is an acceptable length of psychological therapy in a public health care context. Given that there is nothing 'magical' about sixteen sessions, it follows that there is nothing inherently problematic about offering a longer or shorter course of sessions, while retaining the overall DIT focus. However, we would guard against simply extending the contract beyond this number of sessions if this is a way of bypassing the painful reality of ending that has to be faced and processed, which the patient—and sometimes the therapist too—may be unconsciously avoiding. Equally, there might be service pressures that result in a move towards even briefer adaptations of the sixteen-session model. These might prove to be helpful to some patients, but we need to keep in mind that the main randomized controlled trials (RCTs) to date looked at the outcomes for only the original sixteen-session model and not any adaptations, so the efficacy of briefer forms of DIT has not been established (see Chapter 12 for a discussion of research on the outcomes of DIT).

As an approach, DIT is *interpersonal* because it focuses squarely on the patient's relationships, internal and external, as they relate to the problem(s) in the patient's current life that are giving rise to symptoms of depression and/or anxiety. An interpersonal focus is shared with several other modalities, not least interpersonal psychotherapy (IPT) (Weissman et al., 2000), with which, somewhat confusingly, DIT also shares some of its name. Yet the 'interpersonal' in DIT is important because it clearly sets DIT apart from the dynamic models that focus more on intrapsychic variables. Unlike IPT, which does not address internalized object relationships, DIT systematically focuses on the activation in the present of one selected internalized, often unconscious, object relationship that is meaningfully linked to the presenting problems.

DIT is *dynamic* in its focus insofar as it is concerned with helping the patient to understand the interplay between external and internal reality as it relates to a problematic, circumscribed relational pattern. Consequently, it addresses a non-conscious realm of experience, awareness of which is defended against by the patient because it may feel shameful, frightening, or even too exciting. This again distinguishes DIT from IPT, and closely aligns it with other psychodynamic models.

Although there is a substantial overlap in theory between DIT and other psychodynamic models, implementing DIT will, most likely, feel unfamiliar for clinicians trained in long-term psychodynamic therapy or counselling, as it is indeed different in some respects. Thus, the therapeutic priorities singled out in DIT are not typically ones that are taught in training for intensive or open-ended psychodynamic psychotherapy, although they may well turn out to be the ones used by 'good' therapists irrespective of the planned length of therapy (Binder, 2004).

Most psychoanalytic training provides the foundations for long-term, often intensive, interventions. However, once qualified, many therapists find themselves working briefly, without a framework to orient them to the task in hand when a time limit is imposed. The transition from open-ended and intensive work to time-limited, once-weekly therapy is not always a smooth one. No matter how experienced we are in long-term work, we cannot simply export strategies that are helpful in that context and apply them in a brief context without any modifications.

PSYCHODYNAMIC APPROACHES AND DIAGNOSTIC CLASSIFICATION

The development of a protocol tailored to a diagnostic umbrella such as depression or anxiety will be anathema to some psychodynamic practitioners.

Psychiatric classification based on operational criteria, which first entered clinical practice via the third edition of the *Diagnostic and Statistical Manual of Mental Disorders* (DSM-III; American Psychiatric Association, 1980), had advantages, not least that it contributed to convincing decision-makers that psychiatric illness was measurable and predictable. No one would claim that systems are any more than imperfect reflections of psychiatry's aspirations towards measurable observations and the construction of broadly based scientific theories, which might then be testable. Yet, nowadays we operate in a world in which systems such as the DSM-5 (American Psychiatric Association, 2013) or the *International Classification of Diseases, 11th Revision* (ICD-11; World Health Organization, 2019) are reified, shaping how research is conducted and clinical services are configured, and hence how funding is prioritized. This in turn has the effect of making the diagnostic categories seem more 'real', purporting to 'cut nature at the joints' and therefore form a basis for research and treatment.

When psychodynamic therapists engage with and use classification systems, they do so as a concession to pragmatism (records, reporting, reimbursement, research, etc.), but experience the use of diagnostic categories as something with the potential to take the heart and soul out of psychotherapy. Nevertheless, although objections to nosology are common, psychodynamic clinicians may themselves assign individuals to categories such as narcissistic, masochistic, obsessional, and even psychopathic. The tension therefore appears to lie not so much around whether 'diagnosing' per se is helpful or not, but rather around what system is used. There are profound inconsistencies between a psychiatric and a psychodynamic diagnostic approach, many of which are rooted in the respective history of the two disciplines. Psychoanalysts are suspicious of diagnostic systems, believing them to be regressions to a descriptive psychiatry redolent of the end of the nineteenth century and against which Sigmund Freud rebelled by advancing a model of mental disorder based on hypothetical psychological mechanisms (e.g. the diagnosis of neurosis is based on the theories of drive, anxiety, and defence, rather than on a pattern of symptoms).

The difference between the two approaches to classification lies in the logic each one follows to arrive at its conclusions. As Jonathan Shedler, Drew Westen, and colleagues pointed out, the identification of a definitive list of symptoms and signs poorly fits psychodynamic clinical thinking (Shedler et al., 2010; Shedler & Westen, 2004). The latter is based on categories drawing on emergent prototypes and prototypes that reflect the hypothetical underlying mechanisms of disorder, such as unconscious phantasies and defences. Psychotherapists do not think of necessary and sufficient features in arriving at categorical decisions, but rather think of the typicality of an individual relative to an 'ideal type'—which is perhaps never seen but based on the accumulation of clinical cases treated and studied.

Thus, an approach adapted to psychiatric formulation runs counter to the traditional psychoanalytic emphasis on the unconscious and the individual psychodynamics of every case. Our primary interest, as psychodynamic practitioners, is typically the person *in whom* the depression or anxiety is occurring. In other words, we consider it vital in any treatment intervention to understand symptoms in the context of personality structure: for example, panic attacks in a narcissistic individual are lived out very differently from those experienced in a characterologically avoidant individual. The awareness of this context of the wider personality is inherent in DIT.

We are also aware that diagnostic syndromes and their symptoms (e.g. depression) can serve a defensive function. By this we mean not just external secondary gain from illness (e.g. professional and social attention, or avoidance of challenging situations such as needing to work), but also the unconscious, internal purpose within a way of construing the self and the social world. For example, a person who perceives themselves as feeble and others as powerful and exploitative, and who feels helpless and useless as a result, may unconsciously get much pleasure from feeling morally superior to the active others, who inevitably make some mistakes, perhaps occasionally even being 'tripped up' by the patient. They may also sense, as they are supported in their feeble state, that they have tricked the stronger other into protecting them even though they are secretly hostile and contemptuous. In this way, the patient gets to express their competitiveness, envy, and hatred in hidden ways, while feeling helpless, being unaware themself of the 'deal' within which they are living.

Compared with the psychodynamic formulation and the decision about suitability for therapy, diagnosis has been relatively underemphasized in psychotherapy training programmes. It is often claimed that a genuine understanding of an individual's pathology can be reached only at the end of the therapy. While this may be true, it is a false comparison: in all medicine and therapy, the trouble will be better understood after treatment has been given, but systematic, initial diagnosis is a necessary antecedent for a rational choice of physical treatment, and there is a case for it in psychotherapy too.[1]

---

1. Nor was psychoanalysis always opposed to diagnostic labels. Classically, Ernest Jones (1927, p. 183) called for psychotherapists to be trained to distinguish obsessive-compulsive disorder from bipolar illness, paranoid psychotic conditions from phobic disorders, and dysthymia from somatic conditions.

In DIT, we use the initial phase (see Chapter 4) to gather information to be used in a formulation, which is shared with the patient as the basis of the bulk of the work, which may well in turn refine or illuminate the formulation. The defensive function of the pattern of experiencing self, other, and painful affect, in particular, is likely to become clearer and available for work. This is the part that has been unconscious for the patient, which makes it trickier to open up, but actually adds interest and motivation for some patients, who may feel that the self–object–affect part of the formulation is something they already know. In gradually helping the patient to see and feel it, including in the transference, even a brief therapy can be revelatory to the patient and have considerable impact on them.

Unless we adopt a dualist stance, we should feel confident that a reliable and robust psychological-mechanism-based system, which is valuable in establishing suitability for treatment, will also correspond to key brain processes relevant to neuroscience. This is certainly true for two constructs of relevance to DIT, namely attachment (Feldman, 2017; Mikulincer & Shaver, 2016) and mentalizing (Fehlbaum et al., 2022; Frith & Frith, 2021), and is the case for other features of depression and anxiety, for example, memory deficits (Whalley et al., 2009).

Where does DIT situate itself in these debates? The descriptive approach to diagnosis implicitly adopted by us in this book is taken primarily for pragmatic reasons. We recognize that most formal outcome research and some treatment services are organized according to diagnostic categories; hence, we favour an approach to bridging these very different frameworks at a pragmatic level. The diagnosis of major depressive disorder or anxiety disorder, in our view, constitutes only one (small) part of a complete formulation and treatment plan. A judgement about the contribution of interacting psychological, biological, and social systems to the patient's descriptive presentation is a necessary addition to an ICD or DSM diagnosis. The descriptive and psychodynamic approaches to formulation, such as the ones we adopt (with a rather broad brush) in DIT, are not opposed; rather, they are overlapping, complementary, and necessary to each other. We assume—and recommend—an integrated approach in which clinicians implement a research diagnostic and a psychodynamic approach to formulation.

MOOD DISORDERS: DEPRESSION AND ANXIETY

'Depression,' a patient said, 'feels like wearing a beautifully embroidered black veil. I know I can't see things clearly through it, but I don't know that I could reveal myself to the world without it.' This comment captures vividly the complexity of depression: it is a disabling condition and yet the relationship an individual may have with it—that is, its function in the patient's psychic economy—may make the patient fearful of change and hence resistant to being helped. Other patients with both depression and anxiety commonly use metaphors of feeling weighed down, trapped, or deadened to convey the sense of threat and dread (a constricted comfort zone, with fear that change will make things worse) that both conditions tend to bring.

The great majority of patients with mood disorders presenting for psychotherapy in outpatient and primary care settings are troubled by symptoms of both depression and anxiety. In addition, they may have various other diagnosable symptoms, which have sometimes developed alongside the mood disorder. Examples would be disturbances of eating, substance use or abuse (perhaps originally for self-medication), and patterns of dependence, misery, self-harm, or avoidance, which may have become so chronic as to fulfil criteria for a chronic disorder, such as dysthymia or a personality disorder. These clinical presentations pose a challenge to brief interventions. Since the publication of the first edition of this book (Lemma et al., 2011), clinicians using the DIT model have invited us to adapt the model so that it could address more complex cases typically seen in secondary care services. This led to the development of DITCC, in which the length of the treatment is extended to twenty-six sessions spread out over approximately a year (see Chapter 13) and more specific use of mentalizing techniques is made in the therapy. As such, DIT is increasingly developing into a spectrum of interventions, ranging from those for individuals with mild-to-moderate psychological problems to those for individuals with more complex clinical presentations.

In DIT we take the view that patients across the spectrum of mood disorders, with varying combinations of diagnostic labels, have in common a tendency to organize social experiences according to underlying unconscious expectations of self and other that trigger particular affects. Once active in the mind, such (typically unconscious) interpersonal configurations lead to mental and behavioural defensive strategies, which are maladaptive. We apply the structure of focusing on an interpersonal-affective focus (IPAF) across the spectrum, as long as there is not an alternative treatment approach that is needed more immediately (e.g. detoxification, management of suicidal behaviour, or treatment of agoraphobia that would prevent the person from attending therapy sessions).

DIT has been developed to respond to the two predominant types of mood disorders, depression and anxiety, which frequently go together in primary care and outpatient settings. The DIT therapist needs to be conscious that both of these painful states of mind (not only depression) are likely to be consequences of the conflictual unconscious 'script' represented by the IPAF, and that both need to be much improved if the patient is to become well enough to maintain their progress after therapy ends.

DIT formulates the presenting symptoms of mood disorders as responses to interpersonal difficulties or perceived threats to attachments (loss/separation) and hence also as threats to the self. It conceptualizes depression and anxiety with low mood in terms of an underlying temporary disorganization of the attachment system caused by current relationship problems, which in turn generates a range of distortions in thinking and feeling typical of chronically depressed and anxious states of mind. In the therapy, a focus is maintained on this emotional 'crisis' through an elaboration of the thoughts and feelings (conscious and unconscious) most characteristic of the particular patient and relevant to their depressed and anxious mood, as these emerge in the context of the therapeutic relationship. Through the focused exploration of the transference relationship, the patient is helped to develop a better understanding of their subjective reactions to interpersonal difficulties and threats. Making implicit anxieties and concerns explicit through improving the patient's ability to reflect on their own and others' thoughts and feelings, in turn, enhances the patient's ability to cope with current attachment-related interpersonal threats and challenges.

DIT's starting point is rooted in the common clinical observation that patients who present as depressed and/or anxious almost invariably also present with difficulties and distress about their relationships. Although the patient may well experience their problem as 'I cannot sleep or concentrate' or 'I can't face going into crowded places or going to work', the DIT therapist looks beyond such symptoms of anxiety and depression as manifestations of a relational problem, which patients cannot understand, or understand in a maladaptive way, attributing to themselves and others motivations that are unlikely or unhelpful. Once the patient is helped to make some changes in the way they approach their relationship difficulties, the depressive and anxious symptoms are typically alleviated.

There are many features of mood disorders that suggest that a dynamically oriented approach focusing on interpersonal issues is likely to be effective in addressing the symptoms. Interpersonal problems are marked in severe depression and anxiety disorders, and evident even in mild or moderate conditions (Luyten et al., 2005). This seems to be driven not only by the potential of a persistent irrationally depressed and anxious mood to elicit negative responses from others, but also by the inclination of depressed and anxious people to seek and generate interpersonal scenarios with the propensity to evoke distress, such as conflict or resistance to efforts to help, leading to social exclusion and rejection (e.g. Kiesler, 1983; Lewinsohn et al., 1980).

The ground-breaking work of the psychoanalytic researchers Sidney Blatt and Patrick Luyten demonstrates not only that vulnerability to depression is associated with the unconscious generation of interpersonal stress, but also that interpersonal factors explain much current data on the outcomes of treatments of depression (Blatt et al., 2010; Luyten, 2017; Luyten et al., 2006; Luyten & Fonagy, 2018). There is increasing agreement in the field that the interpersonal aspects of depression should be given comparable weight to the normally highlighted intrapersonal dimensions (e.g. McFarquhar et al., 2023). Similarly, the model of 'triple vulnerability' to anxiety disorders posits—in addition to a biological substrate—factors of 'generalized psychological vulnerability', such as experiences of negative parenting and a sense of uncontrollability, coupled with 'specific psychological vulnerability', especially interpersonal triggering events such as the loss of a loved one, relationship difficulties, and trauma such as an assault (Suárez et al., 2008).

While the literature on distorted information-processing in depression and anxiety disorders largely focuses on distortions of conscious cognition (Beck et al., 1979; Clark & Wells, 1995; Kyte & Goodyer, 2008), some concepts in this literature, such as the dominance of a hopeless, helpless attributional style (Abramson et al., 1978), echo classical psychoanalytic writings, which link these observations to unconscious projective and introjective processes (Engel & Schmale, 1967; Luyten et al., 2013).

DIT as an approach includes attention to apparent dysfunctions in interpersonal cognition (mentalizing) concerned with an individual's distorted and inadequate understanding of their own and others' thoughts and feelings. The consideration of mentalizing within DIT, including the use of mentalizing techniques to introduce different perspectives on the selected IPAF, is consistent with data demonstrating theory-of-mind deficits in patients with unipolar and bipolar depressive disorders (Luyten et al., 2019).

Measures of mentalizing in the attachment context also yield indications of a deficit associated with depression (Luyten & Fonagy, 2018; Luyten et al., 2019). This is important as the DIT model assumes that failures of understanding self and other in depression are strongly tied to particular self–other interaction patterns evolved from childhood experiences, whether real, distorted, or imagined (see Chapter 5). Patients with anxiety disorders who are not significantly depressed may have less difficulty with mentalizing; their work on the IPAF may be less interfered with by a conviction that their perception of people's motives is necessary, and even the only one possible. However, anxiety disorders are often motivated by distorted attributions of thoughts and feelings entailed in the threat from and judgements of others, their imagined reasons and drivers, and their possible objectives and aspirations. Proximity to others entails feelings of vulnerability as the possibility of getting closer increases the risk of being 'found out' or 'exposed' in some way.

DIT has a dual focus on interpersonal and affective issues. The affective issues of greatest relevance centre on attachment-related concerns. Compared with securely attached individuals, those who are insecurely attached are more likely to have frequent anxiety states (with a high background level of chronic anxiety), depressive episodes, and residual symptoms, use more pharmacotherapy, and are more likely to be impaired in their social functioning (Conradi & de Jonge, 2009). There is a substantial body of work linking vulnerability to depression to insecure attachment (Bifulco, Moran, Ball, & Bernazzani, 2002; Bifulco, Moran, Ball, & Lillie, 2002; Lee & Hankin, 2009). Blatt's theory of depression identifies two classes of attachment-history-based cognitive–affective schemata most likely to be found in depression: interpersonal dependency and excessive self-criticism

(Blatt, 2008; Blatt & Luyten, 2009), linked, respectively, to preoccupied and avoidant patterns of attachment (Luyten, 2017).

For decades, evidence has been accumulating linking childhood adversity, which is likely to disrupt attachment, to adult vulnerability for depression (Brown & Harris, 1978; Brown & Harris, 1989; Luyten & Fonagy, 2018) and anxiety (Hogg et al., 2023; Torgersen, 1986). The association is increasingly well understood in terms of the effects of attachment experiences on the stress system (Heim et al., 2008) and the moderation of the impact of later stressful experiences by acquiring a secure state of mind in relation to attachment history (Bakermans-Kranenburg et al., 2008).

Attachment experiences also link mentalizing and depression (Luyten & Fonagy, 2018). A reduced capacity to think about mental states may be related to personal histories (e.g. trauma) but may also be a secondary consequence of disordered mood (Luyten et al., 2019). Indications of a failure of mentalizing are not hard to find. There is a re-emergence of a pre-reflective, physical self-experience in place of a psychological self-experience (Fonagy & Target, 2000). Psychological experience is felt to be far too real, with psychological and physical pain and emotional and physical exhaustion commonly being equated (Van Houdenhove & Luyten, 2009). A state of 'hyperembodiment' ensues, in which subjective experiences are primarily felt to be physical in nature. Worries can feel like genuine weights on one's shoulders, and the criticism of others threatens the sense of integrity of the embodied self. The therapeutic task is to help the patient elaborate the state of mind that is experienced as a physical symptom rather than being available for consideration and reappraisal as a belief or a thought. The lack of drive that is at the heart of depression is similarly seen as a regressive embodiment of disempowering thought.

In the formulation of depression and anxiety advanced in support of DIT, distortions of cognitions are considered to indicate varying failures of mentalizing, which may be concrete thinking or indications of pseudomentalizing (also referred to as 'hypermentalizing'). In the latter case, the patient's description of the mental states of others or their own mental state reflects an apparent thoughtfulness, but this lacks some essential features of genuine mentalizing; it is a partial understanding containing some truth, but is excessively detailed and often repetitive. Characteristics include a sense of certainty about mental states, including the unrealistic assumption that one can directly know someone else's mind, and limiting what is attributed to the other's mental state to ideas and themes that reinforce the individual's existing perspective, which, however painful and self-destructive it may be, is held on to for powerful unconscious reasons.

ASSESSING SUITABILITY FOR DIT

If there is an art to psychotherapy, then surely this is most relevant to the assessment for suitability because we are short on science in this domain. Despite the considerable advances we have made in understanding many aspects of the therapeutic process and its outcomes across a range of psychological therapies, our capacity to reliably assess which treatment will work best for which patient remains limited. When it comes to the assessment of suitability, a core competence is the ability to draw on knowledge that pre-therapy patient characteristics are not yet proven to predict outcome in psychodynamic therapy, whatever its particular 'brand' (Lemma et al., 2008).

Notwithstanding this cautionary note, it would be impossible to make any decisions if we were not informed at least by the wealth of practice-based evidence that provides some markers for assessing suitability for a psychodynamic approach. Certain dimensions of the patient's experience (intrapsychic, interpersonal, and pragmatic) are pertinent to assessing when DIT may or may not be indicated for some patients, as well as how it may need to be adapted to meet the patient's needs. Each of the following domains thus provides a partial vantage point from which to consider DIT's suitability. Considered together, they amount to guidelines for assessing suitability rather than evidence-based recommendations (see Figure 1.1).

The patient's response to an exploratory approach

The DIT therapist aims to engage the patient in a process of reflection on their states of mind in the context of relationships, including the therapeutic relationship: hence, DIT makes different demands on the patient relative to, say, cognitive-behavioural therapy (CBT) or IPT. Moreover, despite the greater therapist activity given the time-limited nature of the therapy, there is still a relative lack of directiveness from

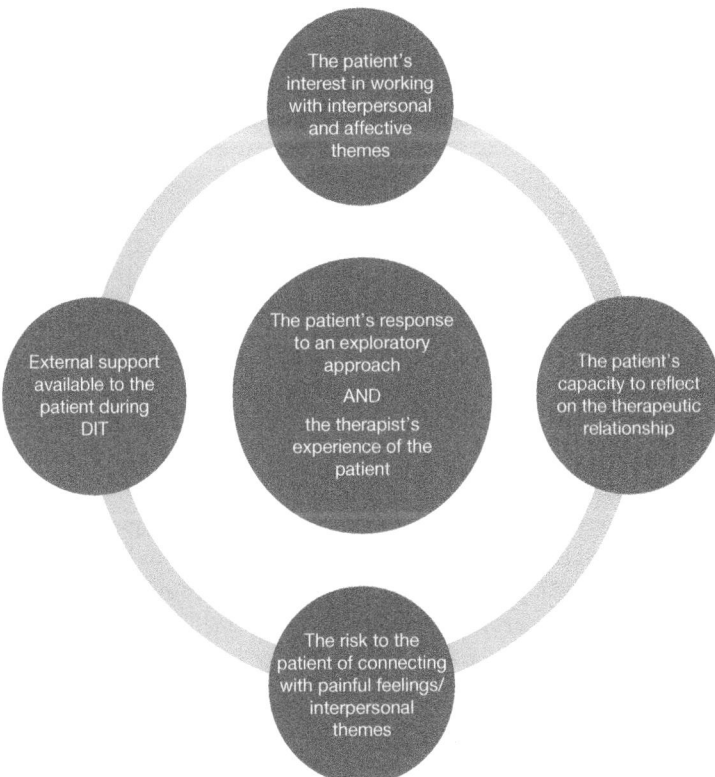

Figure 1.1 Dimensions to be explored when assessing suitability for DIT.

the therapist, compared with other therapies. The therapist approaches the therapeutic situation with an analytic attitude so as to observe the patient's interaction with them and evaluate what adaptations may be necessary to support the patient's capacity to work within an analytic frame. This takes us back to the fundamental importance of adopting a flexible approach that prioritizes meeting the patient where they are, rather than trying at all costs to fit them into a model that is not responsive to their needs.

Having said this, because the DIT therapist adopts an analytic stance, this makes particular demands on the patient, which may render DIT unsuitable or uncongenial for some patients. An important indicator of suitability is therefore the assessment of how the patient manages without systematic therapist-imposed direction in the session (e.g. do they become anxious or paranoid?) and the extent to which the patient is responsive to the invitation to reflect on what is happening in their life, as opposed to primarily seeking relief from symptoms through practical strategies.

The patient's interest in working with interpersonal and affective themes

Every patient comes to an assessment with their own language and frame of reference for emotional distress, and with their own theories, which are often consonant with cultural idioms for the expression of emotional distress. Often the assessment provides an opportunity for sharing different narratives about the problem. The patient may find that DIT's interpersonal and affective emphasis is meaningful and helpful, and they may thus shift, say, from their former physiological or political explanation to a more psychological one. This is not always the case, however. It is therefore important to listen out for whether the patient's own narrative maps comfortably enough on to the DIT one. We are looking for some compatibility between treatment rationale and the patient's own theories. There is little point in offering DIT to a patient who is convinced that their problems are caused by a fixed genetic predisposition or who believes that their depression is a realistic reaction to a global conspiracy, or to an external reality, such as climate change, which is not to do with them individually. The aim of assessment is not to work towards getting the patient to take on our point of view but to find a good-enough fit between our knowledge of the patient's difficulties and the therapeutic approach most congenial to the patient's own way of thinking, or philosophy of life, that could best address those difficulties.

DIT is unequivocally focused on the patient's interpersonal functioning in their current life and in the therapeutic interaction, and on their emotional experience. Given this focus, it is essential to gauge early on the patient's interest in working with these themes. This requires the therapist to engage the patient's interest in DIT by making a trial interpretation (see Chapter 5) that connects the patient's presenting difficulties/feelings/symptoms to their past and current relationships and behaviour.

The patient's capacity to reflect on the therapeutic relationship

We hope that our patients will be able to develop an emotionally 'live' relationship with us that will arouse a host of feelings, positive and negative—some of which could feel terrifying. The patient's grip on reality, and hence their appreciation of the 'as if' quality of the transference, is therefore a vital prerequisite. In order for the patient to use and benefit from DIT, it is important that they can be helped to reflect on the therapeutic relationship while maintaining reality-testing. When this capacity is absent, the patient no longer experiences the therapist, for example, *as if* they were an abusive parent; rather, in their experience the therapist *is* the abusive parent. A symbol is experienced as representing an object. When the symbol and the thing it symbolizes cannot be distinguished, this reflects a breakdown in symbolic functioning, which is psychically devastating—and a contraindication for DIT.

One of the most meaningful indicators of suitability is the patient's response to the therapist's attempts to understand them; for example, does the patient feel relieved or persecuted by the therapist's focus on their mind, or on what may be happening between them in therapy? Interpretations that draw the patient's attention to their unconscious experience of the therapy (e.g. about how the patient may be feeling anxious about the prospect of this kind of engagement) are especially helpful. The patient's response will help the therapist to develop a picture of the patient's current readiness and motivation to engage with the affective and interpersonal focus of the therapy, and, more specifically, to determine the extent to which the patient can:

- Stand back from their experience and observe their own mind
- Receive and make use of what the therapist can offer
- Work to a focus.

The patient's curiosity about their role in their difficulties

DIT therapists are more explicitly supportive than might be the case in other dynamic models, but they are nevertheless also challenging because of DIT's emphasis on supporting the patient to make some actual changes in how they relate to others, and to question their own perspectives. It is never long before the patient realizes, for example, that their narrative about victimization will be gradually challenged by the therapist in order to invite them to reflect on their part in the repetitive pattern that has been selected as the focus of the therapy. This requires considerable motivation on the patient's part, especially when symptoms are ego-syntonic (i.e. they do not generate conflict or self-doubt).

How one assesses motivation is nevertheless complicated because it is a complex, multidimensional concept. There is, in fact, little agreement over the term. It is sometimes defined so broadly that it becomes synonymous with suitability for psychodynamic therapy (Truant, 1999). Clinical work makes one thing very clear, however: motivation does not refer to a static state of mind. Patients will go through periods in therapy when their motivation is high, and at other times the secondary gains from their illness get the upper hand and motivation wanes. The relative predominance of a motivation to change over unconscious gratification from the symptoms, which acts as a resistance to change, is an important factor to assess. DIT will include addressing the defensive function of their way of experiencing themselves, for example, as an innocent victim, or as someone who tries to be helpful but is never appreciated.

The assessment of motivation is of necessity inferential. It can be gleaned from a thorough exploration of the patient's previous experience of therapy, where applicable, and of their expectations of the new treatment. To assess motivation, it is helpful to explore the following areas with the patient:

- What is the patient's relationship to help? What did the patient find difficult or helpful, if anything, in a former therapy or another helping relationship (e.g. with a friend or with their general practitioner)? How realistic are their expectations of therapy? What difficulties do they envisage in relation to the treatment that is proposed? Do they display an active or passive stance? Are they hoping to be 'cured', or do they give some indication of appreciating that therapy will make demands on them and is not just down to the efforts of the therapist?

- Is the patient's relationship to the therapist an overly idealized one? Some positive investment in the person of the therapist and their capacity to relieve suffering is necessary for a working alliance to be established, but this is quite different from the patient who takes a back seat and is expecting a magical transformation at the hands of an all-powerful therapist. Rigid idealization or denigration of a previous therapist should sound alarm bells and can be a poor prognostic sign.
- Is the patient motivated internally or by external sources? This question is typically related to the 'Why now?' question. It is important to explore this because those who enter therapy at the behest of a partner or another mental health professional may establish a weaker alliance or misalliances that can undermine the treatment process. Generally speaking, the patient is motivated to work in therapy if they experience their problems/symptoms at least to a degree as ego-dystonic. It is important here to distinguish between motivation for self-understanding (e.g. 'I want to understand why I always end up feeling humiliated') and a search for concrete relief from symptoms or particular life situations (e.g. 'I want to get out of the council estate I live in, it's getting me down'). Although in both cases the patient will be motivated to get some form of help, it is unlikely that the second patient will find DIT congenial.

The risk to the patient of connecting with painful feelings/interpersonal themes, which could be difficult for them to manage (e.g. increasing risk to themselves), is balanced against the benefits of exploring their issues in therapy.

Although the DIT therapist is encouraged to adopt a more supportive stance than is characteristic of some psychodynamic models, the therapy nevertheless does address unconscious conflict and defences. It is important to assess the risk to which this exploratory emphasis might expose the patient. A key task in the assessment is therefore to consider realistically, with the patient, their capacity to work within a time-limited analytic frame. This requires some knowledge and formulation in the following domains:

- Knowledge of the patient's history of self-harm, violence, neglect, or self-defeating behaviours.

- Assessment of the patient's ego strength. This involves identifying whether the patient's difficulties restrict their self-observational capacity and other executive ego functions, which would contribute to diffuse boundaries and encourage acting out. A patient's ego strength is inferred from the presentation at assessment. It reflects those personality assets that will enable the patient to overcome anxieties and acquire more adaptive defences. At its most basic, ego strength refers to the patient's capacity to be in touch with reality, whereby perception, thinking, and judgement are unimpaired. Ego strength reflects the patient's capacity to hold on to their identity in the face of psychic pain, without resorting to excessive distortion or denial. Ego weakness manifests itself in poor frustration tolerance and impulse control, a lack of tolerance of anxiety, and an absence of sublimatory activity. For example, a patient who is angry and has weak ego strength is less likely to be able to reflect on the source and meaning of their anger and may instead act on it and attack another person. The patient with more ego strength will either be able to think about their anger or might manage to sublimate it and channel it into some other more constructive activity, for example, exercise.
- The patient's capacity to persist with relationships and occupational or vocational endeavours in the face of challenges provides another opportunity to indirectly assess ego strength. This is why it is important to take an educational and occupational history: patients who present with histories of dropping out of education, being fired from jobs, or flitting from one employment to another would raise the question of whether they have a sufficiently well-developed capacity to persevere with stressful situations.

The external resources that could support the patient during the course of DIT

It is important here to keep in mind that we are not assessing whether the patient fits the model but rather the extent to which the model, and the context in which it is provided, can be adapted to meet the needs of the patient. A central feature of the assessment for DIT therefore involves an ability to identify and take account of external resources available to the patient and to the therapist when planning the intervention, so that due consideration is given to the need for additional support through exploring the patient's external resources (e.g. friends and family as sources of support, stability of housing) and the appropriateness of the setting in which the therapy will be offered relative to the patient's needs (e.g. the need for additional support from other professionals).

The therapist's experience with the patient in the session

All the dimensions we have outlined so far will give important clues as to how the patient is likely to respond to DIT. However, the therapist's direct experience of being in the room with the patient is probably the most informative of all. Patients who on paper would seem to be unlikely candidates for DIT may nevertheless convey in their interaction with the therapist some hope that, with careful pacing by the therapist and adequate support both within and outside the therapy, they could make use of DIT. Here it is worth also noting that because of the more explicit supportive stance adopted by the DIT therapist, and its relatively more structured format, DIT might provide a useful bridge into longer-term psychodynamic therapy for patients who are not yet ready to engage with this kind of intervention. The therapist's appraisal of what the patient can tolerate and make use of is also gleaned from the therapist's reflection on the emotional impact the patient's presentation has on them (i.e. the countertransference). This rests on the therapist's ability to appraise the potential significance of their responses to understanding the patient's interpersonal patterns.

As will be apparent from the above list, when assessing a patient's suitability for DIT the therapist will need to appraise several dimensions of the patient's experience, and of their context, and pool them together in order to take a view. As we will repeatedly emphasize throughout this book, a flexible approach is critically important insofar as some patients might at first struggle with some of the demands DIT may make on them, but a therapist who is capable of carefully titrating their interventions could well make it possible for the patient to make use of DIT.

THIS SECOND EDITION

This new edition has two main sections. In the first (Chapters 2 to 9), we update the core approach and techniques of the DIT approach in a way that reflects our experience in treatment, training, and supervising using the first edition. The second section covers new developments that we have undertaken during the intervening years—in particular, research to evaluate the outcomes of DIT (Chapter 12), complex presentations including more elements of personality disorder (Chapter 13), adaptations of the model to work with patients presenting with somatic disorders (Chapter 14), and working via internet-delivered therapy (Chapter 15). It also outlines our experience, from several years of training psychotherapists and getting their feedback as practitioners, of both what can go wrong in implementing DIT (Chapter 10) and what questions are frequently posed to us (Chapter 11). In the final chapter (Chapter 16), we introduce readers to new directions that we are currently working on but have not yet formally integrated into the model in training and practice. We will map out some future directions we see as shaping the future of the DIT model (and which may shape psychotherapy more generally). These include conceptualizations of psychopathology (favouring a general psychopathology factor, or 'p factor', of severity over subcategories of diagnosis as most useful for therapies), and DIT as an evolving spectrum of models with different lengths and modalities of treatment for different situations.

REFERENCES

Abramson, L. Y., Seligman, M. E., & Teasdale, J. D. (1978). Learned helplessness in humans: Critique and reformulation. *Journal of Abnormal Psychology*, *87*(1), 49–74. https://doi.org/10.1037/0021-843X.87.1.49

American Psychiatric Association. (1980). *Diagnostic and statistical manual of mental disorders* (3rd edn.). American Psychiatric Association.

American Psychiatric Association. (2013). *Diagnostic and statistical manual of mental disorders* (5th edn.). American Psychiatric Association.
Bakermans-Kranenburg, M. J., Van Ijzendoorn, M. H., Mesman, J., Alink, L. R., & Juffer, F. (2008). Effects of an attachment-based intervention on daily cortisol moderated by dopamine receptor D4: A randomized control trial on 1- to 3-year-olds screened for externalizing behavior. *Development and Psychopathology, 20*(3), 805–820. https://doi.org/10.1017/S0954579408000382
Beck, A. T., Rush, J., Shaw, B., & Emery, G. (1979). *Cognitive therapy of depression*. Guilford Press.
Bifulco, A., Moran, P. M., Ball, C., & Bernazzani, O. (2002). Adult attachment style. I: Its relationship to clinical depression. *Social Psychiatry & Psychiatric Epidemiology, 37*(2), 50–59. https://doi.org/10.1007/s127-002-8215-0
Bifulco, A., Moran, P. M., Ball, C., & Lillie, A. (2002). Adult attachment style. II: Its relationship to psychosocial depressive-vulnerability. *Social Psychiatry & Psychiatric Epidemiology, 37*(2), 60–67. https://doi.org/10.1007/s127-002-8216-x
Binder, J. L. (2004). *Key competencies in brief psychodynamic therapy: Clinical practice beyond the manual*. Guilford Press.
Blatt, S. J. (2008). *Polarities of experience: Relatedness and self definition in personality development, psychopathology, and the therapeutic process*. American Psychological Association.
Blatt, S. J., & Luyten, P. (2009). A structural-developmental psychodynamic approach to psychopathology: Two polarities of experience across the life span. *Development and Psychopathology, 21*(3), 793–814. https://doi.org/10.1017/S0954579409000431
Blatt, S. J., Zuroff, D. C., Hawley, L. L., & Auerbach, J. S. (2010). Predictors of sustained therapeutic change. *Psychotherapy Research, 20*(1), 37–54. https://doi.org/10.1080/10503300903121080
Brown, G. W., & Harris, T. O. (1978). *Social origins of depression: A study of psychiatric disorders in women*. Tavistock.
Brown, G. W., & Harris, T. O. (Eds.). (1989). *Life events and illness*. Unwin Hyman.
Clark, D. M., & Wells, A. (1995). A cognitive model of social phobia. In R. G. Heimberg, M. R. Liebowitz, D. A. Hope, & F. R. Schneier (Eds.), *Social phobia: Diagnosis, assessment, and treatment* (pp. 41–68). Guilford Press.
Conradi, H. J., & de Jonge, P. (2009). Recurrent depression and the role of adult attachment: A prospective and a retrospective study. *Journal*

of Affective Disorders, *116*(1–2), 93–99. https://doi.org/10.1016/j.jad.2008.10.027

Engel, G. L., & Schmale, A. H., Jr. (1967). Psychoanalytic theory of somatic disorder. Conversion, specificity, and the disease onset situation. *Journal of the American Psychoanalytic Association*, *15*(2), 344–365. https://doi.org/10.1177/000306516701500206

Fehlbaum, L. V., Borbas, R., Paul, K., Eickhoff, S. B., & Raschle, N. M. (2022). Early and late neural correlates of mentalizing: ALE meta-analyses in adults, children and adolescents. *Social Cognitive and Affective Neuroscience*, *17*(4), 351–366. https://doi.org/10.1093/scan/nsab105

Feldman, R. (2017). The neurobiology of human attachments. *Trends in Cognitive Sciences*, *21*(2), 80–99. https://doi.org/10.1016/j.tics.2016.11.007

Fonagy, P., & Target, M. (2000). Playing with reality: III. The persistence of dual psychic reality in borderline patients. *International Journal of Psychoanalysis*, *81*(5), 853–873. https://doi.org/10.1516/0020757001600165

Frith, C. D., & Frith, U. (2021). Mapping mentalising in the brain. In M. Gilead & K. N. Ochsner (Eds.), *The neural basis of mentalizing* (pp. 17–45). Springer International. https://doi.org/10.1007/978-3-030-51890-5_2

Heim, C., Newport, D. J., Mletzko, T., Miller, A. H., & Nemeroff, C. B. (2008). The link between childhood trauma and depression: Insights from HPA axis studies in humans. *Psychoneuroendocrinology*, *33*(6), 693–710. https://doi.org/10.1016/j.psyneuen.2008.03.008

Hogg, B., Gardoki-Souto, I., Valiente-Gomez, A., Rosa, A. R., Fortea, L., Radua, J., Amann, B. L., & Moreno-Alcazar, A. (2023). Psychological trauma as a transdiagnostic risk factor for mental disorder: An umbrella meta-analysis. *European Archives of Psychiatry and Clinical Neuroscience*, *273*(2), 397–410. https://doi.org/10.1007/s00406-022-01495-5

Jones, E. (1927). Discussion on lay analysis. *International Journal of Psychoanalysis*, *8*, 174–198.

Kiesler, D. J. (1983). The 1982 Interpersonal Circle: A taxonomy for complementarity in human transactions. *Psychological Review*, *90*(3), 185–214. https://doi.org/10.1037/0033-295x.90.3.185

Kyte, Z. A., & Goodyer, I. (2008). Social cognition in depressed children and adolescents. In C. Sharp, P. Fonagy, & I. Goodyer (Eds.), *Social cognition and developmental psychopathology* (pp. 201–237). Oxford University Press.

Lee, A., & Hankin, B. L. (2009). Insecure attachment, dysfunctional attitudes, and low self-esteem predicting prospective symptoms of depression and anxiety during adolescence. *Journal of Clinical Child and*

Adolescent Psychology, 38(2), 219–231. https://doi.org/10.1080/153744 10802698396

Lemma, A., Roth, A. D., & Pilling, S. (2008). *The competences required to deliver effective psychoanalytic/psychodynamic therapy.* Research Department of Clinical, Educational and Health Psychology, University College London. https://www.ucl.ac.uk/pals/sites/pals/files/ppc_clinicians_background_paper.pdf

Lemma, A., Target, M., & Fonagy, P. (2011). *Brief dynamic interpersonal therapy: A clinician's guide* (1st edn.). Oxford University Press.

Lewinsohn, P. M., Mischel, W., Chaplin, W., & Barton, R. (1980). Social competence and depression: The role of illusory self-perceptions. *Journal of Abnormal Psychology, 89*(2), 203–212. https://doi.org/10.1037/0021-843x.89.2.203

Luyten, P. (2017). Personality, psychopathology, and health through the lens of interpersonal relatedness and self-definition. *Journal of the American Psychoanalytic Association, 65*(3), 473–489. https://doi.org/10.1177/0003065117712518

Luyten, P., Blatt, S. J., & Fonagy, P. (2013). Impairments in self structures in depression and suicide in psychodynamic and cognitive behavioral approaches: Implications for clinical practice and research. *International Journal of Cognitive Therapy, 6*(3), 265–279. https://doi.org/10.1521/ijct.2013.6.3.265

Luyten, P., Blatt, S. J., Van Houdenhove, B., & Corveleyn, J. (2006). Depression research and treatment: Are we skating to where the puck is going to be? *Clinical Psychology Review, 26*(8), 985–999. https://doi.org/10.1016/j.cpr.2005.12.003

Luyten, P., Corveleyn, J., & Blatt, S. J. (2005). The convergence among psychodynamic and cognitive-behavioral theories of depression: A critical overview of empirical research. In J. Corveleyn, P. Luyten, & S. J. Blatt (Eds.), *The theory and treatment of depression: Towards a dynamic interactionism model* (pp. 107–147). Lawrence Erlbaum Associates.

Luyten, P., & Fonagy, P. (2018). The stress-reward-mentalizing model of depression: An integrative developmental cascade approach to child and adolescent depressive disorder based on the Research Domain Criteria (RDoC) approach. *Clinical Psychology Review, 64*, 87–98. https://doi.org/10.1016/j.cpr.2017.09.008

Luyten, P., Lemma, A., & Target, M. (2019). Depression. In A. Bateman & P. Fonagy (Eds.), *Handbook of mentalizing in mental health practice* (2nd edn., pp. 387–401). American Psychiatric Publishing.

McFarquhar, T., Luyten, P., & Fonagy, P. (2023). A typology for the interpersonal affective focus in dynamic interpersonal therapy based on a contemporary interpersonal approach. *Psychotherapy*, *60*(2), 171–181. https://doi.org/10.1037/pst0000462

Mikulincer, M., & Shaver, P. R. (2016). *Attachment in adulthood: Structure, dynamics and change* (2nd ed.). Guilford Press.

Shedler, J., Beck, A., Fonagy, P., Gabbard, G. O., Gunderson, J., Kernberg, O., Michels, R., & Westen, D. (2010). Personality disorders in DSM-5. *American Journal of Psychiatry*, *167*(9), –1026–1028. https://doi.org/10.1176/appi.ajp.2010.10050746

Shedler, J., & Westen, D. (2004). Refining personality disorder diagnosis: Integrating science and practice. *American Journal of Psychiatry*, *161*(8), 1350–1365. https://doi.org/10.1176/appi.ajp.161.8.1350

Suárez, L. M., Bennett, S. M., Goldstein, C. R., & Barlow, D. H. (2008). Understanding anxiety disorders from a 'triple vulnerability' framework. In M. M. Antony & M. B. Stein (Eds.), *Oxford handbook of anxiety and related disorders* (pp. 153–172). Oxford University Press.

Torgersen, S. (1986). Childhood and family characteristics in panic and generalized anxiety disorders. *American Journal of Psychiatry*, *143*(5), 630–632. https://doi.org/10.1176/ajp.143.5.630

Truant, G. S. (1999). Assessment of suitability for psychotherapy. II. Assessment based on basic process goals. *American Journal of Psychotherapy*, *53*(1), 17–34. https://doi.org/10.1176/appi.psychotherapy.1999.53.1.17

Van Houdenhove, B., & Luyten, P. (2009). Central sensitivity syndromes: Stress system failure may explain the whole picture. *Seminars in Arthritis and Rheumatism*, *39*(3), 218–219. https://doi.org/10.1016/j.semarthrit.2008.08.008

Weissman, M. M., Markowitz, J. C., & Klerman, G. L. (2000). *Comprehensive guide to interpersonal psychotherapy*. Basic Books.

Whalley, H. C., McKirdy, J., Romaniuk, L., Sussmann, J., Johnstone, E. C., Wan, H. I., McIntosh, A. M., Lawrie, S. M., & Hall, J. (2009). Functional imaging of emotional memory in bipolar disorder and schizophrenia. *Bipolar Disorders*, *11*(8), 840–856. https://doi.org/10.1111/j.1399-5618.2009.00768.x

World Health Organization. (2019). *International statistical classification of diseases and related health problems*. World Health Organization. https://icd.who.int/en/

2
Key Analytic Models and Psychoanalytic Concepts Informing Dynamic Interpersonal Therapy

This chapter sets out the four main theories that inform the dynamic interpersonal therapy (DIT) model and the key psychoanalytic concepts that underpin the psychodynamic/analytic competence framework for DIT.

THE THEORETICAL FRAMEWORK OF DIT

DIT is embedded in a range of psychoanalytic ideas that are highly relevant to understanding mood disorders and their impact on an individual's internal and external worlds. We intend that this framework should yield enough common ground to make the model relevant to psychodynamic clinicians with a range of theoretical affiliations.

DIT's principles are rooted in some core psychoanalytic assumptions. These assumptions not only have face validity in the clinical situation, but several of them are also supported by empirical evidence (see, e.g. Fonagy & Target, 2003), namely:

- The impact of early childhood experiences on adult personality and mental health, with particular attention to adult attachment processes and the significance of mental models of relationships

- The internal and external forces that shape the mind, including our perception of ourselves in relationships with others
- The existence of a dynamically unconscious realm of experience that is a motivating force
- The unconscious projective and introjective processes that underpin the subjective experience of relationships
- The ubiquity of the transference, by which patients respond to others, and to the therapist, according to developmental models that have not been updated or challenged.

Although we draw on this shared pool of overarching psychodynamic ideas, we also draw more specifically on object-relations theory, attachment theory, Sullivan's interpersonal psychoanalysis, and mentalizing theory. We will discuss these theories in the following sections.

Object-relations theory

Object-relations theory is too diverse to have an agreed definition (Kramer & Akhtar, 1988), and as object-relations theories have come to dominate psychoanalysis, most theorists have appeared to aspire to this category. Greenberg and Mitchell (1983), in their classic overview, use the term to include all theories 'concerned with exploring the relationship between real, external people and the internal images and residues of relations with them and the significance of these residues for psychic functioning' (Greenberg & Mitchell, 1983, p. 14).

Kernberg (1976b) distinguishes three uses of the term object-relations theory:

1. The understanding of present relationships in terms of past ones, which would include the study of intrapsychic structures as deriving from fixation, modifying, and reactivating earlier internalizations.
2. A specialized approach within psychoanalytic metapsychology, involving mental representations of dyadic 'self'–'object' relationships, which are rooted in the original relation of the baby and mother, and the later development

of this relation into dyadic, triadic, and multiple internal and external relationships.
3. Specific approaches of (a) the Kleinian school, (b) the British Independent tradition, and (c) those theorists who have attempted to integrate the ideas of these schools into their own developmental theory.

In this context, as British analysts, we have been influenced mainly by the third, most limited group among object-relations theories, the 'English' (Kleinian) and 'British' (Independent) schools, and we have tried to integrate their approaches with some concepts of ego psychology (especially in the development of the concept of mentalizing) and the empirically oriented psychoanalytic framework of attachment theory.

The early relationship with the caregiver emerged as a critical aspect of development from studies of severe character disorders by psychoanalysts in the UK. Fairbairn's (1952) focus on the individual's need for the other helped to shift psychoanalytic attention from structure to content, and profoundly influenced both British and North American psychoanalytic thinking. Building on this development, the self as a central part of the psychoanalytic model emerged in the work of Balint (1937, 1968) and Winnicott (1971). The concept of the caretaker or false self as a defensive structure, created to master trauma in a context of total dependency, has become an essential developmental construct. Winnicott's (1965) notions of primary maternal preoccupation, transitional phenomena, the holding environment, and the mirroring function of the caregiver have become widely regarded as useful concepts in understanding the development of self-structure.

During the past half-century, the rise of object-relations theories has been accompanied by a shift in psychoanalytic interest: there has been a reduction of emphasis on the study of intrapsychic conflict, particularly conflicts relating to the sexual and aggressive drives, the centrality of oedipal compromises, and the complementarity of biological and experiential forces in development (Lussier, 1988; Rangell, 1985; Spruiell, 1988). Instead, psychoanalysis has moved increasingly towards an experientially based perspective, emphasizing the individual's experience of being with others and with the therapist in the transference (see e.g. Gill & Hoffman, 1982; Loewald, 1986; Schafer, 1983; Schwaber, 1983). This approach emphasizes phenomenological constructs such as individuals' experiences of themselves (see Stolorow et al., 1987) and of psychic—as opposed to external—reality (see McLaughlin, 1981; Michels, 1985). Patients in treatment commonly express themselves in terms of relationships (Modell, 1990). The move towards an object-relations-based metapsychology could be seen as being led by an increasing cultural emphasis on the point of view of the subject—here, the patient—and the therapist, who learns from their subjective experience of the patient.

Object-relations theories vary along several dimensions. For example, while some move to replace drive theory approaches entirely (e.g. the interpersonal-relational schools, Mitchell & Black, 1995), others are built out of drive theory (e.g. Winnicott, 1962), and others derive drive theory from an object-relations approach (e.g. Kernberg, 1982). Object-relations theories also differ in their focus on mechanisms underlying personality functioning. For example, in general systems theory approaches, the mental mechanism underpinning internalized relationship representations is at the heart of the theory (e.g. Stern, 1985), whereas in self-psychology models, object-relations are merely a route to a psychology of the self (e.g. Bacal, 1990).

Object-relations theories nevertheless share some assumptions. These include that:

1. Severe pathology has pre-oedipal origins (i.e. the first 3 years of life)
2. The pattern of relationships with objects becomes increasingly complex with development
3. The stages of this development follow a sequence across cultures, which may be distorted by personal trauma
4. Early patterns of object-relations tend to be repeated through life
5. Disturbances in these relations developmentally map on to pathology (see Westen, 1989)
6. Transference provides a window on early relationship patterns.

Friedman (1988) differentiates between 'hard' and 'soft' object-relations theories. Hard theories (including those of Klein, Fairbairn, and Kernberg) emphasize hate, envy, and destructiveness, and techniques confronting the unconsciously damaging impulses that result. Soft object-relations theorists, such as Balint, Winnicott, and Kohut, by contrast, see the potential of love, innocence, growth, and creativity, and emphasize techniques that allow progressive unfolding, with acceptance of regression and resistance.

Akhtar (1992) has usefully extended this contrast by using Strenger's (1989) model of the 'classic' and 'romantic' visions of humanity offered by psychoanalysts. The classic view would encompass the traditions of Klein, Kernberg, and some British object-relations theorists. The romantic approach perhaps originates with the work of Ferenczi and is well represented in the work of Balint, Winnicott, and Guntrip in the UK, and Modell and Adler in the USA (discussed in Bateman et al., 2022; Fonagy & Target, 2003). The first approach views psychopathology largely in terms of conflict, the second in terms of deficit. Acting out is seen as an inevitable consequence of deep-rooted pathology in the classic view, whereas the romantic view sees it as a manifestation of hope that the environment may reverse the damage done. There are approaches that combine the classic and the romantic. Kohut and Kernberg propose models of development that are pure representatives of neither tradition, and we also position ourselves between these extremes.

Kernberg's contribution to the development of psychoanalytic thought deserves special mention, as it has informed the way of formulating the focal problem we are following here. Kernberg's systematic integration of structural theory and object-relations theory (Kernberg, 1976a, 1982, 1987) has been highly influential, particularly in relation to personality disorders. His model of psychopathology is developmental, in the sense that personality disturbance is seen to reflect the limited capacities of the young child to address intrapsychic conflict. Neurotic object-relations show much less defensive disintegration of the representation of self and objects into libidinally invested part-object-relations. In personality disorders, part-object-relations are formed under the impact of diffuse, overwhelming emotional states—which may be ecstatic or terrifying and painful—prompting persecutory relations between self and object.

Object-relations theories thus stand against Freud's assumption that psychic structure evolves intrapsychically, whatever the child's relationships. Freud's suggestion that the mind is shaped by frustration of the child's drives allows for only one type of object relationship (where the child's needs are frustrated) to play a part in the creation of mental structures and functions (discussed in Fonagy & Target, 2003; Wolberg, 1995). Freudian and object-relations theories differ in the heterogeneity of possible relationship patterns, seen in the latter as shaping mental structures. The object-relations theories assume that the child's mind is shaped by all early experiences with the caregiver, and our approach follows this assumption. Some theories, for example, attachment theory, which we discuss in the next section, assume an autonomous 'relationship drive', which impels the infant into contact and preoccupation with the caregiver, independent of the gratification of primary needs.

Ego functioning and theories of attachment

Child analysts, such as Selma Fraiberg (1969, 1980) and Anna Freud (1965), helped us to see that symptomatology is not a fixed formation but rather a dynamic entity superimposed upon and intertwined with an underlying developmental process. Anna Freud's studies of children under great social stress led her to formulate a relatively comprehensive developmental theory, where the child's emotional and cognitive maturity could be mapped independently of diagnosable pathology. Her focus on the developmental processes (Freud, 1965) underlying ego capacities, and their relationship to psychological disturbance, is continued in the role of the capacity for mentalizing in our framework.

Another important theorist in the background of our clinical application of attachment concepts is Margaret Mahler (Mahler, 1967; Mahler & McDevitt, 1968; Mahler et al., 1975), who drew attention to the paradox of self-development, namely that a separate identity implies the giving up of a highly gratifying closeness with the caregiver. Her observations of the 'ambitendency' of children in their second year of life were helpful in understanding individuals with chronic problems in consolidating their individuality. Mahler's framework highlights the importance of the caregiver in facilitating separation. A traumatized, troubled parent may hinder rather than help a child's adaptation (Terr, 1983), and an abusive parent may altogether inhibit the process of social referencing (Cicchetti, 1990; Hesse & Cicchetti, 1982). The pathogenic potential of the withdrawing object, when confronted with the child's wish for separateness, was further elaborated by Masten (1982) and Rinsley (1977), and is helpful in accounting for the transgenerational aspects of psychological disturbance.

Joseph Sandler's development of Anna Freud's and Edith Jacobson's (Jacobson, 1964) work represents an early, inspired integration of the developmental perspective with psychoanalytic theory. At the core of Sandler's formulation lies the representational structure that contains both reality and distortion, and is the driving force of psychic life. A further important component of his model is the notion of the 'background of safety' (Sandler, 1987), which is closely tied to John Bowlby's concept of secure attachment and the secure base.

Bowlby's (1969, 1973, 1980) work on separation and loss strongly focused the attention of both clinicians and researchers on the importance of the security (safety, availability, and predictability) of the earliest relationships. His cognitive-systems model of the internalization of interpersonal relationships, that is, internal working models (IWMs), is consistent with object-relations theory (Fairbairn, 1952; Kernberg, 1975). It has been elaborated by other attachment theorists (Bretherton, 1985; Crittenden, 1990; Main et al., 1985), and has been particularly influential as it has a strong evidence base in predicting adult styles of relating, parenting, and mental health. Along with the idea of the secure base, IWMs have been one of the most central concepts of attachment theory (Bowlby, 1973). Bowlby saw the attachment behavioural system as organized by a set of expectations built through experience. This idea has been creatively developed by several major contributors (e.g. Bretherton & Munholland, 1999; Crittenden, 1994; Main, 1991; Sroufe, 1996). Four representational systems are implied in these reformulations:

1. Expectations of how caregivers will interact, beginning in the first year of life and later modified
2. Event representations in which general and specific memories of attachment-related experiences are stored
3. Autobiographical memories connected through personal meaning
4. Understanding of one's own feelings and motives, and those of others.

This concept has had very broad application. Bowlby's developmental model highlights the transgenerational nature of IWMs: that is, our view of ourselves depends upon the working model of relationships that characterized our caregivers. Empirical research has produced very robust findings (see van IJzendoorn, 1995), for example, that an infant's security is well predicted from parental mental representations—coherence of narrative and mentalizing in relation to early experience—assessed before the birth of the child (e.g. Fonagy, Steele, & Steele, 1991; Fonagy, Steele, Steele, et al., 1991).

Although Bowlby recognized that IWMs involved internal objects and object relationships, he thought these were largely formed through external experience: 'The varied expectations of the accessibility and responsiveness of attachment figures that different individuals develop during the years of immaturity are tolerably accurate reflections of the experiences those individuals have actually had' (Bowlby, 1973, p. 235). IWMs of the self and of parents are thus first built on early representations of the relationship, which then evolve into freestanding yet interlocking images of the self and attachment figures (Bretherton, 1985). The term 'interlocking' means that a child who has IWMs of attachment figures as unloving and rejecting will come to hold a model of the self as unlovable, unworthy, boring, and so on. By contrast, a child who holds IWMs of attachment figures as loving and sensitive to their needs will hold a complementary model of the self as deserving of love and care.

Clearly, IWMs will be adaptive for the person holding them provided they enable that person to anticipate how people will behave towards them in future important situations (will loved ones protect them if they are sick, injured, in danger, or simply feeling bad, or will they not notice, not care, be cruel, or misunderstand?). Accurate anticipation requires that earlier experiences, on which prediction is based, have been perceived fairly realistically, and that future relationship contexts are similar. Here, one immediately sees that distorted perceptions (e.g. arising through the operation of primitive defences), and cognitive limitations that are natural at early stages of development, may lead a young child to draw incorrect conclusions from half-understood interactions. If the underlying distortions are not revised, they may be reinforced rather than modified in more realistic directions by later experiences. The protective value of IWMs could then be undermined and replaced by self-defeating misattributions and defensive strategies. These can be seen in the organized but 'insecure' forms of attachment behaviour and representation, described by attachment researchers and summarized later in this chapter, which are familiar to psychotherapists.

Bowlby's development of attachment theory initially drew heated criticism from psychoanalysts (Fonagy, 2001). However, some features that made it anathema at first have gradually come to be seen as advantages: the introduction of biological principles in understanding personality and relationships (really a reintroduction because, of course, Freud began with that framework); a linking of empirical and theoretical evidence, and, related to that, building bridges with a range of neighbouring disciplines; and attention to the non-conscious (procedural or implicit) as well as the dynamically unconscious determinants of feelings, thoughts, and actions. These procedural or implicit determinants of personality structure and affect regulation are seen by us as closely relevant to the understanding of character development and personality disorders, and to the mood disorders of many of our patients (Target, 2005).

Finally, we refer to the work of Daniel Stern, beginning with his 1985 book (Stern, 1985), a milestone in psychoanalytic theorization of development as reflected in the transference. His focus is the reorganization of subjective perspectives on self and other as these occur with the emergence of new maturational capacities. Stern deals with several qualitatively different senses of self, each developmentally anchored. He is perhaps closest to Sandler in his psychoanalytic model of the mind, but his formulation of object-relations also has much in common with Bowlby and Kernberg. Many of Stern's suggestions have proved to be highly valuable clinically, including his notion of an early core self and the role of the schema-of-being-with-another. These concepts, like those of Kernberg's, can be seen to inform the integrative approach we propose in this book.

Interpersonal psychoanalysis: The contribution of Harry Stack Sullivan

Sullivan is a neglected figure within contemporary psychoanalysis. An American psychiatrist working in the 1930s and 1940s, he was one of the main proponents of a particular strand of psychodynamic thinking called interpersonal psychiatry or interpersonal psychoanalysis, which provided an alternative to Freud's drive theory at the time. Although many of his ideas were shared by contemporaries such as Eric Fromm and Karen Horney, Sullivan was a more fervent critic of Freud's emphasis on intrapsychic conflict and the importance of infantile sexuality. Sullivan emphasized the importance of external reality, for example, of the culture and society in which an individual grows up, as well as of interconnectedness, which he understood to be central to understanding the development of an individual's personality and their difficulties.

Sullivan did not disregard the importance of intrapsychic experience, although he has been criticized for this. In his writings, his primary emphasis is on the individual's current relationships and how these impact on evolving personality and psychopathology, perhaps because he had to uphold a contrasting position. Yet, his notion of 'personification' (i.e. the way a person comes to know the world through a set of internal assumptions/'pictures' of the self and others based on developmental experience) is akin to the notion of an internal world. Moreover, there are clear overlaps in his ideas with both attachment theory and object-relations theory, in light of his emphasis on the early mother–child relationship. Consistent with all psychoanalytic models, behaviour and psychopathology were understood by Sullivan in relation to both historical and current interpersonal contexts.

In Sullivan's theory (Sullivan, 1953), depression and anxiety are manifestations of the distortion and complexities of an individual's interpersonal relationships—a conceptualization that also informs DIT. In more contemporary interpersonal models (see Kiesler, 1996), symptoms are seen to result primarily from problematic interactional patterns, which have become entrenched and can lead to extreme interpersonal behaviour. This is simply another way of acknowledging the importance of internalized early interactional patterns, which become dominant and may significantly distort the individual's capacity to appraise what is happening in their relationship with others.

Sullivan's emphasis on actual (i.e. not fantasized) interpersonal exchanges, on how the patient communicates with the other person, and on the assumptions the patient makes about what the other person may be thinking or feeling are all very consistent with the focus in DIT on current relationships and functioning, including our emphasis on underlying attachment models and how they commonly distort mentalizing in relation to external relationships. The indirect, confusing, incongruous, and typically self-defeating communications that transpire in human relationships become the focus of intervention; this helps the patient identify their own contribution to recreating particular interpersonal scenarios, which, despite being deeply distressing, are nevertheless perfectly understandable in light of developmental models that have become internalized. In particular, the relationship that develops between the patient and therapist provides a vehicle for helping the patient to understand some of the more automatic, unconscious assumptions they make about themself and others, and which can give rise to the onset of symptoms.

DIT also borrows from some of the technical principles that guided Sullivan's approach to the therapeutic situation itself. In particular, Sullivan believed that people strive to minimize insecurity. In his view, interpersonal behaviours, even ultimately self-defeating ones, could nevertheless be understood as attempts to avoid anxiety or depression, or to establish and maintain self-esteem. Of particular importance to Sullivan was the psychotherapist's understanding and management of the patient's anxiety, which is present in the form of the patient's expectations and fear of the psychotherapist's disapproval and the interpersonal defences that might be activated to avoid this experience of insecurity. As far as Sullivan was concerned, one of the psychotherapist's primary responsibilities was, as he put it, to 'integrate the situation'—that is, to join with the patient to create an atmosphere of 'interpersonal security'.

Sullivan strongly favoured an engaged, active therapeutic stance that strives to foster this sense of safety. He was very clear that interpersonal learning could occur only in a situation where the patient felt relatively safe, rather than in an atmosphere that was more likely to generate the patient's anxiety, such as being in a room with a relatively uncommunicative therapist. The stance that he therefore advocated was one that he termed 'respectful seriousness'. He believed that empathy was an interpersonal process worked out between the participants during the course of therapy, based on the patient's actual experience.

In accordance with all contemporary psychoanalytic models, Sullivan understood that the patient's perceptions of the therapist were strongly shaped by the patient's experience prior to the treatment (i.e. the transference brought to it). However, he emphasized that they were also shaped by the patient's actual experience during the therapy, and that careful attention needed to be paid to these perceptions. For Sullivan this needed to include an understanding not only of the transference but also of what he termed the 'real' relationship with the therapist, including the impact of the psychotherapist's cultural role, anxieties, foibles, and so on. In other words, Sullivan saw the therapeutic relationship as fundamentally intersubjective.

By paying careful attention to what transpired between the patient and the therapist, the therapeutic situation was thus seen by Sullivan to provide an opportunity for 'facilitating interpersonal learning'. This is one of the core strategies of DIT.

Mentalizing

We have already mentioned mentalizing (Fonagy et al., 2002), another theoretical concept that informs the DIT model. Mentalizing describes the affective, interpretive interface between IWMs that form between self and other. It can be defined as a form of imaginative mental activity about others or oneself, namely perceiving and understanding human behaviour in terms of intentional mental states, for example, needs, desires, feelings, beliefs, goals, purposes, and reasons. Other terms include: mind-mindedness; holding mind in mind; and the ability to see ourselves as others see us, and others as they see themselves. Mentalizing is a metacognitive activity that people do in the background, often implicitly and procedurally, and, as such, it is vulnerable to unnoticed distortions when the person is experiencing emotional arousal and stress. (Mentalizing is described in more detail in Chapters 7 and 13.)

Evidently, being able to mentalize flexibly entails being able to hold several different possibilities in mind at once and to hold multiple perspectives when considering a situation or interaction. We can appreciate that human experience is filtered through the mind, and that therefore our perceptions, desires, and theories are necessarily provisional. The capacity to mentalize begins to develop in the context of early attachment relationships. The parent's ability to effectively 'mirror' the child's internal states is at the heart of early affect regulation (Fonagy et al., 2002). The parent is able to do this through marked and contingent mirroring of the infant's mental states, allowing the infant to recognize their own mental states as separate from the parent's and to develop internal representations of those states (Gergely & Watson, 1996). To do this, the parent needs to be attuned to the infant's mental states and to differentiate their own state from the infant's. Disruption of this process owing to factors such as parental depression, intergenerational transmission of trauma, current trauma, abuse, and neglect will have pernicious consequences for the development of affect regulation. This is of particular significance in patients presenting with depression and anxiety who show deficits in mentalizing. In Chapter 7, we explore how to recognize poor mentalizing and when to employ mentalizing techniques as one of the therapeutic strategies adopted in DIT.

KEY PSYCHOANALYTIC TECHNICAL CONCEPTS THAT INFORM DIT

The Psychodynamic Competences Framework (Lemma et al., 2008)[1,2] describes a model of psychodynamic competences based on empirical evidence of efficacy. It indicates the various areas of activity that, taken together, represent what has been proven to be good clinical practice as observed in outcome trials.

The work to develop the framework began by identifying those psychodynamic approaches with the strongest claims for evidence of efficacy, based on the outcome in controlled trials where a manual was available. In order to determine which studies to select, the reviews of psychological therapies conducted by Roth and Fonagy (2005) were combined with a database of trials and systematic reviews held at the Centre for Outcomes Research and Effectiveness at University College London, as part of scoping work for the UK National Institute for Health and Care Excellence. From the combined lists (with oversight from an expert reference group comprising senior clinicians and

---

1. The full list of competences can be accessed at https://www.ucl.ac.uk/pals/research/clinical-educational-and-health-psychology/research-groups/core/competence-frameworks-6

2. The Improving Access to Psychological Therapies programme in the UK, which was launched in May 2007, provided the backdrop for the first wave of work on the development of competences for the practice of psychological therapies. The cognitive-behavioural therapy competence model was specifically developed to be a 'prototype' for articulating the competences associated with other psychological therapies (Roth & Pilling, 2008).

researchers from a range of analytic traditions), clinical trials of appropriate quality for inclusion in the framework were identified, and the manuals used in these studies were obtained. Only trials for which a manual could be accessed were included. The manuals were then studied carefully, with a focus on what the therapists were expected to do. This qualitative analysis provided the basis for the articulation of the core competences, specific competences, and metacompetences required to practise psychoanalytic psychotherapy (available at https://www.ucl.ac.uk/clinical-psychology/competency-maps/psychodynamic-map.html). These competences, where possible, were peer-reviewed by the originators of the manuals as well as by the expert reference group. To supplement the manuals, several widely cited texts that explicate psychoanalytic terminology and provide clear descriptions of how psychoanalytic concepts translate into clinical practice were also consulted (e.g. Bateman et al., 2000; Etchegoyen, 1999; Greenson, 1967; Lemma, 2003).

We will not elaborate upon the generic psychotherapy competences that are common to different theoretical approaches here. Instead, we will concentrate on the key concepts that underpin psychodynamic work, and DIT in particular. What informs all psychodynamic and analytic psychotherapy is the overarching metacompetence, namely, the ability to approach all aspects of interacting with the patient and managing the clinical setting with an 'analytic attitude' (Lemma et al., 2008). By this, we mean that the therapist is receptive to the patient's unconscious communications and to the unfolding of the transference. This state of mind is no less essential in brief psychodynamic psychotherapy than in longer-term psychotherapy. The following key theoretical concepts constitute the prerequisite knowledge to train in DIT.

Ability to establish and manage the therapeutic frame and boundaries

The *therapeutic frame* refers to the internal and external setting in which therapy takes place, such as the practical arrangements of space and time, and the therapist's attitude. The therapeutic frame forms part of the therapeutic contract and allows us to interpret any deviations from the frame once it is established. The core features of the analytic frame are consistency, reliability, neutrality, anonymity, and abstinence (Lemma, 2016). As therapists, we aim to see each patient at the same time and place each week. We are mindful of the impact on our patients of any breaks in that regularity, both planned and unplanned: in brief psychotherapy the interpersonal pattern can be powerfully activated by such a disruption. We also endeavour to create as reliable a space as possible, free from interruptions and disturbance, so that we can be experienced as fully attentive and trustworthy by our patients. We do not want to be pushed into action, instead aiming to maintain our ability to reflect on what is unfolding in the therapeutic setting—that is, our own capacity to mentalize flexibly. We strive to be as anonymous as possible, while bearing in mind that we are inevitably revealing aspects of ourselves to others and, in any case, our patients are likely to be able to find out information about us outside the setting, for example, from internet or institutional sources. Notwithstanding this, if we reveal too much of our personal tastes and views, we run the risk of disturbing our patients' ability to project whatever they require on to us, thereby restricting the development of the transference. We want to maintain our focus on our patients' internal world and subjective experience. For this reason, we abstain from answering questions about our personal lives (e.g. where we are going on holiday), yet remain open to understanding the importance of such questions (see also Chapter 10). We also want to ensure we are not overly gratifying of our patients, instead occupying a position where we remain affectively engaged with our patients while guarding against retaliating or praising them. In Chapter 3, we will describe the characteristic DIT therapeutic stance, which is a variation of a more classical analytic position.

Managing the therapeutic frame extends to the way we start and end sessions. While there is more structure to a DIT session—particularly during the initial and ending phases, when the therapist has distinct tasks to cover (see Chapters 4 and 9)—we do want to preserve the emergent quality of sessions by allowing space for reflection at the start of the session, rather than rushing in to structure the session for our patients. We would typically end each session by signalling that we have reached the end of the time. This is distinctly different from directive and/or structured therapeutic approaches such as cognitive-behavioural therapy, where the therapist often summarizes the session and usually sets 'homework' for the week ahead. It also diverges from counselling and supportive psychotherapy, where the therapist may give advance warning that the end of time is approaching. The psychoanalytic stance precludes being overly directive, suggestive, or didactic. We can feel challenged by those patients who bring significant issues as the end of the time is approaching, leaving us cutting them off. Yet, this can be understood as a form of resistance, and something we can encourage them to consider in the next session. It is important to hold the boundary of the 50-minute session, and this entails accepting this ending as an expression of our 'hate in the countertransference' (Winnicott, 1949).

Ability to work with unconscious communication

The unconscious refers to that part of the mind that is out of our awareness: to use a common analogy, it is the submerged part of the iceberg. Freud (1900) differentiated between manifest and latent meaning, whereby what is being said overtly in the patient's narrative does not always match the underlying feelings and attitudes that are out of the patient's awareness. This can happen in a variety of ways. A patient may disown their feelings and project them into the therapist so that the therapist becomes aware of powerful experiences that the patient is denying experiencing. The patient may convey their unconscious preoccupations in the way that they segue from one topic to another, suggesting an unconscious connection between these topics. There may be an obvious omission that is worth commenting on, suggesting a possible denial of reality. For example, a patient may never speak about their loving marriage, instead focusing on their problematic relationship with their mother, and in doing so they may be unconsciously splitting good and bad experiences. Alternatively, a patient may change topic to get away from painful feelings or leave the 'meat' of the session until the last few minutes, perhaps unconsciously repeating an experience of feeling cut off. The patient may betray their unconscious feelings and attitudes through their body language rather than their words. For example, a patient may say they do not care about what someone thinks about them, but we witness otherwise through the evident physical tension in the room. The patient's language is often very revealing, in the choice of descriptors, repetition of words, and expressions, as well as slips of the tongue (Freud,

1901) where a patient means to say one thing but substitutes another, perhaps revealing another dimension of their relationship. An example of this is the patient who mistakenly identifies their partner as their parent. Transference (the way the patient transfers earlier relationships on to the therapist) is a further example of an unconscious phenomenon, something we explore later in this chapter. Freud (1900, p. 608) described dreams as 'the royal road to . . . the unconscious', and while we would not expect dreams to feature hugely in brief psychodynamic work, sometimes a patient's dream has helped their DIT therapist to grasp more fully the intensity or focus of the patient's feelings.

The capacity to tune into unconscious communications is a defining characteristic of psychodynamic work and we would expect the DIT therapist to pay attention to this during sessions, tuning into what is being avoided as well as what is being said. The countertransference is one instrument for detecting unconscious processes, albeit one we need to monitor carefully. We are particularly interested in how the unconscious shapes the patient's interpersonal world in DIT, leading to particular attachment strategies. The DIT therapist works within the confines of a focus, a shared aspect of all brief psychodynamic therapies, and hence not all unconscious communication will be addressed with the patient. The therapist should hold in mind the patient's vulnerabilities in titrating how much to interpret at any one time.

The unconscious is at play when it comes to the focus of DIT, the interpersonal and affective focus for the work (i.e. the interpersonal-affective focus (IPAF)). This is a pattern of relating that has become implicit and procedural for the patient in a way that is often out of their conscious awareness. The patient finds it easier to engage with the world in keeping with these repeated patterns of object-relations that allow the patient to anticipate the responses of others. Although this is often self-limiting and painful, it offers a sense of predictability that is strangely reassuring. Part of the work of DIT is drawing the patient's awareness to these unconscious patterns of relating so that they can make more conscious choices about how to respond both interpersonally and internally.

This brings us on to the idea of the *dynamic unconscious*, the way in which material that is painful is pushed out of awareness (repressed) only to force its way back into our mind, often disguised (e.g. reversed), much like the children's game of 'Whack-a-mole'. However much you try to get rid of the mole, in 'the return of the repressed' (Freud, 1896, p. 169) it pushes its way up somewhere else. Another phenomenon is captured by the common expression 'the elephant in the room': we can be painfully conscious of what we are trying to avoid talking about but are often unable even to acknowledge and then think about it in our own mind. Although the dynamic underlying this phenomenon is to avoid pain, as therapists we are working with our patients to help them become more aware of and able to consider these dysfunctional interpersonal ideas and the resultant defence mechanisms.

The DIT therapist should listen to the patient's communications on several levels, to the manifest communication of the interpersonal narratives and their external realities, as well as the unconscious level of what lies behind, including earlier childhood experiences that are embedded in the IPAF. It is challenging for therapists to listen to more than one thing at the same time and to tolerate the dissonance that this can give rise to within them. When conducting a brief psychotherapy such as DIT, it is even more challenging, as there are some aspects of the model that need to be adhered to at certain times, for example, gathering sufficient examples of interpersonal relationships to develop a formulation, or using outcome measures to evaluate the patient's mood and anxiety from week to week. Yet despite this, the DIT therapist should remain true to their psychoanalytic/dynamic background and be actively listening for all levels of communication, manifest and latent. This allows the therapist to remain open to hearing new material without foreclosing understanding. The IPAF is there to be modified rather than become restrictive and fossilized. We want to encourage the patient's capacity to mentalize flexibly by remaining curious in the characteristic 'not-knowing' DIT stance. Rather than assume we already know, it is important to clarify and question what is meant by a particular turn of phrase, as well as to wonder where the patient's missing aggression or anxiety is, for instance.

Ability to recognize and work with defences

Anxiety is inevitable: we are hard-wired with a fight/flight response as part of our survival mechanism to respond to danger. Anxiety is also an integral part of our attachment system, as described earlier in this chapter. We can all anticipate difficulties, as well as ruminate over past events, which can lead to raised states of anxiety. We develop defence mechanisms at an early age as an unconscious way of protecting ourselves from anxiety and in an attempt to bolster our self-esteem. Defences arise in response to intrapsychic conflict (in keeping with drive theory, and creating tension between different internal agencies of the mind), as well as interpersonal conflict when we feel caught between the demands and wishes of different people. Defence mechanisms serve to shield us from painful feelings, a type of character armour. Some defences are adaptive, while others become restrictive and maladaptive. Like a suit of armour, too many defences can leave us feeling weighed down, emotionally restricted, and unable to respond in an agile fashion.

Defence mechanisms are usually categorized as primitive or neurotic, with the distinction relating to the point of development at which they arose. The earlier they occur in development, the more primitive the defences are likely to be, since the infant and the young child have a less sophisticated psychic apparatus, the boundaries of self and other are more diffuse, and there is more distortion of reality at a global and deeper level. Understanding the nature of the defences our patients employ can assist with the question of suitability for brief psychotherapy. As a general rule, the greater and more primitive the defensiveness, the more challenging brief work is likely to be, and the more time is likely to be spent in repairing ruptures in the therapeutic alliance as well as restoring mentalizing in our patients. For some patients, this will mean that the extended model of DIT for complex care (DITCC; see Chapter 13) will be more helpful.

Going into detail about the range of defence mechanisms at play is beyond the scope of this chapter. However, here we include a list of some defences with brief explanations of each.

Primitive defences include the following:

- *Splitting*: separating and compartmentalizing opposing feelings or thoughts (typically good and bad experiences), without ambivalence or nuance. Idealization and denigration exemplify splitting.
- *Denial*: refusing to recognize certain unpalatable aspects of a situation by turning a blind eye.

- *Disavowal*: a more extreme form of denial, whereby the reality of an unacceptable perception is negated.
- *Primitive withdrawal*: retreating into an internal world of phantasy (see Chapter 4) and withdrawing from reality and consciousness.
- *Dissociation*: disconnecting and cutting off from reality. This is seen in trauma, where there can be a cutting off from oneself (depersonalization) as well as from the environment (derealization).
- *Projection*: attributing one's own thoughts, feelings, and motives to someone else.
- *Projective identification*: powerfully evacuating a painful state of mind (e.g. hatred) into someone else who becomes affected by it, then disowning it. It can be used unconsciously to communicate a painful experience, as well as to rid oneself of it, to control the other person, and to avoid separation.
- *Omnipotence* and *manic defences*: viewing the self as special and all-powerful, in a triumphant way that is at odds with reality.

Neurotic defences include:

- *Turning against the self*: taking up the opposite position, including directing aggression and other difficult feelings towards the self rather than others.
- *Reversal*: turning activity into passivity, and vice versa (e.g. sadism/masochism and voyeurism/exhibitionism).
- *Repression*: excluding an anxiety-provoking idea from conscious awareness. Like the 'elephant in the room', these thoughts may not be completely out of mind and keep returning into awareness at some level through the return of the repressed.
- *Regression*: reverting to developmentally earlier psychic functioning, for example, dependency in thinking (as well as action).
- *Undoing*: ways of neutralizing what has been thought or said by taking up the opposite position.
- *Displacement*: shifting unacceptable feelings from one person or area to another.
- *Isolation* and *intellectualization*: separating out feelings from awareness so that an experience can be spoken about

in an unemotional way. Intellectualization is a particular expression of isolation in which there is a focus on cognitions at the expense of affect. This is also known in therapy as *pseudomentalizing*.
- *Conversion*: experiencing psychic pain in bodily, somatic ways, for example, depression expressed as backache.
- *Acting out*: discharging painful feelings through actions in order to get away from them (e.g. shoplifting after a session).
- *Rationalization*: using logic to justify and disguise an unacceptable situation to make it more palatable.
- *Reaction formation*: transforming and inverting a disturbing, intolerable idea, feeling, or impulse into something desirable and acceptable (e.g. reacting to envy of others by being over-nice to them, sabotaging oneself).
- *Sublimation*: diverting unacceptable sexual impulses towards socially valued aims, such as intellectual pursuits, artistic creations, religion, science, or philosophy. It is considered one of the most mature defence mechanisms.

Alongside this list, patients can use any behaviour in a defensive way, such as falling asleep, shopping, eating, sex, exercise, watching TV, or using social media. When exploring our patients' coping strategies in the face of anxiety and low mood, we explore areas such as somatizing, substance abuse, addictive behaviours (e.g. gambling or using pornography), eating disorders, self-harm and risk-taking, perfectionism, body dysmorphia, and body modification through tattooing, piercing, and plastic surgery. All of these can be ways in which our patients respond to painful, unbearable feelings and conflictual interpersonal situations, and so may be defensive responses.

Attachment perspective on defences

In DIT, we conceptualize defences not only as intrapsychic ways to avoid knowing about thoughts and feelings, but also as mental adaptations to recurring interpersonal conflicts or what are felt to be patterns, such as painful attitudes others are believed to hold towards ourselves. Our patients have learned to respond to the interpersonal threats they have encountered in typical ways and have developed internalized procedures for being with others, including defensive secondary attachment strategies that are deactivating or hyperactivating (Shaver & Mikulincer, 2007). Hyperactivation—aligned with Bowlby's protest stage (Bowlby, 1960)—is characterized by increased attempts to establish interpersonal closeness, and manifests in coercion, clinginess, controlling behaviour with up-regulation of emotions, and a wish to merge with the other. Hyperactivation is linked with anaclitic depression, in which emphasis is placed on relatedness (Blatt, 2008; Blatt & Luyten, 2009) and where the self is often experienced as unwanted and unloved in relation to a rejecting, unavailable other. By contrast, deactivation—aligned with Bowlby's (1980) compulsive self-reliance—is characterized by avoidance, distancing from others, self-sufficiency, down-regulation of emotions, and devaluing relationships. Deactivation is linked with introjective depression, in which emphasis is placed on self-definition, and where the self is typically experienced as unlovable and worthless in relation to a critical other.

Each internal attachment strategy is likely to give rise to different interpersonal strategies. Both deactivating and hyperactivating attachment strategies, which lead to affect suppression and intensification, respectively, are opposing defensive responses to the same need to cope with intense feelings of insecurity in relation to key attachment figures (Shaver & Mikulincer, 2007).

Ability to work in the transference

This refers to the way the patient brings their early internalized object relationships from the past ('there-and-then') into the present, 'here-and-now' relationships with other people in their lives as well as in their relationship with the therapist, the primary focus of transference phenomena. Transference is always present, and in the therapy situation it begins before the patient meets the therapist in reality. The patient brings their assumptions to the first meeting, based on their attitudes towards psychotherapy in general, their own ideas about the person they are about to see, and beliefs about what will happen in the initial meeting, all of which have a life of their own that is separate from the actual meeting with the therapist. The transference will manifest in a variety of ways, depending on where the patient finds themself developmentally at that time of their life. They may relate to the therapist as if to their mother or father (maternal or paternal transference), to the wish to be part of a pair (pre-oedipal transference), or in a more triangulated, oedipal configuration. Just as we saw with unconscious processes, there is a compulsion to repeat through the transference the early, repressed experiences with key attachment figures. As such, the transference represents a rich source of information about the patient's IWMs of those interpersonal relationships. The here-and-now relationships are distorted by the earlier internalized object relationships. Rather than seeing transference as an obstacle to therapy, Paula Heimann (1956, p. 307) stressed its value: 'It is the transference interpretation which fully re-instates the past in the present and makes it accessible to the patient's ego.' Thus, we can see the transference as an interpersonal pattern being played out in the consulting room, and it can lend affective power to our formulation because it is a lived, shared experience. By recognizing how early relationships are repeated with the therapist, the patient can gain insight into these unconscious repetitions, which in turn facilitates their making choices that allow for new interpersonal possibilities as well as greater flexibility and emotional intimacy. In DIT terms, this means assisting the patient with stepping outside their IPAF and responding differently. One way we may see this happening is if the patient predicts that they will not get emotional support from the therapist and behaves in a self-sufficient manner, not bringing their concerns to the session. The DIT therapist can interpret this as repetition of an inaccessible other, which is even more painful because it is happening in the context of the therapy where, at a conscious level, the patient entered treatment in the hope of being understood and helped.

One of the adjustments we make to taking up the transference in a brief psychotherapy such as DIT is that we require the existence of a therapeutic alliance to be able to work effectively. We adopt a more supportive and active stance in brief psychotherapy than in longer-term psychotherapy and, as such, it would not be in our interests to sit back and allow the transference anxieties to multiply so we can get a better idea of the patient's difficulties. We also take up those aspects of the transference that may interfere with the therapeutic alliance, as well as manifestations of the transference that exemplify the agreed focus of the work together. At other times, while we may be aware of transferential aspects of our patients' communications, we do not raise them—a selectiveness necessary in all brief psychotherapies.

Ability to work with countertransference

A key psychodynamic competence is our ability to monitor our countertransference, that is, the emotional reaction we are having to our patient, which includes our thoughts, feelings, bodily responses, associations, and actions (e.g. occasionally ending a session early or late). We are aware that we communicate with our patients at both conscious and unconscious levels, in verbal and embodied ways. The transference is a two-way unconscious communication that requires us, as receptive therapists, to receive those communications through our countertransference. This necessitates us being receptive to communications that do not always fit with our self-perception. For example, a patient may see us as cruel or distracted—ego-dystonic qualities that we do not recognize; yet we need to receive these projections and make sense of them in the service of psychotherapy rather than push them back at the patient. Heimann (1950, p. 81) highlighted how 'the analyst's counter-transference is an instrument of research into the patient's unconscious'. Paying attention to our countertransference requires a capacity for self-reflection and self-awareness. It is important for us to differentiate between personal responses that are to do with our own blind spots and difficulties that are responses to our patients. This explains in part the requirement for personal therapy in psychodynamic psychotherapy training so that we are aware of these areas as far as possible, including our own capacity to contribute towards enactments. Similarly, close supervision of our work adds another level of scrutiny to guard against our subjective blocks.

Anna Freud (1954) described the way psychotherapists should strive to find a neutral countertransference position in response to our patients that is equidistant between our id, ego, and superego. We do not want to be overly gratifying to our patients (too aligned with the id), nor do we want to be overly punitive and judgemental (operating from a superego position); we also do not want to be too caught up with real-life solutions and daily functioning at the expense of listening out for unconscious communications (too aligned with ego functioning). This neutrality is important in DIT as we listen to our patient's interpersonal narratives. We are curious about the nature of these interactions and what is being repeated interpersonally. We should be mindful of our neutrality being compromised if we start, for instance, to feel annoyed with our patient's witch of a mother who is portrayed as behaving cruelly at all times. Similarly, we should be on alert if we notice that we are drawn into listening to our patients' narratives uncritically, with great interest or enjoyment.

At times, we may find ourselves pulled into a complementary response in reaction to the patient's projections. Sandler (1976) wrote about therapists' capacity for free-floating responsiveness, the particular way we are unconsciously pulled into enacting a role in relation to our patient. We find ourselves going along with a certain response to our patient as if on autopilot, taking up the role ascribed to us. While we strive to hold the analytic frame, small enactments such as this are an inevitable 'pull' in psychotherapy. When they do occur, they can offer a rich vein of interpersonal information. Sandler described how he repeatedly passed a box of tissues to a tearful patient, until one day he became aware of doing this and decided not to respond as usual. The patient responded angrily at this so-called lapse. In exploring what transpired between them, Sandler was able to understand that he had been drawn into a role-responsive position in his countertransference, whereby he offered the patient the tissues to help 'clean her up', remediating a failure in her early care by doing so. This was happening out of conscious awareness. We can think about the way we are invited to repeat a relationship with our patients and, once aware of this 'role responsiveness', we would then be able to reflect on and interpret it in relation to the agreed interpersonal focus of the work in DIT. As we will see, the IPAF includes a dynamic aspect, a reversed pattern that is defended against in the IPAF (e.g. aggression hidden by over-meekness and fear of the other), and Sandler's concept is useful to pick this up within the transference in DIT.

Ability to make dynamic interpretations

An interpretation is the verbal intervention offered by the therapist to bring aspects of the patient's internal and interpersonal world to their awareness. The timing and content of a psychodynamic interpretation is an art, not a science; it relies on the therapist's ability to intuit how best to reach the patient in that moment. This tends to be a gradual, step-by-step process rather than a single explosion of insight; we start interpreting from areas of conscious awareness before moving into deeper, more unconscious and/or defended areas. Couching our words as hypotheses to be tested out is a helpful way of phrasing our interpretations (e.g. 'It's possible that . . .', 'I wonder if . . .') as well as marking observations as our own (e.g. 'It occurs to me that . . .'), and revealing the way our mind worked in arriving at the interpretation (e.g. 'It brings to my mind the way that . . .').

In DIT, the focal pattern or IPAF guides our interpretations as we bring to the patient's attention the way this pattern keeps repeating itself, including in the transference ('here-and-now'), as well as how the patient's defences both contribute to and are mobilized by this pattern. For example, unconscious aggression can lead to an IPAF in which the patient is weak and threatened, but the fear and expected humiliation may be defended against by suppressing a wish for relationships. We expect therapists in brief psychotherapy to be more supportive and active than in open-ended psychotherapy. However, we want to protect the emergent quality of DIT. Interpretations should be accessible to the patient, and part of our role as DIT therapists is to evaluate whether our interventions are 'landing' with the patient, by considering their response to what we have offered. Does what the patient then says elaborate or deepen their awareness, particularly affectively? Does it open things up further in the patient's and our minds, or does it shut something down?

We need to consider the patient's ego strength and capacity to hear what we say. Sometimes, there is an area of interpersonal vulnerability that leaves the therapist feeling constricted in what they take up with a particular patient. Certain IPAFs, such as those with a hostile or critical other, can leave the therapist feeling as if any interpretation will be experienced as such by the patient, and indeed this may be the case. However, this should not inhibit us from putting forward our thoughts; rather, it is possible to acknowledge the possibility that the pattern could be activated by what we are about to say, yet our hope is that the patient can consider whether there is any validity to what we are observing. We can also couch such interpretations with empathy and validation of the difficult work our patients are undertaking with us.

When it comes to interpreting the transference in DIT, we do so judiciously, bearing in mind its relevance to the therapeutic relationship as well as the focus of our work together. Unlike in transference-focused psychotherapy (see Yeomans et al., 2015), in DIT we take up the transference where it links to the pattern we are addressing as well as in relation to the cautionary tale (Ogden, 1992) (see Chapter 4).

CONCLUSIONS

The four sets of theories that we draw on and have briefly reviewed here reflect certain core assumptions that underpin DIT and its strategies (see Chapter 3). Most notably, these are: (a) the social origins and nature of individual subjectivity, (b) the importance of attachments as the building blocks of the mind, and as the context for developing crucial social-cognitive capacities, (c) the impact of internalized, unconscious 'self' and 'other' representations on current interpersonal functioning, and (d) the importance of the capacity to mentalize experience, without which the individual is more vulnerable to developmentally earlier modes of experiencing internal reality, which, in turn, undermine the capacity to resolve interpersonal difficulties.

We have also set out some of the key competences for psychodynamic psychotherapy that inform DIT, including the ability to establish and manage the therapeutic frame and boundaries; the ability to work with unconscious communication; the ability to recognize and work with defences; the ability to work in the transference; the ability to work with the countertransference; and the ability to make dynamic interpretations.

The following chapters will illustrate how these assumptions and competences translate into technical recommendations and how they give shape to DIT's unifying therapeutic strategy, namely the identification of the IPAF.

REFERENCES

Akhtar, S. (1992). *Broken structures: Severe personality disorders and their treatment.* Jason Aronson.

Bacal, H. A. (1990). Does an object relations theory exist in self psychology? *Psychoanalytic Inquiry, 10*(2), 197–220. https://doi.org/10.1080/07351699009533807

Balint, M. (1937). Early developmental states of the ego, primary object of love. In *Primary love and psycho-analytic technique* (pp. 90–108). Tavistock, 1965.

Balint, M. (1968). *The basic fault*. Tavistock.

Bateman, A., Brown, D., & Pedder, J. (2000). *Introduction to psychotherapy: An outline of psychodynamic principles and practice* (3rd edn.). Routledge.

Bateman, A. W., Holmes, J., & Allison, E. (2022). *Introduction to psychoanalysis: Contemporary theory and practice* (2nd edn.). Routledge.

Blatt, S. J. (2008). *Polarities of experience: Relatedness and self definition in personality development, psychopathology, and the therapeutic process*. American Psychological Association.

Blatt, S. J., & Luyten, P. (2009). A structural-developmental psychodynamic approach to psychopathology: Two polarities of experience across the life span. *Development and Psychopathology, 21*(3), 793–814. https://doi.org/10.1017/S0954579409000431

Bowlby, J. (1960). Grief and mourning in infancy and early childhood. *Psychoanalytic Study of the Child, 15*(1), 9–52. https://doi.org/10.1080/00797308.1960.11822566

Bowlby, J. (1969). *Attachment and loss. Vol. 1: Attachment*. Hogarth Press and Institute of Psycho-Analysis.

Bowlby, J. (1973). *Attachment and loss. Vol. 2: Separation: Anxiety and anger*. Hogarth Press and Institute of Psycho-Analysis.

Bowlby, J. (1980). *Attachment and loss. Vol. 3: Loss: Sadness and depression*. Hogarth Press and Institute of Psycho-Analysis.

Bretherton, I. (1985). Attachment theory: Retrospect and prospect. *Monographs of the Society for Research in Child Development, 50*(1–2), 3–35. https://doi.org/10.2307/3333824

Bretherton, K., & Munholland, K. A. (1999). Internal working models in attachment relationships: A construct revisited. In J. Cassidy & P. R. Shaver (Eds.), *Handbook of attachment: Theory, research and clinical applications* (pp. 89–114). Guilford Press.

Cicchetti, D. (1990). The organization and coherence of socioemotional, cognitive, and representational development: Illustrations through a developmental psychopathology perspective on Down syndrome and child maltreatment. In R. Thompson (Ed.), *Socioemotional development. Nebraska symposium on motivation* (pp. 259–279). University of Nebraska Press.

Crittenden, P. M. (1990). Internal representational models of attachment relationships. *Infant Mental Health Journal, 11*(3), 259–277. https://doi.org/10.1002/1097-0355(199023)11:3<259::Aid-imhj2280110308>3.0.Co;2-j

Crittenden, P. M. (1994). Peering into the black box: An exploratory treatise on the development of self in young children. In D. Cicchetti & S. L. Toth (Eds.), *Disorders and dysfunctions of the self. Rochester Symposium on Developmental Psychopathology* (Vol. 5, pp. 79–148). University of Rochester Press.

Etchegoyen, R. H. (1999). *The fundamentals of psychoanalytic technique* (rev. edn.). Karnac Books.

Fairbairn, W. R. D. (1952). *An object-relations theory of the personality.* Basic Books.

Fonagy, P. (2001). *Attachment theory and psychoanalysis.* Other Press.

Fonagy, P., Gergely, G., Jurist, E., & Target, M. (2002). *Affect regulation, mentalization, and the development of the self.* Other Press.

Fonagy, P., Steele, H., & Steele, M. (1991). Maternal representations of attachment during pregnancy predict the organization of infant-mother attachment at one year of age. *Child Development, 62*(5), 891–905. https://doi.org/10.1111/j.1467-8624.1991.tb01578.x

Fonagy, P., Steele, M., Steele, H., Moran, G. S., & Higgitt, A. C. (1991). The capacity for understanding mental states: The reflective self in parent and child and its significance for security of attachment. *Infant Mental Health Journal, 12*(3), 201–218. https://doi.org/10.1002/1097-0355(199 123)12:3<201::Aid-imhj2280120307>3.0.Co;2-7

Fonagy, P., & Target, M. (2003). *Psychoanalytic theories: Perspectives from developmental psychopathology.* Whurr.

Fraiberg, S. (1969). Libidinal object constancy and mental representation. *Psychoanalytic Study of the Child, 24,* 9–47. https://doi.org/10.1080/00797308.1969.11822685

Fraiberg, S. (1980). *Clinical studies in infant mental health: The first year of life.* Basic Books.

Freud, A. (1954). *The ego and the mechanisms of defence.* Hogarth Press.

Freud, A. (1965). *Normality and pathology in childhood: Assessments of development.* International Universities Press.

Freud, S. (1896). Further remarks on the neuro-psychoses of defence. In J. Strachey (Ed.), *The standard edition of the complete psychological works of Sigmund Freud* (Vol. 3, pp. 157–185). Hogarth Press, 1962.

Freud, S. (1900). The interpretation of dreams. In J. Strachey (Ed.), *The standard edition of the complete psychological works of Sigmund Freud* (Vol. 4–5). Hogarth Press, 1953.

Freud, S. (1901). The psychopathology of everyday life: Forgetting, slips of the tongue, bungled actions, superstitions and errors. In J. Strachey (Ed.), *The standard edition of the complete psychological works of Sigmund Freud* (Vol. 6). Hogarth Press, 1960.

Friedman, L. (1988). The clinical popularity of object relations concepts. *Psychoanalytic Quarterly, 57*(4), 667–691. https://doi.org/10.1080/21674086.1988.11927615

Gergely, G., & Watson, J. S. (1996). The social biofeedback theory of parental affect-mirroring: The development of emotional self-awareness and self-control in infancy. *International Journal of Psychoanalysis, 77*(6), 1181–1212.

Gill, M. M., & Hoffman, I. Z. (1982). A method for studying the analysis of aspects of the patient's experience of the relationship in psychoanalysis and psychotherapy. *Journal of the American Psychoanalytic Association, 30*(1), 137–167. https://doi.org/10.1177/000306518203000106

Greenberg, J. R., & Mitchell, S. A. (1983). *Object relations in psychoanalytic theory*. Harvard University Press.

Greenson, R. R. (1967). *The technique and practice of psychoanalysis*. International Universities Press.

Heimann, P. (1950). On counter-transference. *International Journal of Psychoanalysis, 31*, 81–84.

Heimann, P. (1956). Dynamics of transference interpretations. *International Journal of Psychoanalysis, 37*, 303–310.

Hesse, P., & Cicchetti, D. (1982). Perspectives on an integrated theory of emotional development. *New Directions for Child and Adolescent Development, 1982*(16), 3–48. https://doi.org/10.1002/cd.23219821603

Jacobson, E. (1964). *The self and the object world*. International Universities Press.

Kernberg, O. F. (1975). *Borderline conditions and pathological narcissism*. Jason Aronson.

Kernberg, O. F. (1976a). *Object relations theory and clinical psychoanalysis*. Jason Aronson.

Kernberg, O. F. (1976b). Technical considerations in the treatment of borderline personality organization. *Journal of the American Psychoanalytic Association, 24*(4), 795–829. https://doi.org/10.1177/000306517602400403

Kernberg, O. F. (1982). Self, ego, affects, and drives. *Journal of the American Psychoanalytic Association, 30*(4), 893–917. https://doi.org/10.1177/000306518203000404

Kernberg, O. F. (1987). An ego psychology-object relations theory approach to the transference. *Psychoanalytic Quarterly, 56*(1), 197–221. https://doi.org/10.1080/21674086.1987.11927172

Kiesler, D. J. (1996). *Contemporary interpersonal theory and research: Personality, psychopathology, and psychotherapy*. Wiley.

Kramer, S., & Akhtar, S. (1988). The developmental context of internalized preoedipal object relations. Clinical applications of Mahler's theory of symbiosis and separation-individuation. *Psychoanalytic Quarterly*, 57(4), 547–576. https://doi.org/10.1080/21674086.1988.11927221

Lemma, A. (2003). *Introduction to the practice of psychoanalytic psychotherapy*. John Wiley & Sons.

Lemma, A. (2016). *Introduction to the practice of psychoanalytic psychotherapy* (2nd edn.). John Wiley & Sons.

Lemma, A., Roth, A. D., & Pilling, S. (2008). *The competences required to deliver effective psychoanalytic/psychodynamic therapy*. Research Department of Clinical, Educational and Health Psychology, University College London. https://www.ucl.ac.uk/pals/sites/pals/files/ppc_clinicians_background_paper.pdf

Loewald, H. W. (1986). Transference-countertransference. *Journal of the American Psychoanalytic Association*, 34(2), 275–287. https://doi.org/10.1177/000306518603400202

Lussier, A. (1988). The limitations of the object relations model. *Psychoanalytic Quarterly*, 57(4), 528–546. https://doi.org/10.1080/21674086.1988.11927220

Mahler, M. S. (1967). On human symbiosis and the vicissitudes of individuation. *Journal of the American Psychoanalytic Association*, 15(4), 740–763. https://doi.org/10.1177/000306516701500401

Mahler, M. S., & McDevitt, J. B. (1968). Observations on adaptation and defense in statu nascendi. Developmental precursors in the first two years of life. *Psychoanalytic Quarterly*, 37(1), 1–21.

Mahler, M. S., Pine, F., & Bergman, A. (1975). *The psychological birth of the human infant: Symbiosis and individuation*. Basic Books.

Main, M. (1991). Metacognitive knowledge, metacognitive monitoring, and singular (coherent) vs. multiple (incoherent) model of attachment: Findings and directions for future research. In C. M. Parkes, J. Stevenson-Hinde, & P. Marris (Eds.), *Attachment across the life cycle* (pp. 127–159). Tavistock/Routledge.

Main, M., Kaplan, N., & Cassidy, J. (1985). Security in infancy, childhood, and adulthood: A move to the level of representation. *Monographs of the Society for Research in Child Development*, 50(1–2), 66–104. https://doi.org/10.2307/3333827

Masten, A. S. (1982). *Humor and creative thinking in stress-resistant children*. University of Minnesota.

McLaughlin, J. T. (1981). Transference, psychic reality, and countertransference. *Psychoanalytic Quarterly*, 50(4), 639–664. https://doi.org/10.1080/21674086.1981.11926976

Michels, R. (1985). Introduction to panel: Perspectives on the nature of psychic reality. *Journal of the American Psychoanalytic Association*, *33*(3), 515–519. https://doi.org/10.1177/000306518503300301

Mitchell, S. A., & Black, M. (1995). *Freud and beyond*. Basic Books.

Modell, A. (1990). *Other times, other realities*. Harvard University Press.

Ogden, T. H. (1992). Comments on transference and countertransference in the initial analytic meeting. *Psychoanalytic Inquiry*, *12*(2), 225–247. https://doi.org/10.1080/07351699209533894

Rangell, L. (1985). On the theory of theory in psychoanalysis and the relation of theory to psychoanalytic therapy. *Journal of the American Psychoanalytic Association*, *33*(1), 59–92. https://doi.org/10.1177/000306518503300104

Rinsley, D. B. (1977). An object relations view of borderline personality. In P. Hartocollis (Ed.), *Borderline personality disorders: The concept, the syndrome, the patient* (pp. 47–70). International Universities Press.

Roth, A., & Fonagy, P. (2005). *What works for whom? A critical review of psychotherapy research* (2nd edn.). Guilford Press.

Roth, A. D., & Pilling, S. (2008). Using an evidence-based methodology to identify the competences required to deliver effective cognitive and behavioural therapy for depression and anxiety disorders. *Behavioural and Cognitive Psychotherapy*, *36*(2), 129–147. https://doi.org/10.1017/s1352465808004141

Sandler, J. (1976). Countertransference and role-responsiveness. *International Review of Psychoanalysis*, *3*, 43–47.

Sandler, J. (1987). *From safety to superego: Selected papers of Joseph Sandler*. Guilford Press.

Schafer, R. (1983). *The analytic attitude*. Basic Books.

Schwaber, E. (1983). Psychoanalytic listening and psychic reality. *International Review of Psychoanalysis*, *10*, 379–392.

Shaver, P. R., & Mikulincer, M. (2007). Adult attachment strategies and the regulation of emotion. In J. J. Gross (Ed.), *Handbook of emotion regulation* (pp. 446–465). Guilford Press.

Spruiell, V. (1988). The indivisibility of Freudian object relations and drive theories. *Psychoanalytic Quarterly*, *57*(4), 597–625. https://doi.org/10.1080/21674086.1988.11927223

Sroufe, L. A. (1996). *Emotional development: The organization of emotional life in the early years*. Cambridge University Press.

Stern, D. N. (1985). *The interpersonal world of the infant: A view from psychoanalysis and developmental psychology*. Basic Books.

Stolorow, R., Brandschaft, B., & Atwood, G. (1987). *Psychoanalytic treatment: An intersubjective approach*. Analytic Press.

Strenger, C. (1989). The classic and the romantic vision in psychoanalysis. *International Journal of Psychoanalysis, 70*(4), 593–610.
Sullivan, H. S. (1953). *The interpersonal theory of psychiatry.* W. W. Norton.
Target, M. (2005). Attachment theory and research: A bridge from psychoanalysis joining normal and abnormal development. In E. S. Person, A. M. Cooper, & G. Gabbard (Eds.), *The American Psychiatric Publishing textbook of psychoanalysis* (pp. 159–172). American Psychiatric Publishing, Inc.
Terr, L. C. (1983). Chowchilla revisited: The effects of psychic trauma four years after a school-bus kidnapping. *American Journal of Psychiatry, 140*(12), 1543–1550. https://doi.org/10.1176/ajp.140.12.1543
van IJzendoorn, M. H. (1995). Adult attachment representations, parental responsiveness, and infant attachment: A meta-analysis on the predictive validity of the Adult Attachment Interview. *Psychological Bulletin, 117*(3), 387–403. https://doi.org/10.1037/0033-2909.117.3.387
Westen, D. (1989). Are 'primitive' object relations really preoedipal? *American Journal of Orthopsychiatry, 59*(3), 331–345. https://doi.org/10.1111/j.1939-0025.1989.tb01669.x
Winnicott, D. W. (1949). Hate in the counter-transference. *International Journal of Psychoanalysis, 30,* 69–74.
Winnicott, D. W. (1962). Ego integration in child development. In *The maturational processes and the facilitating environment* (pp. 56–63). Hogarth Press, 1965.
Winnicott, D. W. (1965). *The maturational processes and the facilitating environment.* Hogarth Press.
Winnicott, D. W. (1971). *Playing and reality.* Tavistock.
Wolberg, L. R. (1995). *The technique of psychotherapy* (4th edn.). Jason Aronson, Inc.
Yeomans, F. E., Clarkin, J., & Kernberg, O. F. (2015). *Transference-focused psychotherapy for borderline personality disorder: A clinical guide.* American Psychiatric Publishing.

3
Core Features and Strategies

The techniques used in dynamic interpersonal therapy (DIT), which we will outline in detail in Chapter 7, are by no means exclusive to this approach and will be familiar to psychodynamically trained clinicians. DIT, however, distinguishes itself at the level of its overall strategy because it is a time-limited therapy consisting of sixteen weekly sessions structured around the formulation and working through of a problematic, recurrent interpersonal-affective pattern that becomes the focus of therapy (the interpersonal-affective focus (IPAF)) (see Box 3.1). In Chapter 13, we outline an adaptation of the model for complex cases (DIT for complex care; DITCC), which extends the therapy to twenty-six sessions.

DIT can be conceptualized as having three phases, each with distinctive aims and strategies. In this chapter we will give an overview of the three phases to sketch out the trajectory for the therapy. In subsequent chapters we will then go into the detail of each phase.

AIMS

DIT has been developed to meet the needs of patients who are depressed and/or anxious. It primarily targets the patient's interpersonal functioning and capacity to think about, and understand, changes in mood triggered by the activation in the mind of a particular self–other representation as the medium through which to reduce symptoms of depression and/or anxiety.

DIT thus has two primary aims:

1. To help the patient understand the connection between their presenting symptoms and what is happening in their relationships, through identifying a core, unconscious,

> **Box 3.1**
>
> **CORE FEATURES OF DIT**
>
> - Works on a circumscribed interpersonal-affective focus (IPAF)
> - Focuses on the patient's mind rather than their behaviour
> - Time-limited (16 sessions)
> - The therapeutic relationship is addressed and used to help the patient explore their IPAF
> - Makes use of expressive, supportive, mentalizing, and, when appropriate, directive techniques to maximize change within a brief format
> - Primarily targets enhanced interpersonal functioning and capacity for understanding self and other, rather than character change

repetitive pattern of relating that becomes the focus of the therapy (the IPAF).

2. To expand the patient's capacity to reflect on their own states of mind and so enhance their ability to manage interpersonal difficulties, that is, to mentalize more flexibly about self and others.

It is important to keep in mind DIT's dual aims because they will provide an orienting internal frame of reference for the therapist, which is especially helpful during the middle phase of the therapy when the therapist may struggle to stay focused (see Chapter 6).

TRAJECTORY OF THE THERAPY

We conceptualize DIT as consisting of three phases. Many brief psychodynamic models also structure the therapy in a similar way: an *initial phase* concerned primarily with engaging the patient and assessing their difficulties, a *middle phase* during which the therapist focuses on an identified problem or pattern, and an *ending phase*, which reviews the progress made and helps the patient prepare to leave by focusing on the conscious and unconscious meaning for them of separation from the therapist.

The three phases in DIT and their related aims and strategies are somewhat artificially divided and 'timed' for the sake of clarity. In practice we would expect there to be some flexibility in how and when the various strategies linked to each phase are implemented. For example, although we suggest that the formulation is shared with the patient in session 4, this may well be possible only in a later session, and very occasionally a little sooner.

The initial phase (sessions 1–4)

Broadly speaking, the first four sessions are devoted to the assessment of the problem and its dynamic formulation—which we refer to as the IPAF—and to engaging the patient through working in an explicitly collaborative way and involving them in refining the formulation (see Table 3.1).

Table 3.1 INITIAL PHASE: SESSIONS 1–4

Aims:
• Engagement
• Exploration of depressive/anxiety symptoms (including risk factors) with an emphasis on the origins and psychological meaning of the symptoms
• Identification of strengths/resources in the patient and in their wider interpersonal network
• Formulation of focal area of work

Strategies:
• Identify the patient's 'interpersonal map', which includes a detailed picture of the patient's significant relationships and their connection with presenting problems
• Use attachment self-descriptions to characterize the patient's basic attachment style
• Focus on interpersonal circumstances and significant life events preceding the onset of depression/anxiety and modulators of mood and/or anxiety
• Assess the patient's current and past interpersonal functioning to identify recurring interpersonal pattern(s) that inform the patient's experience of their relationships
• Discuss and agree with the patient the formulation, treatment rationale, and goals

This initial phase is fundamental to the subsequent course of DIT, because the remainder of the therapy is structured around the exploration of the specific IPAF that emerges from this assessment. In our experience, this is the phase that clinicians new to DIT find the most challenging, but also the most helpful because the practice of explicitly formulating a focus then provides an invaluable compass for the therapist's interventions during the subsequent two phases. The IPAF provides the spine for the work of the middle phase. However, it is important to keep in mind that the IPAF is an ongoing formulation that will be revised and refined as the work progresses, up until the very last session.

The middle phase (sessions 5–12)

The primary aim during the middle phase is simple: to intervene, using a range of techniques (see Chapter 7), to facilitate the working through of the mutually agreed IPAF (see Table 3.2). The therapist's central therapeutic strategy is their unwavering attention to the IPAF and to unpacking it, as it were, by helping the patient to consider its contribution to maintaining the problem/symptom(s) they

Table 3.2 MIDDLE PHASE: SESSIONS 5–12

Aims:
• Working through of mutually agreed interpersonal-affective focus
Strategies:
• Help the patient to stay focused on the exploration of narratives about relationships (real or imagined)
• Keep the focus on the patient's state of mind, not their behaviour (link interpersonal processes with the patient's mental states)
• Help the patient to discover what they currently feel and how this relates to current and past interpersonal experiences, including in the relationship with the therapist
• Help the patient to make connections between symptoms and interpersonal events
• Adopt an active, supportive stance to encourage the patient to try out new ways of resolving their difficulties (e.g. trying out new ways of communicating with others)

are experiencing, its function in the patient's mind (including what it defends against), and its 'cost' (i.e. the impact it has on their relationships, symptoms, etc.), as well as encouraging the patient to make changes in relation to the pattern and the agreed goals of treatment.

Sessions during this phase, in common with other psychodynamic approaches, have a more emergent quality, to allow space for the elaboration of the patient's affective experience and of their imaginative life. Silence therefore has a place in DIT. A common mistake is to assume an overly active stance, with the attendant risk that the sessions become too directive and too cognitive, thereby losing their psychodynamic focus. Nevertheless, relative to longer-term psychodynamic models, in DIT the therapist is more active, inviting the patient, where possible, to gradually try out different ways of approaching interpersonal difficulties.

The ending phase (sessions 13–16)

Given DIT's emphasis on the importance of attachments, the meaning of the loss of the relationship with the therapist is focused on in the final sessions (see Table 3.3). Endings can mobilize particular feelings and fantasies very powerfully, and the therapist needs to help the patient to make sense of their experience of ending. Often the IPAF that has been worked on is relevant to understanding the patient's particular experience of separation.

Table 3.3 ENDING PHASE: SESSIONS 13–16

Aims
• To enable the patient to explore conflicts concerning loss, separation, and independence triggered by anticipated separation from the therapist • To take stock of what has been achieved and plan for the future
Strategies
• Facilitate expression of the patient's anxieties and fantasies about ending • Review the work that has been accomplished • Acknowledge the progress made • Anticipate future difficulties/areas of vulnerability • Write a 'goodbye' letter summarizing the work

Alongside the exploration of the experience of ending, the therapist also uses the last few sessions as an opportunity to engage the patient in reviewing the work on the IPAF (which includes writing a 'goodbye' letter to the patient, which recapitulates the IPAF) and consolidating the gains made, as well as anticipating future vulnerabilities.

Our experience of training and supervising clinicians offering DIT suggests that this phased protocol enables dynamically oriented clinicians to achieve good results. Drawing on their established experience of working psychodynamically, therapists structure their interventions guided by five relatively simple strategic steps in the course of a brief therapeutic engagement (Lemma et al., 2010):

1. Identify an attachment-related problem with a specific relational emotional focus that is felt by the patient to be currently making them feel depressed and/or anxious.
2. Work with the patient collaboratively to create an increasingly mentalistic picture of interpersonal issues raised by the problem.
3. Encourage the patient to explore the possibility of alternative ways of feeling and thinking ('playing with a new internal and external reality'), actively using the transference relationship to bring to the fore the patient's characteristic ways of relating.
4. Ensure the therapeutic process (of change in self) is reflected on.
5. Near the end of treatment, present the patient with a written summary of the collaboratively created view of the patient and the selected area of unconscious conflict, for them to hold on to, to reduce the risk of relapse.

In later chapters we will describe these strategies in more detail, but for now we will focus in broader terms on the three foci that are central to DIT and on the therapeutic stance characteristic of DIT.

THE DIT FOCI

The interpersonal-affective focus

DIT adopts an idiographic approach to formulation that emphasizes the dynamic specificity of the patient's experience of depression and/

or anxiety. This distinguishes it from other brief models, for example, interpersonal psychotherapy (IPT), that accommodate the patient's experience into pre-established focal problems.

The primary task of the initial phase, which organizes DIT's therapeutic thrust, is to identify typically one dominant and recurring unconscious interpersonal pattern, which in DIT is called the IPAF (see Chapter 5). This pattern is nested within an unconscious approach to attachment, dependence, and possible intimacy, which is captured by a broad description of the patient's dominant attachment style. The specific pattern that is agreed with the patient as a focus for work is underpinned by a particular representation of self-in-relation-to-another that characterizes the patient's interpersonal style and leads to difficulties in their relationships because it organizes interpersonal behaviour. These representations are typically linked to one or more particular affects. Affects are understood to be responses to the activation, in the patient's mind, of a specific self–other representation (Kernberg, 1980).

Past experiences, while clearly informing current functioning and internal object-relations, are not the major focus of DIT. They may be included in the formulation shared with the patient so as to meaningfully frame the patient's current difficulties in the context of their lived experience over time, but they are not a central component of the therapeutic process. Rather, given the brief nature of the therapy, the focus is on a core segment of the patient's interpersonal functioning that is closely connected with the presenting symptom(s) and is informed by early developmental experiences as well as other factors.

The IPAF guides the therapist's interventions during the middle phase and provides the focus for helping the patient to begin to make some changes. It is through small changes in one circumscribed interpersonal area that shifts in functioning can often occur and symptoms are alleviated. These developments rely on the therapist's unwavering and empathic attention to the IPAF. In practice this means that the therapist will actively redirect the patient back to the focus if the patient digresses from it and will actively work to understand with the patient why they might feel the need to avoid the IPAF. Occasionally, the therapist will find that more than one interpersonal pattern needs to be addressed. Where this is the case, the therapist will discuss and agree this with the patient. When deciding what to focus on, it is important to bear in mind that DIT is a brief therapy that is not aiming to facilitate broad character change. Rather, the IPAF is selected in terms of its most immediate relevance to the onset of the patient's depression and/or anxiety.

Here-and-now focus

The 'here-and-now' focus is central to DIT and denotes three related activities, namely the focus on *current affect*, on the patient's *current difficulties*, and on their *current relationship with the therapist*. We will now look at each of these in more detail.

FOCUS ON AFFECT
Affect is a distinctive feature of psychodynamic therapy (Blagys & Hilsenroth, 2000). Emotional expression is related to better treatment outcome, irrespective of therapeutic modality. Throughout the therapy careful attention is devoted to the patient's affective state during the session, not least their pattern of affect regulation. The cognitive–affective structures of self and other representations regulate the patient's interpersonal exchanges, especially with significant attachment figures in the present. Helping the patient to become cognizant of what they feel, of the interpersonal triggers for particular feelings, and of how they manage these feelings is a core feature of DIT. Some patients may feel the need to avoid emotions, denying them or playing them down to protect themselves from underlying attachment needs (e.g. to be loved) that expose them to interpersonal risks. Others, instead, may up-regulate their emotions, to feel that they are getting through to the other (e.g. the patient who presents in very dramatic ways, 'catastrophizing' their emotions in order to divert the therapist's much-needed attention towards them).

As this affective exploration takes place, emotional communication by the therapist is important to the patient's own emotional state. This is not through a passive process such as habitual mirroring. Rather, it results from the patient's active use of the therapist's emotional expression in forming their appreciation of an event and using it to guide behaviour. For example, a patient who was in thrall to a harsh superego, and who became very caught up in their mind with self-destructive accusations, responded with significant relief when a 'confession' about a sexual transgression was normalized and responded to by the therapist with empathy and curiosity rather than admonishment. The function performed by the therapist here is that of transforming the patient's experience into something emotionally digestible. The therapist provides the patient with an experience of being understood that enables them to gradually build up a sense that their own behaviour is meaningful and communicative. The quality of these exchanges can contribute to laying the foundations for the patient's capacity to recognize and regulate affects, which will be less well developed in some patients.

The capacity to reflect on what we are feeling underpins the capacity to regulate affect (Fonagy et al., 2002). Each patient's pattern of affective arousal is different. The therapist's understanding of this pattern rests on a careful tracking of the patient's emotional state during the session. This tracking involves a number of related interventions, as follows:

- *Help the patient to recognize their feelings as their own*: many patients come into therapy without any real sense of what they really feel. Helping them to label their feelings is often an essential first step in the process. This requires a shift away from the 'why' of experience (often of concern to psychodynamic therapists) to the 'what' of experience.
- *Help the patient to differentiate feelings from actions*: some patients, particularly those who struggle to represent their experience in their minds, can all too readily experience feelings as actions. The failure of the capacity to symbolize, to interpose thought between feeling and action, may render some feelings terrifying.
- *Facilitate discussion of the connection between feelings and actions*, which in turn facilitates self-understanding and awareness of motivations attributed to others (e.g. 'When I feel anxious I want to avoid being with you . . . I missed last week's session because I think you find me boring').

FOCUS ON EXPLORATION OF CURRENT DIFFICULTIES

DIT focuses on the exploration of current difficulties in the patient's life rather than trying to establish links to the childhood origins of these difficulties. Although some reconstructive interpretations are made during the course of DIT, these are not considered to be a primary vehicle for facilitating change. Rather, the emphasis is placed on interventions that help the patient to feel they are working on difficulties that are 'live' and current (in their current relationships, including their relationship with the therapist) and to which they can bring about a degree of change. The aim is thus to review the patient's experience related to the IPAF as much in the present as possible—that is, what the patient feels and is struggling with *right now*.

Focus on the therapeutic relationship

An important current relationship that is focused on in DIT is the relationship with the therapist. DIT makes active use of the patient–therapist relationship to help the patient to explore the IPAF in the immediacy of this relationship (see Chapter 8). The relative balance placed in DIT between transference interpretations and other kinds of interventions is primarily dictated by the patient, moment by moment, since this kind of interpretation is a 'high-risk, high-gain phenomenon' (Gunderson & Gabbard, 1999, p. 691).

With some patients, for example, those who have few current relationships or those who struggle to report on their relationships outside therapy for defensive reasons, the transference relationship becomes a primary entry point into the patient's affective experience and their imaginative life (that is, their fantasies). For others, however, the report of their current relationships outside therapy will be affectively charged and will provide sufficient immediacy for the therapist to be able to engage the patient in a live exploration of the IPAF without needing to systematically elaborate these patterns at the level of the transference. The interpretation of the transference is thus guided by the extent to which the exploration of the IPAF is rendered more emotionally 'persuasive' by this focus as opposed to a focus on what is happening in the patient's relationships outside the therapy.

Focus on the patient's mind

A distinguishing feature of DIT is that it approaches the exploration of problematic interpersonal patterns not by addressing the patient's behaviour, but through its consistent focus on the patient's conscious and unconscious mental states (beliefs, feelings, wishes, and thoughts)—both their own and what they imagine or believe to be going on in the minds of others. The capacity to mentalize supports the daily struggle with what it means to have a mind. In some patients this capacity is severely undermined, and this deficit may be regarded as central to their psychopathology, as in the case of patients with borderline personality disorder (Bateman & Fonagy, 2016). In depressed and anxious patients, even if this deficit is not central to their psychopathology in quite the same way, these patients do demonstrate failures of mentalizing that contribute to their difficulties in relationships.

A central aim in DIT is to provide the patient with an experience of being with another person who is interested in thinking with them about what distresses them, so as to stimulate the patient's own capacity for reflecting realistically on their own experience. The goal is thus not only to work on an unconscious conflict, but also to use the focus on the IPAF to stimulate the patient's own capacity for thinking and feeling about their experience.

This focus on the patient's state of mind is fundamental to DIT and it informs technique insofar as the helpfulness of the therapist's interventions (e.g. the interpretation of transference) is evaluated against the criterion of whether they help to stimulate the patient's capacity to represent their own subjective experience in relation to that of others, in the context of a problematic interpersonal relationship.

The DIT therapist is particularly interested in making explicit what has effectively become procedural so that the patient is then better able to effect change in how they manage their relationships. Working through the IPAF therefore involves not only challenging unthinking patterns of relating in attachment situations, through the central example of the IPAF, but also enhancing the patient's awareness of how their behaviour and affective states are driven by conscious and unconscious mental states. That is, the patient's social interactions and expressions of feeling will crucially depend on how they understand their own and others' motivations.

The IPAF is a particular locus of fixed interpretation. So, for example, there is in the patient's mind an unconscious expectation that: 'I am an unlovable person condemned to loneliness; the person I want to be with is contemptuous of me; I will always be ashamed and humiliated; I need to protect myself by keeping my distance and pretending not to want a relationship.' This will loosen its grip as the patient's mentalizing capacity increases through trying out different perspectives on the 'evidence' in current, 'hot' examples, especially through looking at sensitivities in relation to the therapist.

THERAPEUTIC STANCE

The so-called analytic attitude is a core distinguishing feature of a psychodynamic approach. To a large extent—and we will qualify this shortly—this is also true of DIT.

Nowadays there is no consensus on psychodynamic technique (Gabbard & Westen, 2003); even definitions of the analytic attitude vary across different schools of psychoanalysis. There is nevertheless some agreement about the importance of the therapist being as unobtrusive as possible and retaining a more neutral, relatively anonymous stance towards the patient that prioritizes reflection and interpretation over action. Such an attitude, of course, is in itself an intervention because patients will react differently to, for example, the therapist's interest in the meaning behind the patient's request for advice rather than providing the advice requested. The patient's reactions to the therapist then become the focus of exploration and provide opportunities for understanding the transference and, through this, the patient's internal world of relationships.

Keeping to an interpretive mode conveys to the patient, even if painfully, that difficult states of mind can be reflected upon with another person. This way of working has contributed to a caricature of the psychodynamic therapist as aloof and unemotional. This caricature is common and, while it may be true of some individual therapists, this is by no means the majority, and it does not fit the supportive, collaborative stance adopted by the DIT therapist. Aloofness is unhelpful here. Striving for neutrality and relative anonymity are important but should not result in emotional detachment. On the contrary, the therapist should be actively engaged and emotionally attuned to the patient's subjective experience: the therapist is also a participant in the therapeutic process and will experience strong feelings in response to the patient's communications.

The analytic attitude at its best—and what we aspire to in DIT—rests on a particular way of listening (see Chapter 7): the therapist empathizes with the patient's subjective experience while at the same time being curious about its unconscious meaning, rather than directly correcting it or giving advice. The therapist also needs to be able to stand back from the interaction with the patient so as to reflect and comment on it, thereby helping the patient to gain understanding of how they relate to others while at the same time modelling a reflective stance. In all psychodynamic work, this requires the therapist's capacity to alternate between the temporary and partial identification of empathy and the return to the position of an observer of the interaction. It also requires a well-developed capacity for self-monitoring and self-scrutiny in order for the therapist to reflect on and modify their responses in the moment and to note their own contribution to therapeutic impasses or enactments (see Chapter 10).

The DIT therapist thus adopts an involved, empathic, 'supportively frustrating' manner. In other words, the core principles of an analytic attitude are adhered to but sometimes the therapist will contextualize their approach. For example, if the patient reacts to the therapist's silence by feeling that the therapist is sitting in judgement over them, the therapist would acknowledge and convey interest in the patient's experience of their silence, and might even explain (particularly in an early session) that the silence is giving the patient space to say what is on their mind (a supportive intervention). The therapist would simultaneously remain focused on engaging the patient in identifying and exploring the state of mind triggered by their silence (an exploratory intervention that may be experienced as frustrating of the patient's wish to simply be rescued from what the silence exposes them to in their mind). Thus, the therapist shows and encourages mentalizing, with its respect for the patient's position while including other points of view, such as their own intention.

The therapist strives to adopt a 'not-knowing' but curious stance that prioritizes the joint exploration of the patient's mental states as they relate to the identified interpersonal process that has been agreed as the focus of the therapy. Interpretations of deep unconscious material are generally avoided in favour of facilitating and supporting the patient's own capacity to stand back from their own immediate experience in order to be able to reflect on it.

From the outset, the emphasis is on working collaboratively with the patient, especially in arriving at a formulation that provides a productive focus for the therapy. The therapist is explicit about the nature of DIT (the therapist might, for example, also suggest to the patient that they read the DIT patient information leaflet; see Appendix 1) and about their understanding of the patient's problems, openly checking it out with the patient, and jointly elaborating it in their formulation (the IPAF; see Chapter 5). The aim is to create the opportunity for the patient to actively participate in arriving at and understanding a focus for the work.

The patient's conscious as well as unconscious feedback on the therapy is important. This is provided through different 'modes': concretely and directly through outcome monitoring forms, through conscious feedback, and indirectly through the narratives the patient brings that provide vehicles for unconscious communication about the therapy and the therapist. It is important for the therapist to be receptive and responsive to the patient's conscious and unconscious feedback and aware of the relationship between the two. If the patient questions the therapist's understanding or perception of the treatment, the therapist responds non-defensively, providing a clear, unambiguous account of how they have arrived at their understanding. The aim is to be as transparent as possible while being attuned to and working with the patient's need, where it arises, to control the therapist through projective processes.

Although the basic stance in DIT is thus an analytic one, rooted in attunement to the patient's conscious and unconscious communications and in using the transference, the brevity of the treatment requires more activity on the part of the therapist. This might sometimes include, for example, 'normalizing' experience by disclosing what (hypothetical) other people's thoughts and feelings might be in similar situations, or through acknowledging the patient's progress and communicating hopefulness. The therapist's self-disclosure is, however, generally discouraged. For example, the therapist might say that many people feel anxious in big groups of people (keeping the focus on the patient's anxiety), but would *not* say that they hate parties, which would bring the focus on to themselves.

REFERENCES

Bateman, A., & Fonagy, P. (2016). *Mentalization-based treatment for personality disorders: A practical guide* (2nd edn.). Oxford University Press.

Blagys, M. D., & Hilsenroth, M. J. (2000). Distinctive features of short-term psychodynamic-interpersonal psychotherapy: A review of the comparative psychotherapy process literature. *Clinical Psychology: Science and Practice, 7*(2), 167–188. https://doi.org/10.1093/clipsy.7.2.167

Fonagy, P., Gergely, G., Jurist, E., & Target, M. (2002). *Affect regulation, mentalization, and the development of the self.* Other Press.

Gabbard, G. O., & Westen, D. (2003). Rethinking therapeutic action. *International Journal of Psychoanalysis, 84*(4), 823–841. https://doi.org/10.1516/002075703768284605

Gunderson, J. G., & Gabbard, G. O. (1999). Making the case for psychoanalytic therapies in the current psychiatric environment. *Journal of the American Psychoanalytic Association, 47*(3), 679–704.

Kernberg, O. F. (1980). *Internal world and external reality: Object relations theory applied.* Jason Aronson.

Lemma, A., Target, M., & Fonagy, P. (2010). The development of a brief psychodynamic protocol for depression: Dynamic interpersonal therapy (DIT). *Psychoanalytic Psychotherapy, 24*(4), 329–346. https://doi.org/10.1080/02668734.2010.513547

4
The Initial Phase

In any brief intervention the initial sessions are critical to the final outcome. The therapist not only has the task of engaging the patient so that they stay the course of treatment, but also needs to do so relatively rapidly, given the brevity of the therapy. In large part, engagement is facilitated through formulating a focus for the work that is meaningful enough to the patient to engage them with the goals of treatment, and can also be realistically addressed within the time limit.

The first four sessions in dynamic interpersonal therapy (DIT) are therefore devoted to identifying a focus for intervention that engages the patient to work actively on an area of their interpersonal functioning (the interpersonal-affective focus or IPAF) to alleviate their more acute symptoms of depression and anxiety. In Chapter 5 we will focus in detail on how to formulate the IPAF. In this chapter we will review the aims and strategies of the initial phase of DIT, that is, typically sessions 1–4.

ENGAGEMENT

In the initial phase, one of the therapist's priorities is to work to engage the patient actively, by developing a good therapeutic alliance. It can be all too easy to forget that initial sessions can be potentially 'traumatic' for many patients, as Klauber (1981) observed, since the patient takes stock of painful aspects of themselves and of their current predicament, sometimes for the first time. This is all the more so when the focus of the therapist's exploration is on the patient's relationships and their states of mind. This focus is invariably felt by the patient, even if only unconsciously, to direct attention implicitly to their contribution or responsibility for their situation. By contrast, labelling the patient's difficulties as an 'illness' (e.g. as an interpersonal psychotherapy therapist might do) is often experienced as a relief for the patient, who is then helped to feel that their difficulties are not their 'fault'.

If we accept that an assessment is inherently 'traumatic' in this sense then it becomes incumbent on the therapist to create the conditions within which this trauma can be borne without the patient needing to take flight. This involves the therapist offering the patient a measure of support and 'orientation', as advocated by Sullivan (1953) (see also Chapter 2), in order to foster 'interpersonal security'.

In order to minimize the likelihood of the patient's anxiety undermining the rapid development of the therapeutic alliance (which is crucial in a brief intervention), the DIT therapist provides some orientation to the patient by welcoming them and introducing the aims of the initial sessions. The therapist will also ask questions more frequently than might be the case in more standard psychodynamic assessments. Although this stance is therefore more explicitly active and supportive, and hence provides structure, the fundamental aim is one shared by all psychodynamic approaches: to help the patient gradually shift from a position where they are seeking help and relief from their symptoms to one where they are interested in meaning, particularly regarding what is going on in their mind and in their relationships.

At this early stage it is important to assess whether the patient might require an explicit strengthening of the supportive aspects of the therapeutic relationship to engage them. The patient's responses to the therapist's interventions, to the silences, and to the more emergent quality of the sessions are all informative here. Assessing the patient's situation in relation to the feasibility of their participating in a short-term treatment is important, as is ensuring that there are no significant implicit threats to the treatment being offered (see Chapter 1).

We use our experience of the qualities of the patient's responses to us in the session to identify what adaptations might be necessary to meet the needs of a patient who might have difficulty engaging with therapy. For example, some patients might have had little, if any, experience of another person helping them to make sense of what they feel. With these patients, initially, the work is often not about uncovering meaning; rather, it is about helping the patient to build a relationship within which they can articulate *what* they feel before they can begin to explore *why* they feel in a particular way. The provision of more, or less, structure in the session will therefore be informed by the live experience with a particular patient, at a given point in time, and is reviewed, in the therapist's mind, in every session.

Engaging the patient involves communicating our respect for, and acceptance of, their position. The therapist responds to the patient's presenting problems in a concerned and non-judgemental manner. This will be conveyed through the more prosodic features of speech, such as tone of voice, and also through:

- Asking clarifying questions so as to understand the patient's perspective without making assumptions: 'You said the relationship with X was "less of a burden". What do you have in mind when you say that?'
- Communicating empathic observation and understanding in response to the patient's conscious and unconscious communications: 'When I just asked about your mother your whole demeanour changed: you stiffened and you began to speak very fast, as if you felt pressure to answer me and at the same time wanted to get away from considering this with me. I wonder if this is a difficult relationship for you?'
- Respecting the patient's need for defences: 'Ensuring you insulate yourself from others is a way of protecting yourself from this feeling of rejection. Given what you have been through in your life I can see that this feels essential.'
- Maintaining an engaged, active, and realistically optimistic attitude that conveys support for the patient's development and therapeutic goals: 'As I listen to you talking about what you want for yourself, I can sense your commitment to making some changes in your life. Even though we both know that this will be challenging, your motivation to do so comes across and is a real strength.'
- Using collaborative language: '*We* will work on this together and I will do my best to keep us to this focus.'
- Validating the patient's experience as understandable given their circumstances: 'It is understandable that you should feel so mistrustful and alert to danger since your assault—it was a deeply unsettling experience.'

LISTENING OUT FOR 'CAUTIONARY TALES'

The initial sessions are critical to the course of DIT as unless the patient stays, there is no therapy. There is also the risk that a compliant or desperate patient will stay, but will avoid talking about some areas that they expect will cause difficulty or misunderstanding. Unless this is noticed and worked on by the therapist, it could greatly limit the benefit the patient might receive from the therapy. An important way of fostering the therapeutic alliance is through containing the patient's anxiety about engaging in therapy and the threats it is felt to pose to them.

Communicating clearly at the outset the boundaries and frame of the therapy, and its nature, is necessary to give the patient a sense that they can understand what is being offered, and so that they can give meaningful consent to it. This is the basis for a collaborative relationship. For some patients, though, the nature of their anxiety about starting therapy may not be contained sufficiently by clarifying these important parameters. Some patients will need more explicit indications from the therapist that we understand just how fearful they feel at the prospect of therapy—for example, through acknowledging the challenge that making adjustments implies (e.g. 'It's not easy to change and I can understand why you might not want to do it at all').

More importantly, however, the anxiety becomes manageable if the patient can be helped to reflect on their conscious—and especially unconscious—anxieties about the therapy and the therapist, and if the therapist is experienced by the patient as being capable of tolerating those anxieties:

> T: You have clearly conveyed to me that your experience of being helped has always been negative: you trust another person, then invariably feel exposed and then somehow neglected.
> P: Yes.
> T: Even though you keep reassuring me—and yourself too—that talking to a therapist will be different, I could well understand if in fact you were feeling very concerned that what is supposed to be a helpful relationship will end up in the same painful pattern.

A key task in the initial sessions is therefore to listen out for the patient's 'cautionary tales' (Ogden, 1992), that is, their unconscious anxieties about developing a relationship with the therapist that will reflect particular expectations of themselves and of other people[1]. The patient's anxieties are typically communicated through the interpersonal narratives that they bring. The quality of the phantasies the patient has about us as therapists is vitally important to the viability and outcome of DIT. The term 'phantasies' is derived from classical psychoanalysis and is used to indicate constructions and beliefs of which the patient is unaware: these are unconscious wishes that are defended against. This contrasts with 'fantasies', which are in conscious awareness. For example, a patient might have an unconscious phantasy that the therapist will exploit and harm them, turning what they say against them. Consciously they might think the therapist probably will not be able to understand them because they are so different, so there is not much point in coming to therapy.

At the outset, many prospective patients are likely to turn to us with a mixture of fear and hope that activates latent phantasies regarding authority figures and caregivers—phantasies into which we will be unconsciously fitted. The patients who are most difficult to help in a time-limited therapy such as DIT are those with persecutory phantasies that shape virtually all aspects of their mind because they relate to the world with phantasies organized around controlling, tormenting, or rejecting the object before they then run the risk of becoming the victim of phantasized retaliatory attacks.

More typically, the patient's anxieties will variously reflect their belief that relationships will inevitably become painful, disappointing, unreliable, and so on. Many, but by no means all, patients arrive for the initial consultation in a state of need (and fear that this need might not be met), looking for an authoritative person to relieve their distress. The underlying initial transference may therefore be to

---

1. 'The patient unconsciously holds a fierce conviction (which he has no way of articulating) that his infantile and early childhood experience has taught him about the specific ways in which each of his object relationships will inevitably become painful, disappointing, annihilating, lonely, unreliable, suffocating, overly sexualized, etc. There is no reason for him to believe that the relationship into which he is about to enter will be any different. In this belief the [patient] is of course both correct and incorrect.' (Ogden, 1992, p. 235)

a powerful, omniscient parental figure. In turn, this may set up a conflict between the wish for, and the fear of, a dependent relationship, as it immediately establishes the therapeutic relationship as unequal in the patient's mind.

Being able to accurately identify these concerns and convey understanding of them to the patient early on in therapy draws the patient's attention in an immediate way to their anxieties. Very importantly, it also allows the therapist to give the patient an experience of the kind of reflection that will take place within the therapy while testing out the patient's capacity to make use of it (see also Chapter 3).

It is helpful and containing for the patient if the therapist is able to articulate these anxieties early on. We take up the cautionary tale with the patient before we have arrived at the IPAF, and it may inform that formulation or even capture the essence of the self–other–affect configuration; it may also point to the patient's defences. In the following clinical vignettes, we will see how for each patient an important dimension of their internal experience emerges through the narratives that they recount and how the therapist's understanding leads to the articulation of distinctive cautionary tales.

Case examples of 'cautionary tales'

Mr F arrived for his first session late and very flustered. He complained about the traffic and was evidently angry with a driver who had taken his place at a parking space. He referred to the driver in derogatory terms. Although he was apologetic about his lateness, the therapist nevertheless immediately felt on guard, as if she was somehow being blamed.

Mr F was one of five children. He spoke about a rather deprived early childhood; both parents had been unemployed and the family struggled to make ends meet. Mr F's depression coincided with a stressful work situation in which he was 'moved sideways'. He felt bitter about this decision and had since lost all interest in his work. He thought that he had been discriminated against because he had not gone to a good university.

As the therapist listened, she thought that Mr F's narrative about the difficulty with parking contained an important 'caution', namely about the extent to which he was preoccupied with how much space she would have in her mind for him. This alerted the therapist to the likelihood that he might experience her, in the transference, as favouring another in her mind who would be seen as taking up the space that should rightfully belong to him. The therapist was also alert to the underlying grievance and the patient's difficulty in taking any responsibility for his part in this dynamic. This, in turn, helped the therapist to speak with the patient about this core anxiety as he approached the prospect of therapy.

Another patient, Ms Y, who was referred because she was seized by panic when she had to present her work in public, also arrived late for her first session. She was very apologetic, and the therapist sensed Ms Y's considerable unease in the session, as she could barely look at the therapist. Early on in the session, Ms Y recounted an incident from her university days when she had agreed to present her work to her peer group, but when she arrived at the seminar she felt 'frozen' and had stammered, which had only made her feel worse. She had then withdrawn to her room for weeks, feeling as if she had 'leprosy', as she put it.

Towards the end of the session, after picking up further confirmatory evidence both from the stories the patient recounted and from the therapist's own countertransference, the therapist retuned to this story as a marker for how exposed the patient was feeling in the session. She said that one risk they both needed to keep in mind was that the patient might experience the therapy a bit like the seminar and might fear being similarly exposed and humiliated by the therapist. If that were the case then the patient's only solution might be to withdraw from the therapy—as she had perhaps done by arriving late and hence limiting her exposure to the therapist's evaluation of her.

WHAT DO WE NEED TO KNOW IN ORDER TO FORMULATE A DYNAMIC FOCUS FOR INTERVENTION?

Before we turn to how to formulate, we need first to establish the range of information that the therapist is interested in so as to arrive at a formulation (i.e. the IPAF) that can then be shared with the patient.

History-taking versus history-making

Psychiatric and psychotherapeutic assessments are both structured around eliciting a patient's history, but they do this in different ways. Psychiatrists typically question the patient systematically about their childhood, sexual and relationship history, their work trajectory, and their previous treatments. A great deal of information is thus collected. Asking about a patient's occupational background or knowing about the patient's sexual history might yield valuable information that will inform the psychiatrist's understanding of the problem. Nevertheless, when reading through standard psychiatric reports and then meeting the patient in question, it soon becomes apparent that this type of detailed, factual information tells us comparatively little about the patient's capacity to use therapy or, indeed, about the patient's problems and their dynamic meaning.

To gain a more in-depth perspective of the patient, we as therapists need to pay attention to the *process* of the assessment with this patient. In other words, we must be attuned to how the patient constructs their narrative (i.e. the form as opposed to the content of what the patient communicates) and what use the patient makes of us in doing so. Throughout the early stages of DIT, it is therefore important for us to reflect on what is happening between us and the patient and to consider some of the following questions: How does the patient relate to us? How does the patient describe their experiences? What feelings are triggered in us during this process? The answers to these questions are as important as, and often far more telling than, the biographical information collected.

The relationship that evolves during the initial sessions between patient and therapist is important on practical and epistemological grounds. From a purely practical point of view, no meaningful assessment or formulation of the patient's difficulties could be arrived at without devoting attention and effort to establishing a good working alliance with the patient. If the patient cannot trust the therapist or sense empathic concern from them, the patient is unlikely to engage fully in the initial sessions or in the subsequent therapy.

There are also theoretical reasons for the privileged space accorded to the relationship between therapist and patient. Contemporary epistemologists argue that all knowledge acquisition is a process by which the knower actively organizes and shapes what is perceived and thought, and thereby constructs what is known (Berger & Luckmann, 1996). Knowledge of a patient thus represents the outcome of a dynamic interaction between knower and known, between subject and object. Most of this dynamic construction will be unconscious, outside the full awareness of either participant. The therapist needs to be mindful of the fact that the knowledge gathered in these early sessions is inevitably subjective and arises from the meeting of two particular people; thus, the patient would not be the same with another therapist.

What is being described here is not 'history-taking' as such; rather, the emphasis is on 'history-making' (Hirschberg, 1993), that is, on the importance of addressing how the patient organizes and constructs their account of their difficulties as they engage with the therapist. It can indeed be helpful to comment explicitly on this during early sessions. For example, as well as commenting on any contradictions or omissions in a patient's account, the therapist might take note of how much or little detail is offered, whether the narrative is difficult or easy to follow, or whether the patient appears preoccupied with particular relationships that cause their presenting concerns to be conveyed in an incoherent fashion.

The way the patient presents their history will provide important clues about their capacity to think about themself in relation to others and about others in relation to them; that is, it tells us something about the patient's capacity for self-reflection and mentalizing. When we listen to the way the patient constructs the narrative, we are paying attention to how they present their relationships with the significant figures in their life. For example, if there are difficulties in a relationship we note whether the patient seems aware that how they feel about the difficult situation may be different from how the other person feels about it.

Coherent narratives, which have been shown to be associated with secure attachments, tend to include an acknowledgement of conflict, pain, and mixed feelings; in speaking about such difficulties the patient demonstrates an appreciation of the complexity of their own and other people's motivations. By contrast, the narratives typically associated with a 'preoccupied' insecure attachment status reveal more unnoticed contradiction, denial, confusion, or overwhelming negative affects such as anger or fear. The patient might leave us feeling that they are still in the thick of negative emotional experience and cannot take a step back from it to gain perspective. Alternatively, with a more 'dismissing' style of insecure attachment, the patient might, for example, recount painful, neglectful, or even abusive experiences and yet talk about them in a very cut-off manner, minimizing the significance of these experiences and perhaps responding to the therapist's empathic interest with further dismissiveness: 'I don't remember much but it was definitely normal,' or 'Spare the rod and spoil the child'.

Listening in this way is very different from 'taking a history'. The skill lies in managing to combine this very specialized type of attention, which is the hallmark of analytic listening (see Chapter 7), with a capacity to weave in and out of the patient's narrative and cover certain areas of the patient's life and functioning that the therapist needs to know about to meaningfully assess the patient's capacity to make use of DIT. For example, the patient might well respond to an interpretation about their internal world, and this may lead us to conclude that they could use DIT. However, if we know little or nothing about who is actually in the patient's current life and who could support them through the demands of therapy, we may be arriving at a wrong conclusion. Some patients are unable to manage the space between sessions if they have few or no support systems. It is therefore imperative that by the end of the initial phase we know something not only about the primitive figures that populate the patient's internal world, but also about who exists in the patient's external world, and the quality of those relationships (see below).

In order to be in a position to formulate we need to gather relevant information in the following domains.

History of the presenting problem: the symptom/problem from the patient's point of view

To begin with we need to take a history of the problem and its timeline (see Box 4.1). The aim is to create an understanding of the onset of the difficulties that have brought the patient to therapy. For many patients the problem will have developed gradually, with a succession of events contributing to their recognition that there is a problem. Others might recognize that there is a problem that is getting worse, but be unclear how it started or why a preferable situation may have deteriorated. In such cases there may be stressful life events or major changes associated with the onset of the problem, as well as changes in its intensity. In many cases, the problem that is ostensibly the reason why the patient

> **Box 4.1**
>
> **ASSESSMENT OF THE PROBLEM/SYMPTOMS**
>
> This will include:
>
> - Its nature as perceived by the patient (e.g. is it experienced as 'symptoms' that need managing, or as a problem in relationships?)
> - Its origins (when did it start?)
> - Its course over time, bearing in mind modulating and exacerbating variables (what makes it better or worse?)
> - Its interpersonal context (how do the patient's relationships affect the problem/symptoms, and how are they affected by it/them?)
> - Its severity (what are the risks to the patient and/or others?)

has been referred or has actively sought therapy may not in fact be the source of their distress. Rather, it acts as a distraction or screen.

The answer to the question 'Why now?' is very important. It is useful to establish why a patient is presenting for help at this particular time, as this might give some indication as to what other difficulties may be occurring in their lives. These difficulties might otherwise remain in the background—for example, children leaving home or a change of job or partner precipitating depression, or awareness of a developing addiction. This exploration is important not only because it provides the therapist with information relevant to the eventual formulation, but also because the process of examining the course of their difficulties over time can implicitly help the patient gain some perspective about their problem and, to an extent, perhaps increase its predictability and so the patient's sense of perceived control over their life.

Family history

The patient's family history includes information about the composition of the patient's family of origin, as well as their extended family.

Information about the extended family is often very important as it can lead to an exploration of how particular patterns or dynamics may be repeating themselves across generations. The information typically includes information about who is in the family; their ages and occupations; births and deaths (including miscarriages, terminations, and stillbirths); marriages and divorces or separations; and any major illnesses, including mental health conditions.

Medical history and the patient's bodily self

If the patient presents with some physical problems that appear to be connected to depression and/or anxiety, taking a very brief medical history will be important to ascertain exactly what is happening in relation to the patient's experience of their physical self. However, such a history should not overshadow the more important exploration of the meaning attributed by the patient to any physical problems, and how these problems affect the patient's perception of themselves or how they might be used interpersonally (e.g. to ensure proximity to an attachment figure: 'If I'm ill then she won't leave me').

Our patients bring their minds *and* their bodies to psychotherapy, yet it is surprising how often we neglect the body both in ongoing therapy and at the assessment stage. A rich source of information about the patient's experience of themselves can be found in how they relate to their physicality because the actual or phantasized limits of the body influence how we relate to ourselves and to others. Visual or auditory impairment, for example, might not only affect an individual on a pragmatic level but also profoundly influence the confidence with which they approach the world and, importantly, the way others relate to them.

We can begin to reflect on the patient's subjective experience of their body by observing their use of the physical space in the consulting room and the way they experience themself in their body. For example, a very tall patient might walk into the room stooped, whereas another might walk into the room and bump into the furniture. It is seldom appropriate at the assessment stage to comment on striking features of someone's physicality because at this early stage any thoughts we will have about the matter are likely to be highly speculative. Referring to such features may also feel very intrusive or critical to the patient. However, feeling free to note in our own mind these perceptions and reactions to the patient's physical presence may provide yet another source of information that can assist us in the task of formulating.

Mapping the interpersonal landscape

THE PATIENT'S INTERNAL WORLD OF OBJECT RELATIONSHIPS

An important task in these early sessions is to map out the patient's characteristic interpersonal style through closely exploring their experience of significant relationships, past and present (see Figure 4.1). The therapist's basic stance during these early sessions is one of curiosity about the patient's subjective experience of their interpersonal world, to tease out recurring relational and affective patterns that are typically structured around a 'self' and 'other' representation. The richest source of information about the dominant qualities of these unconscious representations can be gleaned from the stories the patient tells about their relationships, which we refer to here as interpersonal narratives.

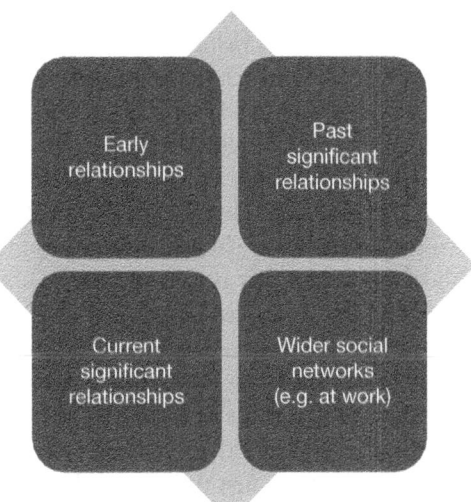

Figure 4.1 The interpersonal map.

From the outset, the emphasis in DIT is on trying to locate the problem in an interpersonal context, that is, to understand how the manifest problem (e.g. depression) can be seen as a manifestation of a circumscribed recurring interpersonal pattern. This requires focused attention on helping the patient to report interpersonal narratives, which will allow the therapist eventually to formulate the patient's internal world of relationships as the basis for helping them to understand their subjective experience of relationships. Here, the focus is placed on *recurring interpersonal scenarios* rather than on the details of the people involved and of the situation.

Therefore, to assess the quality of the patient's relationships, the therapist encourages the patient not only to describe the problem from their point of view, but also to provide narratives about their relationships, past and present. For example, if the patient is focusing narrowly on a description of symptoms, the therapist sensitively acknowledges the distressing nature of these symptoms but also enquires about the interpersonal context in which they occur or fluctuate. This might also bring in the reported opinions of others, which can be telling and might be important in the patient's experience of the situation: 'My wife thinks I exaggerate everything'; 'My parents always warned me about letting people be nosy or get close'.

As the patient tells us their story we begin to listen out for patterns in their relationships that will assist us in building a schematic picture of their internal world. It is helpful to note what repetitive conflicts emerge as we explore these relationships—for example, whether the patient repeatedly engages in relationships in which they are submissive or in which they feel secretly triumphant over other people. Likewise, we note which dynamics are absent—for example, whether relationships are reported to be always conflict-free. Omissions and emphases are often telling. Some patients display from the outset reluctance to talk about a particular period of their lives. For example, the patient's narrative may be skewed in favour of detailed accounts of their childhood experiences, or the patient may talk only about their present life and gloss over their history. Omissions or cursory descriptions should always alert us to the operation of resistance. In these situations, the patient might be helped to explore a difficult period in their life if we can recognize first that they feel they are in danger if, for example, they reveal things about—or even think about—their early childhood.

There are two key questions that we need to be able to tentatively answer in the lead-up to negotiating the IPAF:

- What kind of relationship(s) does the patient typically create?
- How does this relate to the presenting symptoms?

We are therefore interested in formulating the relationship models that organize the patient's experience, modulate their affect, and direct their behaviour, and that are meaningfully connected with the onset and maintenance of symptoms. Recurring interpersonal configurations alert us to internalized object relationships that have taken root in the patient's internal world. The patient's pattern of relating can become entrenched such that they can function only by adopting a very specific role in relation to the other, or they filter what they perceive in highly predictable ways—for example, the patient who always hears criticism even when praised, or who invariably sets up the other as neglectful.

In asking the patient questions about a range of relationships (see Figure 4.2), one of our aims is to gain some sense of who the patient identifies with, both consciously and unconsciously, focusing on building a preliminary sketch of those qualities that have been assimilated or repudiated. A helpful question in this respect is to ask the patient what their father and mother are (or were) like. If the patient gives a very global reply, for example, 'They were good parents', we can prompt them to be more specific—perhaps to think of a few adjectives that best describe each parent. This exploration not only begins to put some flesh on the bones of the various significant figures in the patient's life, but the quality of the patient's descriptions is also informative because it gives some clues as to whether we are dealing with a predominantly borderline or neurotic personality organization. See Chapter 13 for a discussion of DIT for complex care (DITCC), an extended form of DIT designed for work with patients with these more complex or severe mental health presentations.

In these early sessions we are therefore simultaneously thinking about the quality of the patient's object relationships and making inferences about the level of maturity of these relationships, that is, whether the patient relates to whole or part-objects and the patient's

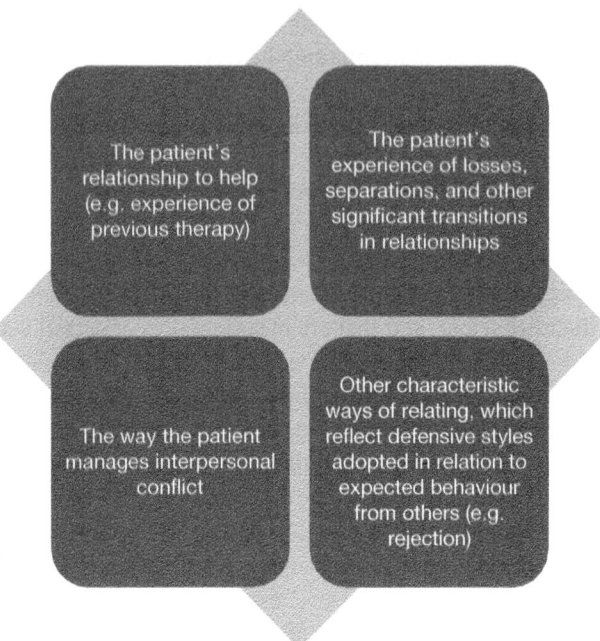

Figure 4.2 Interpersonal contexts yielding information about key attachment patterns.

capacity to be separate from others. In this respect, it is important to make a distinction between a 'narcissistic involvement', where the other is an appendage or extension of the self, and a mature 'object relationship', where the other is seen as separate from the self (Mason, 2000). It is helpful to consider, too, whether the self is experienced as cohesive or vulnerable to fragmentation if others are not available.

As we listen, we are looking for evidence of the patient's ability to confide, to trust, and to see others as potentially helpful, as opposed to feeling paranoid and mistrustful of others' intentions towards the self. Having friends is an encouraging sign, but it does not guarantee a capacity to genuinely engage with others as separate from the self. For example, the patient may relate internally to their so-called friends as no more than 'cloned confirmations of the self' (Bolognini, 2012)—that is, narcissistic satellites that hold the self together but do not allow for the other's separate existence.

Keeping in mind the external reality of the patient's interpersonal context

DIT's emphasis on the importance of the individual's actual attachments to their mental well-being orients the therapist to the importance of the patient's *current* external context. This will include their social networks, work, and/or education. It also includes attention to the impact of factors such as race, culture, disability, sexuality, class, education, and (un)employment on people's experience of themselves with others.

In addition to eliciting a relationship history, which will enable us to build a picture of the patient's internal world, it is therefore important to also assess the patient's wider social networks (including their educational and/or employment interpersonal contexts) and the quality and pattern of the interactions between the patient and their friends/acquaintances/colleagues/bosses (e.g. issues of relationship to authority, dominance and submission, dependency and autonomy, intimacy, trust, etc.). This provides yet another source of information to assist us in identifying recurring interpersonal configurations, and hence a possible focus for the work.

The patient's external relationships, and the availability (or lack) of support for the patient's wish to engage in therapy—or even hostility in relation to their wish to engage in therapy—also deserve consideration. With more psychically fragile patients, the question of who will support them during breaks in the therapy (e.g. over holidays) needs to be carefully considered. Lack of support from colleagues or family members might undermine further a fragile therapeutic alliance and tenuous motivation for change. For the most disturbed patients who show a proneness to acting out, special provision may need to be made to ensure they have additional professional support for the duration of their psychotherapy.

Using the relationship questionnaire

In the second or third session (depending on the patient's degree of distress and the detail they provide in the immediate presentation), the exploration of the patient's characteristic stance towards relationships is opened up and facilitated by suggesting that they read the attachment style statements (Hazan & Shaver, 1987, supplemented by Bartholomew & Horowitz, 1991) shown below. This can be done along with any other measures that the patient might be asked to fill

Table 4.1 RELATIONSHIP QUESTIONNAIRE RATING SCALE

	Not at all like me	Somewhat like me					Very much like me
Style A	1	2	3	4	5	6	7
Style B	1	2	3	4	5	6	7
Style C	1	2	3	4	5	6	7
Style D	1	2	3	4	5	6	7

in as part of outcome monitoring (see later in this chapter for a discussion of the use of outcome monitoring in DIT).

The patient is asked to rate each statement on the scales (Table 4.1). Their ratings can then be used to begin a discussion with the therapist about their usual behaviour in, and feelings about, close relationships. These ratings are revisited in the ending phase (see Chapter 9). The review of the ratings provides an opportunity to reflect on the change that has occurred (which may well be outside awareness, as pervasive attachment assumptions or attitudes are usually more implicit than conscious) and any further changes that the patient would like to work towards in the future. For the most part, the scores on these attachment descriptors unsurprisingly show little change over the course of sixteen sessions, but what can—and often does—change is the patient's appraisal of their characteristic patterns (i.e. less distorted by defences and more awareness of their attachment style) and of how they would like to change.

The statements are:

A. It is easy for me to become emotionally close to others. I am comfortable depending on them and having them depend on me. I don't worry about being alone or having others not accept me. [This corresponds to a 'secure' tendency in relation to adult attachment, where the person is relatively positive about both self and other.]

B. I am uncomfortable getting close to others. I want emotionally close relationships, but I find it difficult to trust others completely, or to depend on them. I worry that I will be hurt if I allow myself to become too close to others. [This corresponds to a 'fearful' stance, where the person is relatively negative about both self and other and, while feeling vulnerable, feels unsafe in a dependent relationship.]

C. I want to be completely emotionally intimate with others, but I often find that others are reluctant to get as close as I would like. I am uncomfortable being without close relationships, but I sometimes worry that others don't value me as much as I value them. [This characterizes a 'preoccupied' attachment style, with the patient being negative about self and ostensibly positive about the other; it would be expected to be associated with intense but anxious relationships, which may also be ambivalent and unstable.]

D. I am comfortable without close emotional relationships. It is very important to me to feel independent and self-sufficient, and I prefer not to depend on others or have others depend on me. [This captures a 'dismissing' attachment style, with the patient being ostensibly positive about the self and negative about the other; it suggests distance and an unconsciously defensive stance of self-sufficiency. It may be associated with denigration of others and relationships, or an apparent lack of interest in them.]

The patient is asked to rate how like them each statement is. This creates a profile across the four prototypical stances that delineates the patient's predominant approach to relationships and closeness.

- Relationship patterns dominated by Style A (secure attachment) are characterized by being balanced (selective and flexible), reversible, and stable (consistent over time and progressive, developing positively over time).

The other patterns are typically inflexible in structure within a relationship and repetitive across different contexts.

- Style B relationships (fearful attachment) are characterized by perceived dangers and risks: the patient is fearful of intimacy and can be quite socially avoidant, or they can be volatile as the conflict between getting close and having to escape is repetitively played out.

- Style C (preoccupied attachment) is characterized by a preoccupation with relationships, bringing others too close to the self, and generating unstable and self-focused structures where the patient imagines knowing more about the feelings of others than is justified by the circumstances. This can be seen as an effort to feel more in control of and less confused by intense involvements, with 'overthinking' in the absence of a real understanding of the feelings and motivations of self or other, despite a continual need to engage.
- Style D (dismissing attachment) relationships are distancing and often quite stable but inflexible. There can be considerable selfishness and thoughtlessness, where others are rarely seen clearly as 'three-dimensional' real figures and there is little conscious emotional investment.

The therapist should be particularly wary of problematic combinations of styles. For example, a style that combines preoccupation with relationships and fearfulness of them often characterizes individuals who are exceptionally vulnerable to rejection. Other unhelpful 'combined' styles include that of distancing with preoccupation, where the strategies dictated by these styles contradict each other. Combinations of Style A with other styles are more positive. In the circumstances of clinical depression, an endorsement of Style A and denial of affinity to the other styles is likely to reflect an idealized pattern of denial of interpersonal difficulties.

During the remainder of the therapy, the patient's attachment styles can be linked to the IPAF—and particularly to the defensive function of the IPAF—if we take into account the attachment strategy that the patient is employing. Hyperactivating attachment strategies may function to keep the other engaged by amplifying distress and remaining in a passive, helpless position. Deactivating attachment strategies can operate to downplay the significance of relationships and minimize their importance to the patient. The more complex attachment style, which combines hyperactivation and deactivation and is seen in some patients with personality disorders, can be linked in the psychoanalytic literature to Glasser's core complex (Glasser, 1979, 1992), in which there are claustrophobic and agoraphobic anxieties at play. This complexity can be reflected in the dynamic of the IPAF and its reversal; for example, the patient might consciously be preoccupied with a fear of being trapped in a stifling relationship pattern, but during the treatment it can emerge that there is a resistance to change based on the avoidance of rejection and being alone.

THE PATIENT'S CULTURAL CONTEXT

We do not develop in isolation. From the moment of birth we are part of a family system, and also of wider systems, such as the culture into which we are born. This wider system needs to be integrated into the therapist's understanding of the patient's presenting problem and of their relationships.

The internal world is always in a dynamic interaction with the external world. Although there is never a direct correspondence between the external and the internal, as what is internal reflects the operation of defensive processes that distort what is taken in from the outside, our assessments and formulations need to reflect the reality of our patients' lives just as much as what they idiosyncratically make of this reality. To have the best possible understanding of our patients and their needs we need to be curious about the external world in which they live. If we do not ask about it, we may never know and we can jump to erroneous conclusions.

Culture is especially important because the notions of self, of separation, and of individuation that are so commonplace in Western models of therapy might not be as relevant for other cultures. In the West, the individuated self is the goal of therapy. It is a self that values differentiation. In the East, the relational self is more permeable and we encounter more fluid self–other boundaries; the unit of identity is not an internal representation of the other but of the family or community (Pande, 1968).

The relationship with the therapist will also be influenced by cultural factors (Kareem, 1999). By virtue of our own cultural identifications or our race, we may find it easier to relate to some patients than others, and the same will apply to our patients. Being open and receptive to these transferences and countertransferences is essential to a good assessment. Patients do not always seek likeness in their therapists with respect to cultural background. Instead, some actively seek difference and in so doing may be communicating something very important about their own cultural identifications. For example, one biracial young woman specifically requested a white therapist. In the therapy it soon became clear that the patient perceived her 'white' self as good and her 'black' self as bad, hence she defensively wanted to identify herself with the white therapist.

Diversity and difference are often thought and spoken about in terms of difference residing in the other: 'they' are different. This is certainly the case when the subject is a member of the dominant group. Individuals from the dominant culture tend to view the world from the perspective of their identity representing the norm and perceive those with non-normative identities as the ones who are different. We become like fish that cannot see the water in which we are swimming. In DIT, we are curious about the patient's internal and external world, including culture and points of difference that exist between the patient and the therapist. It is not that the patient is different and the therapist is not (or vice versa). The therapist and patient both have socially constructed identities that differ from each other and need to be taken into account when exploring the IPAF, including how this plays out in the transference. Tang and Gardner (1999, p. 8) make the point that 'As a person of color and of a different culture, the minority therapist is more than just a blank screen, and his or her color will pull forth a rich variety of projections and stereotypes.' We may focus our attention on one aspect of perceived difference without giving much attention to the various points of difference and sameness that exist between two people (age, sex and gender, sexual orientation, class, ethnicity, political views, and so on). Cultural neutrality is the therapist's capacity to remain equidistant from the values, ideals, and mores of the patient's culture and our own, much as Anna Freud recommended finding a position of analytic neutrality in relation to our patients (as we described in Chapter 2).

Some therapists have not explored their own feelings about their ethnicity and culture, which can lead to blocks in clinical work. Personal therapy and supervision can be particularly beneficial in thinking through these issues to avoid becoming defensive or collusive, thereby circumventing considering the impact of cultural norms and social mores on the transference and countertransference. We can also maintain cultural neutrality and avert countertransference pitfalls by studying the interface between social anthropology and clinical work; by treating patients of many cultures; by avoiding the pitfall of being excessively curious about the patient's culture; and by leading an open and cosmopolitan life that exposes us to different cultures (Akhtar, 1999).

HOW MANY RELATIONSHIPS NEED TO BE EXPLORED BEFORE SHARING A FORMULATION WITH THE PATIENT?

As a general rule, all significant attachments, past and present, deserve exploration. It is best to start with an exploration of the patient's significant current relationships and work backwards to the patient's early experiences. For each relationship, the therapist engages the patient in thinking about the perceived quality of these relationships and how they impact on the patient's experience of themselves.

It is important to elicit at least one detailed account of some important current interpersonal interactions in which the patient's attachment system has been activated, for example, an argument with a partner. In this context the therapist can focus on identifying common communication difficulties; explore any open conflict with intense affect and understand its outcomes; identify and point to ambiguous, indirect non-verbal communication; point to dramatically distorted assumptions in the patient's belief that they have communicated (even when they may have not done so very clearly) and that they have understood what has been said to them (when in fact they have not); highlight problematic communication patterns (e.g. silence to close off communication or repetitive statements such as 'I know that I am no good'); and point to risky communication by listening for the assumptions that the patient makes about the thoughts or feelings of others, including the therapist.

NEGOTIATING THE THERAPEUTIC CONTENT AND GOALS FOR THERAPY

All the information that is gleaned from exploring the various dimensions of the patient's experience, as outlined earlier in this chapter, contributes to the formulation of the IPAF. In Chapter 5 we will focus exclusively on how this is done in DIT. Here, though, we want to continue sketching out the overall trajectory of the initial phase, where, once the focus has been agreed with the patient, an important task during session 4 is to engage the patient in articulating the aims for the therapy. This may not be familiar territory for some psychodynamic clinicians, but the identification of meaningful and realistic goals is important in a time-limited intervention. It creates a helpful opportunity for the therapist to engage the patient at the outset in working towards change, and promotes hopefulness.

The process of identifying aims begins with the therapist enquiring explicitly about what the patient hopes to achieve in relation to the agreed IPAF—that is, in what way the patient would like to step out of their characteristic relational pattern. Many patients will give very diffuse, general answers to this question, such as 'I want to be happy'. The challenge is to help the patient to translate this general wish into something more specific and interpersonal, such as 'I want to be able to communicate to others what I need from them'—a capacity that would contribute to their sense of happiness.

When discussing aims, the patient's resources need to be considered along with their vulnerabilities, to help the patient to reflect on their expectations of therapy and introduce some realism about what might and might not be achievable. It is also timely to acknowledge the patient's strengths here.

With some patients the most realistic goal is to set in motion a process of understanding or of 'working towards' some change in relationships rather than achieving an observable change in their relationships over the sixteen sessions. Such goals may involve the patient relating differently to others (e.g. asking for clarification rather than jumping to conclusions) or responding differently (e.g. expressing their needs more clearly); being more aware of affects; and/or dropping some of the defensive coping strategies they typically employ. For other patients, one or more stated aims might well conflict with unstated ones. Where this is the case, the therapist also needs to communicate understanding that, in addition to the stated aims, there might be less conscious aims that oppose change. For example, a patient might say that they would like to get a better understanding of why their marriage is failing, but the unconscious aim is to recruit the therapist into supporting the patient's position against their spouse.

HOW MUCH INFORMATION DOES THE PATIENT NEED ABOUT DIT IN ORDER TO CONSENT TO IT?

Therapy is not the place for a seminar on how therapy works, but neither is it unreasonable for patients to want to find out what we think about their difficulties and how we think we can help them. During the initial sessions some patients will ask about the therapy and how it works. Such questions may, of course, mask anxiety about engaging in the process, and this needs to be explored, but we have a duty to inform our patients of the service they are receiving, just like any other service. Patients both have a right to know and are possibly anxious for their own individual reasons.

Some patients may well be preoccupied with whether they are 'mad' or 'bad', or whether we think they will get better or not. It is important to avoid colluding with the patient's wish for a definitive answer or reassurance by offering detailed replies on this front, which in any event could be only partial and tentative at such an early stage of therapy. Nevertheless, it is part of the therapist's responsibility to convey to the patient an understanding of their predicament and how the proposed therapy might help them. Interpreting the patient's questions as simply reflecting anxiety about the process, or their fear that they might be going mad or are a 'bad' person, is unhelpful, although such speculations will be true for some patients. In our responses we can both acknowledge the actual question and give some opinion as well as attend to the anxiety that may lie behind the question.

In DIT, the therapist is direct and transparent about their understanding of the patient's difficulties and how the therapy will help. Early on in therapy, the therapist will provide the patient with sufficient direct information about the therapy (including its risks and benefits) so as to make consent meaningful (a sample patient information leaflet about DIT is provided in Appendix 1).

It is helpful to personalize the explanation of the treatment rationale by linking it to the patient's own history and current experiences. This minimizes the risk of becoming unhelpfully intellectual and increases the likelihood of engaging the patient in the treatment process. It is also helpful to manage the patient's expectations by stressing the difficulties involved in changing long-established patterns and pointing to the challenge that the patient is about to undertake.

At the start of therapy, the therapist will also agree a verbal contract with the patient, which will include specification of the following:

1. The affective–interpersonal context of the intervention (namely, negotiating the IPAF).

2. The short-term duration of the therapy (sixteen weekly sessions, each of about 50 minutes), including agreement about planned breaks.
3. The problem area that will be targeted.
4. The crisis management plan, where appropriate.
5. The agreement to complete the relationship questionnaire (discussed earlier in this chapter) and any other forms of outcome monitoring used within the service, which might happen at the start of each session.

Some patients passively accept what is offered. In such instances, the therapist encourages the patient to reflect on their reactions to the proposed therapy and its general focus on feelings and relationships, to enlist more active participation in the process.

As we mentioned earlier, it is not necessary to enter into lengthy explanations about how DIT aims to help the patient, but it is essential to provide some brief guidance on the expectations of both therapist and patient to orient the patient to the particular style of therapy in the sessions to come. Once the IPAF has been negotiated, the therapist might say something along these lines:

> Now that we have agreed a focus for our work I want to tell you about how we will work together. Each week you will have time to talk about the things that are on your mind. We have already identified a specific area in your relationships where there is room for change, and I will try to keep us focused on this because we will be meeting for another twelve sessions. I am interested not only in what happens in your relationships between sessions, but also in your feelings about these events. This includes feelings about me, our relationship, or the therapy. It may feel difficult to raise this with me, but it will be important for us to think together about what may be on your mind about how this is going.

MANAGING RISK AND SELF-HARM

The management of risk in DIT is no different from what all therapists do when faced with a patient who is at risk of harming themself and/or others: the priority is to ensure safety. If the patient presents with a risk of self-harm, it is important to engage them, from the first session, in jointly identifying how they will access help when in a crisis and putting into place additional support as necessary. The risk of self-harm is not constant and may fluctuate over the course of the therapy in a way that requires a continuous, session-by-session assessment of the patient's state of mind. With more disturbed patients, it is vital to carry out an assessment of risk ahead of any breaks in the treatment and to make arrangements for additional support when required.

Having stressed the importance of ensuring the patient's safety, it is also the case that in the area of mental health we inhabit a risk-averse culture in which the need to act so as to pre-empt the patient's acting out can sometimes unhelpfully preclude reflection on the conscious and unconscious meaning of the patient's suicidal thoughts or violent fantasies (i.e. their interpersonal function) (see Briggs et al., 2008). It is therefore essential to consider not only how to keep the patient safe but also what might be giving rise to an increase in risk: is the therapist pushing the patient too much? Is the patient trying in some way to attack the therapist? Is the patient's self-harm a response to a separation? So, while complying with the service's governance structures for the management of risk, the DIT therapist should not abandon their capacity to reflect on the unconscious meaning of the risky behaviour and try to engage the patient in reflecting on it.

When working with patients who pose a risk of self-harm or acting out, it will be helpful to refer to Chapter 13, which offers a model for working with patients requiring complex care.

MANAGING THE FRAME AND THE SETTING

The therapist strives to establish and maintain a consistent therapeutic frame, setting out clearly at the outset the parameters within which the treatment will take place (the setting; the frequency and length of sessions; the limits of confidentiality; expectations of the patient; and arrangements/cover over breaks). Sometimes there will be pressure from the patient to change the frame. It is important to evaluate the meaning of the patient's requests for modifications to the parameters of the therapy as the basis for responding to them.

The therapist endeavours to be receptive to the patient's conscious and unconscious experience of the setting and its boundaries, and to help them to articulate this experience. This is to ensure that the agreement to the therapy and its boundaries is rooted in an exploration of the patient's conscious and unconscious feelings and fantasies about the therapy.

When managing forms of acting out in relation to the setting (by the patient, the therapist, or both), the therapist strives to maintain (or regain) a reflective stance, but may also need to set clear limits where necessary (e.g. if the patient's behaviour undermines the viability of the treatment). Managing the frame involves managing interruptions in the therapy by preparing the patient for planned interruptions (e.g. holiday breaks) and, once again, helping them to explore their conscious and unconscious responses to both planned and unplanned breaks. This exploration needs to be linked to the IPAF, where relevant, and is not carried out for its own sake.

THE USE OF OUTCOME MONITORING AND VIDEO/AUDIO RECORDING OF SESSIONS

In developing DIT, originally for use in the Improving Access to Psychological Therapies (IAPT) programme in the UK and now used within primary care in the NHS, we have been pragmatic in a number of ways. One of these is to embed the protocol in the discipline of routinely measuring outcomes as required in IAPT to allow comparisons of outcomes across different treatment modalities. This is by no means standard practice within psychodynamic approaches. Along with manuals and competences, we can also add outcome monitoring to our list of 'non-analytic-self' antigens, which are experienced as intruders and are repudiated by the 'psychic immune system' (Britton, 2003). At its best, this kind of monitoring is construed as an intrusion into the therapeutic process or is felt to be irrelevant because the measures used are often (and with good reason) considered inappropriate to the process of change that dynamic approaches try to support: the measures focus on mood symptoms as opposed to, for example, relationships or self-perception. At worst, the antipathy of psychoanalytic therapists to outcome monitoring results from their conviction that the treatment they are offering is effective (Busch et al., 2009), which does not need to be evidenced beyond the clinical observation of the clinician and other like-minded colleagues. But, as Busch and Milrod (2010) observe:

> Clinical lore and observation can be highly biased, as the subjectivity of the observer can override an accurate assessment of a patient's improvement. . . . Psychoanalysts pride themselves on their awareness of the impact of fantasy and wishful thinking during their treatments, but minimize the impact of such factors on their subjective assessment of their own clinical outcomes. Identification with powerful and respected leaders and theoreticians in the field can colour a more objective assessment of treatment effectiveness. In our wish to be therapeutic and our belief in our treatment, it is all too easy to disregard patients who were treatment failures. (Busch & Milrod, 2010, p. 310).

The aversion to outcome monitoring is also fuelled by our narcissism: outcome monitoring can understandably feel like a kind of personal monitoring, and a deterioration in the patient's scores on outcome measures can feel like a crushing judgement of our competence (Okiishi et al., 2003). But to insist that only the therapist treating the patient can evaluate the results of a psychodynamic treatment is to propose a closed-loop system and ignore basic awareness of narcissistic and other biases. Sophistication is necessary to evaluate patient reports in the consulting room, as well as part of conducting outcome research. However, if sophistication becomes a euphemism for insistence that outcomes can be accurately judged only by those committed to a particular form of treatment, the confidence of the patients, the general public, and the scientific community will be eroded.

We take the view that despite the limitations of questionnaires in detecting meaningful and sometimes subtle changes, it is nevertheless good practice to monitor treatment outcomes, just as it is to audio or video record sessions and have a supervisor listen to or watch the recordings. This kind of 'monitoring' could be more helpfully construed as additional feedback for the therapist and, as such, another form of support for the therapist to help them to reflect on the course of therapy. Our experience 'on the ground' has been that after some initial anxiety therapists have actually welcomed recordings and use them to reflect on sessions, often identifying subtle enactments that they had not been consciously aware of at the time.

The inclusion of outcome monitoring in routine practice makes pragmatic sense because DIT can then be compared with other psychological interventions, particularly in a climate of evidence-based practice where lack of evidence is often erroneously construed as evidence of ineffectiveness. Just as important, provided the measures are meaningful to the changes DIT is trying to support, continuous monitoring also serves to focus both patient and therapist on how the work is progressing. If the patient's scores remain static, or even worsen, over the course of the therapy, this can helpfully raise the question of why this is happening. A deterioration in scores on questionnaires should never be taken as absolute evidence that the therapy is failing, but neither can it be dismissed as irrelevant to what is transpiring between the therapist and patient. It should at the very least give pause for thought and lead to a review of what may not feel—and may indeed not *be*—helpful to the patient.

In DIT used within the IAPT programme, therapists are encouraged to administer measures at the start of each session. Although we recognize that this practice may be felt to be intrusive to the therapeutic process (and sometimes may turn out to be so with some patients), experience shows that this intrusion is typically felt more acutely by the therapist than by the patient. In practice, completing the forms takes up the first few minutes of every session, and can feel awkward for the therapist as they sit and observe the patient filling in the forms. It is important, however, not to split off the questionnaires from the interaction with the therapist by asking the patient to complete them before coming in to the session. Integrating this activity within the session ensures that the therapist can monitor and respond to the patient's communication through the questionnaires. Indeed, once the therapist is acculturated to the routine of outcome monitoring, the 'use' made of the questionnaires by the patient becomes grist to the therapeutic mill. For example, one patient reported significant improvement in the sessions, but her scores on the questionnaires remained very high (i.e. clinically severe). When this discrepancy was picked up on by the therapist, it made it possible to understand at the level of the transference the patient's wish to 'punish' the therapist and deprive her of evidence she might share with others that the therapy was of help—an enactment of the grievance the patient harboured towards her mother.

We may note the way in which patients respond to the outcome measures with hyperactivating or deactivating attachment strategies, respectively elevating or downplaying their scores. This can be brought to the patient's attention as another way in which they may unconsciously contribute to keeping the IPAF going, this time in the transference to the therapist.

During training, DIT sessions are also recorded and evaluated by the supervisor. As with outcome monitoring, this practice can at first feel threatening to the therapist. The impact it might have on the patient is often cited as the reason for not making recordings. In our experience, very few patients refuse recording of their sessions or find it intrusive, although the meaning of being recorded is invariably worthy of exploration. Some patients regard it as an expression of their 'specialness', while others may at times fear that what is on the recording may be seen or heard by others who would be critical of the patient. The patient's fantasies about being recorded always warrant the therapist's acknowledgement, interest, and exploration with the patient.

From the therapist's point of view, we have found that once the initial anxiety about making recordings of sessions is overcome, they experience access to the recordings as helpful in reviewing their work. Not uncommonly, as a recording is replayed, the therapist notices a particular quality in the exchange that had not been apparent or consciously registered at the time—in other words, the recording itself functions as an adjunct to supervision even before the supervisor has listened to it and made comments. The recorded sessions also play an important part in the use of the competence framework (see Appendix 3) to evaluate whether the therapist is being faithful to the DIT model, and to provide guidance about areas for improvement.

REFERENCES

Akhtar, S. (1999). *Immigration and identity: Turmoil, treatment, and transformation*. Jason Aronson.

Bartholomew, K., & Horowitz, L. M. (1991). Attachment styles among young adults: A test of a four-category model. *Journal of Personality and Social Psychology, 61*(2), 226–244. https://doi.org/10.1037/0022-3514.61.2.226

Berger, P. L., & Luckmann, T. (1996). *The social construction of reality: A treatise in the sociology of knowledge*. Penguin.

Bolognini, S. (2012). The profession of ferryman: Considerations on the analyst's internal attitude in consultation and referral. In B. Reith, S. Lagerlöf, P. Crick, M. Møller, & E. Skale (Eds.), *Initiating psychoanalysis: Perspectives* (pp. 148–166). Routledge.

Briggs, S., Crouch, W., & Lemma, A. (Eds.). (2008). *Relating to self-harm and suicide: Psychoanalytic perspectives on practice, theory and prevention*. Routledge.

Britton, R. (2003). *Sex, death, and the superego: Experiences in psychoanalysis*. Karnac Books.

Busch, F. N., & Milrod, B. L. (2010). The ongoing struggle for psychoanalytic research: Some steps forward. *Psychoanalytic Psychotherapy*, 24(4), 306–314. https://doi.org/10.1080/02668734.2010.519234

Busch, F. N., Milrod, B. L., & Sandberg, L. S. (2009). A study demonstrating efficacy of a psychoanalytic psychotherapy for panic disorder: Implications for psychoanalytic research, theory, and practice. *Journal of the American Psychoanalytic Association*, 57(1), 131–148. https://doi.org/10.1177/0003065108329677

Glasser, M. (1979). Some aspects of the role of aggression in the perversions. In I. Rosen (Ed.), *Sexual deviation* (2nd edn., pp. 278–305). Oxford University Press.

Glasser, M. (1992). Problems in the psychoanalysis of certain narcissistic disorders. *International Journal of Psychoanalysis*, 73(3), 493–503.

Hazan, C., & Shaver, P. (1987). Romantic love conceptualized as an attachment process. *Journal of Personality and Social Psychology*, 52(3), 511–524. https://doi.org/10.1037/0022-3514.52.3.511

Hirschberg, L. (1993). Clinical interview with infants and their families. In C. Zeanah (Ed.), *Handbook of infant mental health* (pp. 173–191). Guilford Press.

Kareem, J. (1999). The Nafsiyat Intercultural Therapy Centre: Ideas and experiences in intercultural therapy. In J. Kareem & R. Littlewood (Eds.), *Intercultural therapy* (2nd ed., pp. 14–38). Blackwell Science.

Klauber, J. (1981). *Difficulties in the analytic encounter*. Jason Aronson.

Mason, A. (2000). Bion and binocular vision. *International Journal of Psychoanalysis*, 81(5), 983–989. https://doi.org/10.1516/0020757001600327

Ogden, T. H. (1992). Comments on transference and countertransference in the initial analytic meeting. *Psychoanalytic Inquiry*, 12(2), 225–247. https://doi.org/10.1080/07351699209533894

Okiishi, J., Lambert, M. J., Nielsen, S. L., & Ogles, B. M. (2003). Waiting for supershrink: An empirical analysis of therapist effects. *Clinical Psychology & Psychotherapy*, 10(6), 361–373. https://doi.org/10.1002/cpp.383

Pande, S. K. (1968). The mystique of 'Western' psychotherapy: an Eastern interpretation. *Journal of Nervous and Mental Disease*, *146*(6), 425–432. https://doi.org/10.1097/00005053-196806000-00001

Sullivan, H. S. (1953). *The interpersonal theory of psychiatry*. W. W. Norton.

Tang, N. M., & Gardner, J. (1999). Race, culture, and psychotherapy: transference to minority therapists. *Psychoanalytic Quarterly*, *68*(1), 1–20. https://doi.org/10.1002/j.2167-4086.1999.tb00634.x

5
The Interpersonal-Affective Focus

Arriving at a psychodynamic formulation, and explicitly sharing this with the patient in order to negotiate the focus of the work, represents the final outcome of the initial phase. As we saw in the previous chapter, a core strategy in the initial phase involves identifying interpersonal and affective patterns in the patient's past and current relationships to formulate a recurring configuration of 'self' and 'other' representations that will become the focus for the remainder of the therapy. In this chapter, we will describe how we formulate in dynamic interpersonal therapy (DIT) to arrive at a focus for the therapy. It is this focus that will orient both the therapist and the patient in the middle phase sessions, ensuring that some meaningful work and change can be achieved within the time limit.

WHAT IS A PSYCHODYNAMIC FORMULATION?

A formulation bridges theory and practice. It ensures that therapy is mapped to the needs of the individual patient and provides a focus for the work. The formulation will thus also inform the direction and goals of treatment.

In a general sense, a psychodynamic formulation strives to identify both the external and the internal factors that have contributed to and/or are maintaining the problem. This formulation is a provisional hypothesis, which will most likely be refined in collaboration with the patient as the work progresses. It is all too easy to become attached to our hypotheses, but it is incumbent on us to monitor whether we become so married to our hypothesis that we no longer remain alert to what the patient may be trying to communicate that is incongruent with it.

Because it is explicitly shared with the patient, the formulation gives the patient a chance to respond to it and to work with the therapist to refine it so that there is a good fit between the formulation and the patient's current difficulties. This process is important because if the formulation makes sense to the patient they are more likely to be engaged with the therapy.

The choice of framework for formulating is a question of personal preference, which invariably reflects the therapist's own theoretical allegiances. This is true of DIT, but, besides our own theoretical preferences, we also wanted the framework for formulation to be as simple as possible while doing justice to the complexity of an individual's mental life. This is why we opted for the interpersonal-affective focus (IPAF), to which we will now turn.

THE INTERPERSONAL-AFFECTIVE FOCUS: AN OVERVIEW

By session 4, the therapist will have elicited several interpersonal narratives (INs) and sketched out the patient's interpersonal map. The therapist will also have identified the relational anxiety embedded in the 'cautionary tale'. Taken together, these sources of information help the therapist to formulate the IPAF, that is, the dominant internal relationship that is linked to the manifest problem.

Our starting point for formulating in DIT is that to understand how the patient relates to others, we have to gain a detailed picture of their internal world of relationships and of the states of mind that this internal world of loving and hating figures—and of loved and hated figures—gives rise to. The internal world, as we conceptualize it in DIT, consists of prototypic schemas involving invariant dimensions of early affectively charged relationships (e.g. experiences of union and separation). In early life, heightened affective exchanges are psychically organizing: they allow the infant to categorize and expect similar experiences. For example, a 'negative' experience may be internalized as a working model of an 'ugly' self relating to a 'humiliating' other. Once learned, a relational working model sets a template for interpreting later events in a similar way; that is, it generalizes.

External relationships at any stage of life may then trigger the affects associated with particular relationship constellations and the associated relational phantasy (e.g. 'If I get close to another person they will see my ugly self and humiliate me, so it's best to keep to myself'). These mental representations of 'self' affectively interacting with 'other' therefore contain both conscious and non-conscious cognitive and affective components deriving from significant interpersonal experiences with key attachment figures. Although the experiences that contributed to these schemas remain for the most part inaccessible to conscious memory, they nevertheless structure how we think and feel about ourselves and about others. This is why, even though we may not be able to recall early events, we nevertheless continue to organize the present according to developmental models. In our view, a useful way of formulating these dominant internal relationships is found in Kernberg's (1980) distinctive integration of object-relations theory and ego psychology, which focuses on prototypes of positive and negative relationships that become internalized. Following on from this, we conceptualize unconscious conflict as resulting from a clash between particular self and other representations (Kernberg, 1980), resulting in a recurring interpersonal pattern and expectation of others. The IPAF thus consists of four dimensions (see Figure 5.1):

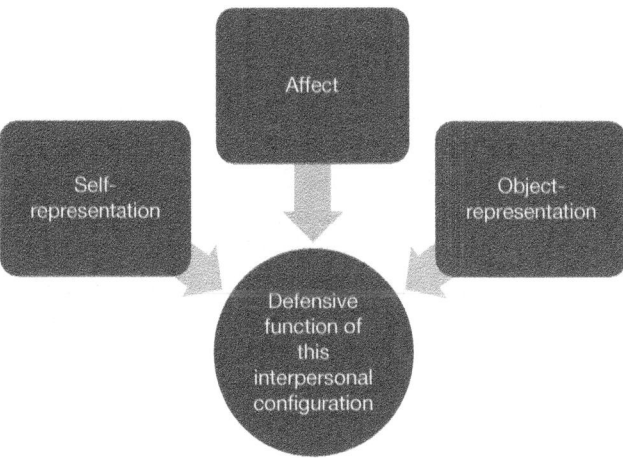

Figure 5.1 The IPAF dimensions.

1. A self-representation (e.g. a demanding infant: 'I always ask for too much')
2. An object-representation (e.g. a rejecting mother: 'No one is there for me when I need them')
3. An affect linking the two (e.g. terror: 'The worst moments are when I feel in pain and there is no one to turn to')
4. The defensive function of this configuration (e.g. avoidance of own aggression; by maintaining the other in one's mind as 'always rejecting', the patient can remain in the victim position and avoids reflecting on their own tendency to reject).

The elaboration of the self and object descriptors is a vital component of the formulation of the IPAF (see below). This requires a systematic testing-out of the descriptors across a range of INs. For example, if the patient's self-representation is 'demanding' we would expect to see this experience of the self manifesting across a range of interpersonal scenarios, including in the transference.

At this stage of the therapy, the therapist needs to ensure that the formulation does not become overloaded, potentially losing focus if it embraces too many self and object descriptors. The key is to anchor the identification of the descriptors by ensuring that (a) they are relevant to more than one relationship or situation that is problematic and (b) they help the patient to understand the link between their current symptoms and the IPAF.

The self and object descriptors are an attempt to capture the patient's experience of the self in relation to the other. Problems with identifying the descriptors often result from two sources. First, there may be confusion between a recurrent affective experience (e.g. the patient often feels 'angry') and the descriptor. 'Angry' is not a self-representation, even if the patient may feel this is a defining feature of how they see themself. The self-descriptor aims to get behind the anger, as it were. For example, the patient may often feel angry because they see themself as 'useless'. Second, there may be confusion between the self-representation and the patient's characteristic defence. For example, if we consider a patient who characteristically tries to appease others as a way of averting confrontation, their descriptor would not be 'appeasing' because this is the defence.

THE PATIENT'S EXPERIENCE OF THE IPAF

To begin with, the description of the self- and other-representation is just that: a *description* that aims to capture the quality of the patient's experience of themself when they relate, in their mind, to an other to whom particular qualities have been (rightly or wrongly) attributed. Typically, the patient finds this kind of conceptualization relatively unthreatening, as it describes their experience without any suggestion of the part they may also play in keeping alive this version of reality. The latter is for the most part the work of the middle phase, when the IPAF is 'unpacked' and its various nuances and defensive dimensions are explored. Not uncommonly, the affect that is identified at this early stage is conscious affect. It is only as the IPAF is worked on that the unconscious affect that is defended against is gradually brought to the patient's conscious attention (e.g. panic that defends against rage).

In our experience of practising DIT and of supervising our colleagues we have been repeatedly struck by the powerful impact that the articulation of the IPAF has on the patient. Often the patient is deeply affected as they listen to the therapist offering an account of how they have understood the patient's experience. When the IPAF has face validity, and this can be illustrated to the patient through examples of how this pattern is manifest across different domains of the patient's life (e.g. in intimate and work relationships) and how it is also connected with the onset of symptoms, this can help the patient to feel that there is some underlying 'sense' to their predicament.

Of course, for some patients, being understood is not a straightforward experience, however benign the therapist's intentions. It may instead feel very exposing or humiliating, as if they have been 'caught out'. This is especially so because implicit in the IPAF is an invitation to the patient to consider their own role in their predicament. For most patients the challenge arises when the defensive function of the self–other configuration is added to this description of the 'internal state of affairs', as it were. This is because now the patient is invited to take some responsibility for also 'doing' something to their objects; for example, the way a patient may have a particular investment in seeing themself as someone who is forever being disappointed. In other words, the therapist attends to the role of the defensive function in maintaining the patient's psychic equilibrium. The therapist will be guided by their assessment of what the patient can bear to hear in the initial phase: there is no value in naming a descriptor that may be unpalatable to the patient even if it is likely to be correct. The work of the middle phase (see Chapter 6) will involve helping the patient to face a potentially more unpalatable version of the self and what they do to others, in their minds and in actuality.

In the middle phase of the work, the way in which the self may also identify with the object becomes more apparent. The patient may enact a role reversal such that, returning to the example given above of an 'ugly self' felt to be relating to a 'humiliating other', the patient may, in turn, become the humiliating other in their relationships, locating in someone else the pain of being the undesirable one—not infrequently locating it in the therapist through a process of projective identification. The therapist's task then becomes that of helping the patient to consider their investment in maintaining the internal status quo, sensitively pointing out its apparent benefits alongside the heavy interpersonal costs and symptomatic expressions.

Inviting the patient to consider the ways in which they may be contributing to their difficulties in this way is more or less easy depending on how capable the patient is of reflecting on their experience and the impact they may have on other people in their life. For this reason, we suggest that the comprehensiveness of the IPAF that is shared with the patient in session 4 is guided by what the patient appears capable of taking in at that point, and is accordingly titrated in terms of its content so as to ensure that the patient is not unduly persecuted by it.

It is not uncommon for the defensive function of the IPAF, and the unconscious affect that links the self–other representation, to be addressed only in later sessions. By then, the patient will, it is hoped, have developed a solid working alliance with the therapist and will have been helped sufficiently to develop a mentalizing stance, such that they are now better equipped to reflect on their contribution to the relational impasse captured in the IPAF and how this is connected to their presenting difficulties. It is important to keep distinct the defensive function of the IPAF (i.e. the specific self–object–affect configuration) from the patient's use of defences more generally (see Chapter 6).

The therapist needs to be receptive to the patient's conscious and unconscious experience when hearing the IPAF for the first time, so as to tease out the multilayered nature of the patient's experience of being understood or of realizing how much they have actively, albeit unconsciously, participated in the creation or maintenance of their difficulties.

Case example

Carol, a 27-year-old woman, was referred because of panic attacks and eating problems, which consisted of erratic bingeing but without vomiting. She binged as a way, as she put it, 'of shutting down my feelings'. It was only when she ate that she felt as if 'nothing matters'. Her depression had worsened after the break-up of a relationship six months previously. Since then she had felt very worried about the future, fearing that her life was going nowhere. She said that she felt very lonely. She added that she feared loneliness the most.

As the therapist explored her relationships it soon became clear that Carol found it difficult to sustain relationships; she felt that people were often trying to get away from her and she had been told by friends and a previous partner that she could be 'too much'. She feared this was true. If she was in a relationship, she recognized her heightened sensitivity to feeling easily rejected, for example, if friends did not *always* invite her to join them. When she was not with her boyfriend she called him several times a day and would worry if she could not get hold of him.

Carol described a close, yet anxious, attachment to her mother, whom she praised for her commitment to charity work and emotional resilience. Her father had died when she was very young. She described her mother as coping very well with raising her as a single parent. As Carol got older, her mother developed a very successful business and worked long hours.

In the first session, the therapist experienced Carol as anxious to rapidly establish a closeness with her. Prior to the initial session Carol had phoned several times to confirm that she was coming. The therapist was struck by this behaviour and thought that it communicated Carol's anxiety about whether she was kept in mind, but it also gave the therapist a more direct experience of how controlling she could be.

In the first session, the therapist invited Carol to think about why she had sought help. Carol had had some prior therapy while at university; she had been told then about intensive therapy and wondered whether she should come several times per week because she recognized that her problems were severely restricting her life. The therapist was struck by what she experienced as Carol's over-eagerness to come into therapy, to have sessions all the time, as if she could not bear to be left alone with any gaps when she might have thoughts that could be too disturbing.

To begin with, Carol described her mother as a very self-sufficient woman, whom she admired greatly. She had berated herself by comparison because she could not 'get her act together' as her mother had done after her father died. In the second session, Carol spoke some more about her mother. She said that she had missed her mother a great deal as she was growing up. The woman who the week before had been presented as the perfect role model now took on a qualitatively different appearance: her mother was now described as unavailable, at times even selfishly pursuing her own career. When the therapist asked her how she had managed when her mother was away, Carol replied that she did not think about her any more and she just got on with her life.

The therapist tracked this sequence to get a picture of what would happen when the mother came home: Carol said that at first, she felt distanced from her and could be quite rejecting of her, but it was not long before she reconnected with her longing for her. She would then turn to her mother for comfort, only to feel dismissed by her (her mother would, for example, tell her not to cry, and Carol recalled her 'physical coldness'). At least, this was how she experienced it consciously: it became apparent over the ensuing sessions that Carol could be rather unforgiving and hostile towards others if they were not available to her when she needed them, and yet she struggled to see how punishing she could be of them. The therapist therefore wondered about Carol's unconscious investment in keeping the other as 'rejecting' as a defence against knowing about her own aggression.

On the basis of this additional information about Carol's experience of her relationship with her mother, the therapist began

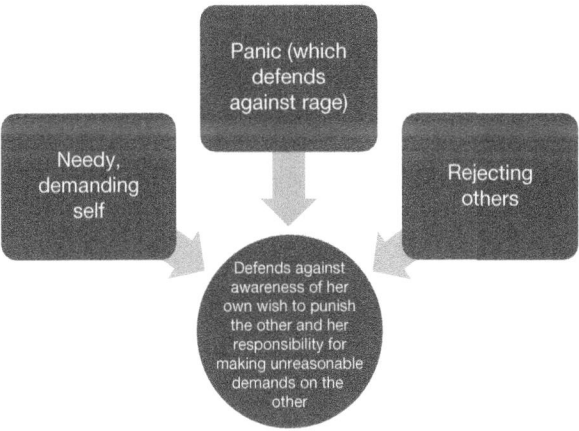

Figure 5.2 Carol's IPAF.

to formulate that one significant internalized object relationship might be as follows: a needy, deprived self relating to a dismissive, unavailable other. The conscious affect associated with this was, in fact, a lack of affect: Carol described dissociating herself from her feelings, retreating into a 'nothing matters' state that she recreated in her binges. However, she had also told the therapist that what she feared most was 'loneliness'. The therapist hypothesized that the defended-against feeling was that of loneliness and even panic, which she managed by retreating into binges. This was not an unconscious affect because Carol knew this is what she sometimes felt: what she was not aware of was how she used bingeing as a defence against this internal state of mind (see Figure 5.2).

This formulation could then be applied to the emerging transference and Carol's wish for a very intensive therapy—a theme to which she returned several times in the first few sessions and to which the therapist felt under pressure to respond. This wish suggested that in coming into therapy the internal model that was activated was one in which Carol felt like a very needy, deprived child who needed to secure as many sessions as possible with her therapist as a way of controlling her because she anticipated in her mind an unavailable mother/therapist.

CONSTRUCTING A FORMULATION: A STEP-BY-STEP GUIDE

A DIT formulation has several components:

- It describes the problem as seen by the patient.
- It contextualizes the problem in a developmental framework taking into account temperamental dispositions, physical factors, traumatic experiences/life events, past and present relationships, and sociocultural factors.
- It pulls together this information into an account that meaningfully links the patient's difficulties with a psychological, dynamic process.

Using the psychodynamic formulation aide-mémoire in Box 5.1, let us return to Carol and formulate her problems using this model.

Step 1: Describe the problem

Carol presents with panic and bulimic symptomatology. She uses eating, according to her, as a way of not feeling anything. She also describes relationship problems: she fears that she is not kept in mind and seeks constant reassurance from others.

Step 2: Describe the cost of the problem

Carol acknowledges that she has problems in establishing relationships and that she can be suffocating. This alienates others and makes her feel lonely.

Step 3: Contextualize the problem

Carol reports a difficult early life. Her father died when she was very young and she subsequently lived with her mother. Her mother was a single parent and a busy professional woman who had to leave Carol in the care of nannies. Carol therefore often felt lonely, longing for

Box 5.1

DIT FORMULATION AIDE-MÉMOIRE

Step 1: Describe the problem
Ask yourself: How does the patient view the problem: what or who is the patient reacting to?

Step 2: Describe the cost of the problem
Ask yourself: What limitations in the patient's functioning or distortions in their perception of others and self have resulted from the problem?

Step 3: Contextualize the problem. Identify relevant predisposing factors and current external factors (e.g. unemployment) that are relevant to understanding the onset and course of the symptoms/ difficulties
Ask yourself: How do environmental (e.g. history of trauma, developmental factors influencing the processing of trauma, family system, other relevant life events) and/or biological factors (e.g. disability) relate to the presenting problem?

Step 4: Describe the patient's recurring object relationship that is meaningfully connected to the presenting symptoms/ difficulties
Ask yourself: How does the patient experience themself in relation to others?

- Identify who does what to whom and the associated affect.
- How is this internalized object relationship manifest in the patient's current life?
- How might the representations of self/others influence and be influenced by current relationships?
- How do these internalized object relationships manifest themselves in the patient's relationship with you?

Step 5: Identify the defensive function of the recurring pattern
Ask yourself: What is the patient afraid of/trying to avoid in themself? What are the possible consequences of change?

her mother's return, but then resenting her mother, and needing to punish her when she returned.

She describes her mother telling her not to cry. Carol thus learned early on that the best way to manage her affects was to switch herself off from them, so that she did not have to feel her mother's absence and her loneliness.

In her adult life, Carol encounters more loneliness because she appears incapable of establishing intimacy without taking over the other person in an attempt to control an object whose attention she internally fears she cannot sustain.

Step 4: Describe the recurring object relationship that is meaningfully connected to the onset and/or maintenance of symptoms and the affect that is linked with the activation of the pattern

Carol experiences herself as needy and sensitive to feeling too much for others. She needs constant reassurance in her relationships because she does not trust that she is kept in mind by the other. She experiences the other as unavailable to her, such that she has to chase them—as with her boyfriend, whom she phones several times a day—to concretely reinforce her presence in their mind. In the assessment relationship these patterns manifest themselves in her need to confirm the time of her appointment and in her wish to have intensive therapy, as if anything less would expose her to the experience of not being kept in mind (i.e. that another patient will replace her in the therapist's mind). The perceived loss of the object's undivided attention elicits overwhelming anxiety in the form of panic attacks.

Step 5: Identify the defensive function of the recurring pattern

Carol's experience of her self as needy and demanding, and of the object as rejecting and unavailable, is not a pleasurable one—it causes her significant levels of distress. Yet, to relinquish this version of reality would also mean having to face her own rage towards the object and not only her tendency to control the object (of which she had some awareness) but also her wish to punish the object, and hence she would have to take responsibility for her own aggression.

THE TRIAL INTERPRETATION: WORKING TOWARDS SHARING THE IPAF

In the initial sessions the therapist will make a trial interpretation both to elaborate the evolving formulation in the light of the patient's response to the interpretation and to assess the patient's capacity to make use of such interventions. Returning to Carol, before sharing a possible IPAF, in session 3 the therapist took up Carol's interpersonal pattern in the transference. The therapist proceeded gradually, mindful that Carol was highly sensitive to feeling 'pushed out' by the other, so here she raised the less contentious 'rejecting other' pole of the experience (rather than Carol's self-representation as needy and the demanding way in which she defends against being dropped from the mind of the other):

> You have mentioned several times your sense that what you need is an intensive therapy. You may well be right about that. I don't yet have a clear view of that myself, but what I have been thinking as we talk together is that you are very anxious about starting this therapy and you may be worried about whether I will be available to you when you need me to be, about whether I will keep you in mind when we are not meeting. Wanting more sessions may be your way of ensuring that you are firmly in my mind and that no one else can take up your place in my mind.

Carol was silent and then started to cry. She recognized that this was what she always did in her relationships: she couldn't bear to not be 'central' to the other person. Carol's response to the transference interpretation gave the therapist the confidence to share the emerging IPAF and to engage Carol in refining it. The therapist shared the IPAF along these lines:

> One of the things that I have been really struck by over the past few sessions is that you seem to be very preoccupied with whether, as you put it, you are 'central' to the people you want

to be close to, with whether they keep you in mind. It's been the case here too, between us, with you feeling very worried that unless you book yourself in to see me several times a week you will drop out of my mind and you will find yourself on your own—an experience that is familiar and terrifying for you. It seems to me that as you approach a relationship you typically feel yourself to be very needy, demanding even, and expect the other to be unavailable to you. You are terrified of being left on your own and so you try to find ways of minimizing the likelihood of this happening and, as you helpfully recognize, this can paradoxically have the opposite effect to the one you are hoping for: the other person may feel controlled and then they may pull away. And then this only confirms your worst fears and the cycle begins again.

Having put it this way, the therapist and patient could then return to the IPAF when exploring particular INs in the course of therapy, inviting the patient to stand back from her immediate experience and engaging her in thinking about this pattern. The IPAF can also be shared bit by bit, starting with the part of the pattern that is easiest for the patient to hear before agreeing on the descriptor and image that best captures the interpersonal dynamic.

USING THE PATIENT'S LANGUAGE AND METAPHORS

When formulating and constructing the IPAF it is very helpful to personalize it so as to capture the patient's immediate affective experience. This requires paying careful attention to the patient's choice of words, the imagery associated with their descriptions of feeling states, or the metaphors they use. The therapist's attunement to these idiosyncratic terms often also serves to convey to the patient that the therapist has listened to them carefully. There can be a significant affective gap between describing the self as, for example, 'unattractive' and using the patient's more idiosyncratic self-descriptor, which often carries greater valence in the internal world, as in the case example below. Particular words or expressions then become shared markers for the recognition of the self- and/or other-representations. We cannot stress enough how important it is to devote time to the identification of the patient's more idiosyncratic descriptors.

Case example

Timothy, a 30-year-old man, was referred for help with recurrent depression. He presented as likeable and eager to please. He was the youngest of ten children and said he had been severely bullied by his older brothers. He described himself as 'crafty' and told the therapist stories of conning or reacting aggressively to others. However, he also described feeling 'like a loser'.

In session 3, the therapist formulated an IPAF that proposed Timothy's self-representation as 'a loser' in relation to an object who treats him badly or humiliates him. This particular configuration left him feeling humiliated and aroused in him a need to seek revenge, triumphing over others through various forms of 'crafty' behaviour so as to reverse the representation of self and other and to thereby triumph over the felt-to-be-humiliating object. This included the development of a false self—a 'Jack the lad', cheerful chap persona—and the denial of more vulnerable, sensitive aspects of the self. The overarching impact of all his defensive strategies was to keep the object at a distance and to be responsible for repeatedly losing potentially enriching interpersonal experiences.

Timothy found the IPAF helpful and agreed to work on this focus. The sessions with Timothy in the earlier part of the middle phase focused on the mechanisms by which he kept the object at a distance and, indeed, kept his 'true' (more vulnerable, pained) self at a distance via a 'false' pleasing, 'cheeky chappy' presentation. He and the therapist noticed his rivalrous relationship with others—his need to be the favourite and most liked—but how this presentation belied more real feelings of being left out and vulnerable. This experience was presented as making sense in view of his being one of ten children, vying for parental attention, but emphasis was placed on the fact that his strategies for coping with this had now become problematic for him. It was then possible to look at the ways in which he attempted to triumph over others as a way of managing a very painful sense of himself as 'a loser'.

For some time, the therapist struggled to take anything up in the transference. In thinking about this the therapist became aware that Timothy's interpersonal strategies of keeping others away from his vulnerable, 'true' self were very seductive and compelling. The therapist had to work hard not to be pulled into his central self–other dynamic and to thus maintain her ability to think and to notice his avoidance of 'real' feeling and his manipulation of the truth. The therapist had to stand back from the way in which Timothy used somewhat glib, emotionally flat, or clichéd reporting of the week's events to keep her at a distance from the more painful feelings that he was unable to bear. This involved managing her own countertransference so as to not be overwhelmed, confused, irritated, or made to feel 'mad' by the manner in which his accounts became elusive and 'slippery' as a result of him providing her with slightly differing facts and emphasis at different points.

Using the experience in the transference, the therapist was able to make more productive inroads into reaching Timothy and helping him to make sense of the INs he was bringing. Earlier narratives of rivalry, his own 'craftiness', and being treated badly began to be replaced by ones of loneliness and isolation.

In the middle stages of the work with Timothy, he began many sessions by recounting how 'lonely' he felt. Of course, this had a meaning within the session as well as beyond, and enabled useful work around his desire for closeness with the therapist, combined with his ways of avoiding this. In the later middle part of the work, Timothy was more able to grasp his avoidance of emotional relating and the ways in which his more narcissistic 'best beloved' requirements interfered with this. As Timothy became more in touch with his own pain, vulnerability, and need, he was able in a more real way to focus on his need to triumph over others, often in quite aggressive and destructive ways. Earlier in the work he could see the impact of such behaviour on himself, but in the later stages he was also able to feel some shame and to acknowledge the impact of his devious or aggressive behaviour on others.

In the middle to end stages of work with Timothy, the therapist, together with Timothy, was able to productively utilize some of the quippy phrases that he used in the earlier stages to distance her and himself from his emotions. Particularly useful was a throwaway phrase he brought into an early session—DTA (don't trust anybody)—and his initially proud descriptions of himself as 'Jack the lad' and as a 'honey monster'. All of these phrases became invaluable to the work, as they were used as signifiers of the central, identified interpersonal dynamic.

The ending phase of work was defined by sadder feelings and a sense of mourning for the more 'real' self that Timothy had so effectively denied. He was able to manage working with some of his frustrated feelings about ending and his fear of, combined with an excitement about, a referral for longer-term group work.

USING THE TRANSFERENCE AND COUNTERTRANSFERENCE TO INFORM THE FORMULATION

Three sources of information are available to assist us in the process of formulating self–object representations: the patient's narrative account of their childhood history with significant others, the patient's current relationships, and the relationship the patient develops with us. To arrive at an IPAF the therapist actively draws not just on the content of the patient's narratives, but also on the experience and observation of the patient's ways of relating within the session.

The transference is what makes it possible for us to be drawn into the patient's world so that we may experience it ourselves rather than relying on the patient's report of their relationships. For Freud the transference was a form of remembering, but, as Lear (1993) puts it, this is a highly particular kind of remembering, moreover one that:

> is not a form of recollection, but of memorialisation; an enactment designed to make the present into an artefact of the past . . . the aim of the enactment is to endow the world with comprehensible meaning (Lear, 1993, p. 745).

Here Lear highlights two very important functions of the transference: the way in which it creates a familiar, 'known' (at an unconscious level) road map for how to relate and what to expect from others, and how this map performs a vital function in the patient's internal world. This is why the therapist can often reliably anticipate the patient's fierce investment in keeping alive the unconscious pattern that is also part of their problem.

The therapist makes use of their understanding of the transference and countertransference to develop hypotheses about problematic interpersonal patterns. At this early stage transference interpretations are kept to a minimum, but the therapist's understanding of the developing transference is central in helping to generate hypotheses about the patient's interpersonal functioning.

Not all patients are overly preoccupied in an obtrusive manner with the therapist at the very outset, and so for some, the transference may be less obvious and/or intrusive. For others, however, the anxieties about starting therapy are acute. If, from the outset, the patient is very preoccupied with the therapist (which is more likely if they have a comorbid personality disorder), the therapist engages the patient in elaborating a description of what preoccupies them about the therapist and about what they are feeling.

Case example

> Ms A, who was referred for social anxiety and mild depression, arrived for the first session apparently very anxious, and found it hard to speak. The therapist noted that the patient could barely establish eye contact and that she looked noticeably stiff in her posture while the therapist set out the boundaries for the initial consultation.
>
> The therapist asked Ms A how she was feeling, to which Ms A replied that she had not wanted to come and had come only because her general practitioner (GP) had sent her. The therapist invited Ms A to tell her a bit about how the consultation with the GP had gone. The patient spoke about how she had felt that the GP dismissed her problems, and, with conviction, she added that the GP thought that she was to blame. The therapist enquired about what it was that had made her feel so sure that this was what the GP believed. The patient said that the GP was rushed in her manner and had barely asked her any questions, and that she looked disapproving.

Having explored this exchange, focusing in particular on what the patient was feeling and thinking, and what she imagined the GP was feeling and thinking, the therapist abstracted the underlying relational pattern and acknowledged that the patient had felt both neglected and disapproved of, and asked Ms A whether this was a familiar feeling for her. The patient replied that people were not interested in her and that she often felt looked down on by others. The therapist then linked this to how the patient had started the session feeling anxious, and that perhaps she was now worried about what the therapist was thinking about her. The patient replied that when the therapist had described what was going to happen, and that they had only 50 minutes, this had made her feel that the therapist was just going through the motions and that she was not really interested. The therapist said that this seemed to be a familiar experience, just like with the GP. The patient agreed. The therapist tentatively added that the patient seemed to expect that others would be dismissive of her and that, from this perspective, the therapist stating the length of the session no longer felt like a fact that she might or might not like, but instead she heard it as a confirmation that the therapist was simply not interested in her. The therapist added that if this is how she felt, then she could understand why the patient was finding it hard to open up.

The intervention illustrated in this case example is characteristic of how the DIT therapist engages with an interpersonal scenario and illustrates of some of the key features of a DIT transference interpretation in these early sessions:

- It deconstructs an IN (the story about the GP) in order to abstract an implicit relational pattern.
- It links this pattern to the here-and-now relationship with the therapist.
- It frames it in the context of current triggers (starting therapy).
- It validates the patient's experience and conveys that the patient's response is understandable given the version of self and other that has been activated.

HOW TO SELECT A FOCUS

By the third or fourth session, the therapist will have a working hypothesis about the most salient IPAF that is meaningfully connected to the symptoms. As we described in Chapter 4, testing out the emergent patterns across a range of INs is essential to this process. The formulation of the most relevant IPAF is probably the most challenging juncture for the therapist, not least because patients will present with a number of interpersonal patterns that are more or less adaptive and reflect particular qualities of self- and other-representations. The therapist therefore has to decide between a number of relational constellations to arrive at the most productive route through which to understand, and work on, the patient's current difficulties.

In selecting a focus, we are looking for a *specific* interpersonal constellation that sheds some light on the onset and/or maintenance of the patient's symptoms/difficulties. Here the timeline of the symptoms is helpful because we are trying to distil what pattern was activated in the patient's mind around the time of the onset of symptoms.

In practice, the descriptors of the self–other poles of the IPAF need to be specific and distinct. For example, during the initial sessions with one patient the therapist was able to identify with the patient that he often felt 'defective' and 'a burden'. Alongside this, they established together that the patient frequently experienced other people as 'critical, patronizing, and unpredictable'. In order to arrive at an IPAF, the therapist had to do more work because 'being defective' and 'being a burden' are not the same experiences. It was possible that the patient's self-representation as 'defective' exposed him to the experience of feeling that he was a burden, which is quite different from a self-representation of 'being a burden'. Similarly, there are potentially significant differences between an object experienced as critical or patronizing and one felt to be 'unpredictable'. Faced with this not uncommon potential multitude of possible self–other constellations, when selecting a focus, the therapist is guided by three considerations (see Figure 5.3):

1. The connection between the IPAF and the presenting symptoms needs to be meaningful and have face validity for the patient (i.e. temporal contiguity).

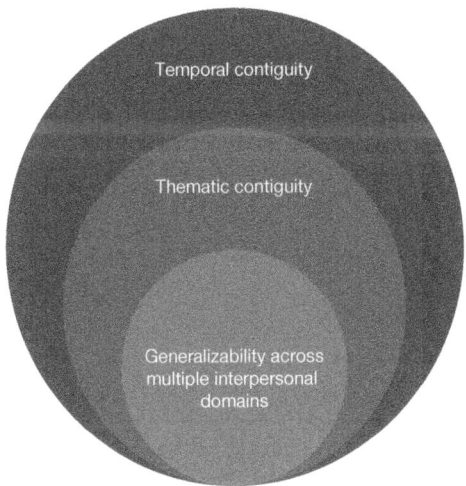

Figure 5.3 Criteria for selecting an IPAF.

2. The validity of the IPAF is supported by a goodness of fit with the patient's patterns as evident through their INs (i.e. thematic contiguity).
3. The IPAF is recurring and manifests itself across a number of the patient's relationships (i.e. its generalizability across multiple interpersonal domains).

SHARING THE IPAF WITH THE PATIENT

Once the therapist has developed some ideas about the IPAF these are shared with the patient in a tentative manner that clearly communicates the therapist's interest in the patient's own views about it. For example, the therapist might say:

> Having listened to what you have told me over the past few sessions about how you are feeling and what you are most concerned about in your life right now, I have some ideas about what's been going on for you and how this might help us to make sense of the symptoms that have brought you here. I would like to share these with you to see what you think so that we can see whether this might be of help in finding a focus for our work.

The therapist can then present the patient with their understanding of how the patient's difficulties have developed, the relational pattern that appears to be connected to the onset and/or maintenance of these difficulties/symptoms, and the impact this has on the patient's current relationships.

Especially in the early stages of learning the DIT model, therapists who are not used to sharing formulations tend to over-saturate the formulation and/or deliver the IPAF 'in one go'. When this happens, the patient often feels overwhelmed and the exchanges between patient and therapist lose the emergent and collaborative qualities that are central to DIT. The key is to remember to present the IPAF in a piecemeal manner, ensuring the patient is engaged with how resonant the various components feel and explicitly inviting the patient to fine-tune the various dimensions of the IPAF. It is helpful to make reference to some of the INs to help the patient to trace how you arrived at the IPAF.

Throughout this process, the therapist is alert to the patient's response to the formulation, to ascertain its relevance and/or perceived threat to the patient's equilibrium. This is very important because, as we noted earlier in this chapter, the IPAF describes an interpersonal pattern that (although distressing to the patient, i.e. it is ego-dystonic) may nevertheless serve a protective function and therefore may be felt to be psychically necessary.

The aim is to work *collaboratively* with the patient to promote a sense of agency and participation in arriving at a formulation that is meaningful to them. In one sense all psychodynamic approaches, at their best, are collaborative. In DIT we use this term not only as a reminder of this important feature of the therapeutic encounter, but also to underline that the DIT therapist is *explicitly* collaborative insofar as they actively seek out the patient's view of the formulation and engage the patient in refining it.

It is very important to approach the task of formulating in an open, tentative manner that invites the patient to comment and express any anxieties or disagreement they have about the suggested focus. The discussion of the IPAF should provide the patient with an opportunity to ask questions and to clarify and agree therapeutic aims so that they feel engaged with the work. A formulation is a working hypothesis and, as such, requires regular revision in light of patient feedback and the therapist's evolving understanding of the patient over time.

A question frequently asked by therapists learning the model is what they should do if the patient disagrees with the IPAF. If the therapist has actively engaged the patient in developing the IPAF, if it meets the three criteria listed above (thematic contiguity, temporal contiguity, and generalizability), and if the therapist has been responsive to the patient's feedback, it is very unusual for the IPAF to become a source of conflict and disagreement because it is the outcome of the patient's and the therapist's joint efforts. The IPAF, as we have seen, may feel very challenging, and the patient may struggle to work on it during the middle phase, but in our experience this kind of natural resistance to taking responsibility for what we do to ourselves and to our objects is far more common than disagreements over the actual content of the IPAF.

Case example

Marc is in his mid-twenties—a rather small, studious-looking man, with an intense frown that had a peculiarly distancing effect on the therapist on first meeting him.

His GP referred him after having signed him off work for two consecutive weeks due to stress, following a difficulty with his boss. Marc had been in this job for just under a year when he started to feel bullied by his boss.

Marc is the older of two brothers. His father died unexpectedly of a heart attack when Marc was five years old. Following the father's death, his mother appeared to have sunk into a very depressed state of mind from which she never fully emerged. Marc still lives at home with his mother, while his younger brother left home to move in with his girlfriend just under a year ago.

Marc presents as rather subdued, and on first meeting him, the therapist found it hard to engage him. She felt that he was depressed and his social withdrawal was marked. As he described his relationships, he conveyed a sense that he was always on guard, as if he could never quite let himself relax. He was very anxious in the first session.

Marc explained that he had never taken to his boss because the boss was 'loud' and 'brash'. A few months prior to being signed off work by his GP, Marc had felt particularly humiliated by his boss after he was openly critical of one of Marc's reports in front of other colleagues. At the time, Marc had barely spoken, feeling himself immediately to be 'stupid', and he felt that he had not defended his position. Subsequently, he felt that everyone viewed him differently and he found it increasingly hard to even look people in the eye when he was at work. He ruminated over this exchange in his mind, and the more he did so the angrier he became. He spoke about the 'injustice' of it all, as he was hardworking and diligent.

As Marc spoke about his difficulties, the therapist became aware that Marc was having a particular impact on her: she felt she was being recruited into siding with him against the boss, who had become the personification of evil. The therapist made a mental note of this, but said nothing at this stage. This feeling nevertheless grew stronger as he described in more detail his relationship with his younger brother. He felt that his brother had acted selfishly, leaving home just when Marc had taken up a new job and their mother had become more severely depressed. Consequently, Marc had felt that the burden of care for his mother had fallen on him, as he felt it had always done since his father's death.

The description of his brother bore an uncanny similarity to Marc's hated boss. His brother was described as loud, unthinking, and selfish. They had never been close, and he reluctantly acknowledged that his brother was very successful in life. He spontaneously recounted that as they were only 18 months apart in age, they had shared many friends and had gone to the same school, but he felt he was always in his brother's shadow because of his more outgoing personality. When the therapist invited him to elaborate on this, Marc gave a very detailed account of his brother's superior physical achievements. In this respect he thought that his brother had taken after their father, who had been an excellent runner in his youth. He added, somewhat pointedly, that his brother had been fortunate to inherit his father's height and strength, whereas he had followed in the maternal footsteps: he described his mother's family as 'clever thinkers prone to depression'. Marc's current interpersonal world was very impoverished and had been so for many years, not just since he had become more evidently depressed. He had one close male friend who, based on Marc's description, struck the therapist as also quite a fragile, anxious individual. Nevertheless, they did meet every few weeks and shared an interest in film.

Marc had not had any girlfriends in the past five years. His only relationship of note had lasted a few months. He had met his then girlfriend when he had just started university. The relationship ended unhappily when the girlfriend complained that he never wanted to go out. Marc justified this in terms of prioritizing his studies at the time because he wanted to get a good degree.

The therapist enquired about how Marc had felt when his brother left home to live with his girlfriend. He replied dismissively that he did not care about what his brother did with his life, but that he certainly would never choose a girl like his brother had done. He described the girlfriend as an 'airhead' who enjoyed clubbing and clothes.

The therapist spent some time exploring Marc's relationship with his parents. Marc said he did not really feel that he knew his father except through his mother's rose-tinted glasses. He had grown up hearing what an impressive character he had been, and he mentioned twice the way his mother referred to his father's 'stature'—both concretely, as he had indeed been tall and strong, and because of his standing in the world of work. As he spoke he conveyed a sense of hopelessness about his own capacity to be impressive, and the therapist reflected this back to him.

By the end of session 2, the therapist had become conscious of a pattern in the room: whenever she tried to be empathic or made some observation, Marc either appeared to ignore it or typically replied that 'It was not quite like that.' The therapist began to feel that she was being carefully scrutinized and duly criticized, as if in the room the roles had been reversed: it was now Marc who was in some way criticizing her reports, just as he said his boss had done to him. By now the therapist also hypothesized that Marc had probably always felt second best in relation to both the idealized father figure in his mother's mind and the younger brother who had become his living embodiment.

In session 3, the therapist explored further the circumstances around the time when Marc's brother had left home. It became clear that the onset of a more insidious state of depression dated back to that time, and that it had then been further aggravated by the more recent incident at work. It emerged that the mother had felt bereft by the brother's decision to move away from the family home. She appeared to have been stuck in an unresolved grief reaction following the death of her husband, which was fuelled with new impetus by the departure of her younger son. All this appeared to have deeply angered Marc, who had seemingly always felt in the shadow of both his father and his brother's greater stature in his mother's eyes. The incident at work had been the final blow for him, as he had somehow always managed to reassure himself of his superior intellect as a defence against his deep-rooted conviction that he was simply not good enough for his mother. To be attacked publicly, as he saw it, for producing a bad report reduced his intellectual stature, and he felt profoundly humiliated and exposed to the critical eyes of others. His anxiety indeed had a distinctly paranoid flavour. His basic response to this interpersonal scenario was one of passive aggression, where he said nothing, withdrew into himself, and internally remained locked in a grievance against the other person. His most profound grievance was towards the parental couple in his mind, by whom he felt painfully excluded.

In approaching a possible focus, the therapist began by summarizing the way in which Marc had conveyed to her his long-standing experience of not having any stature in his mother's eyes, and that this characterized more generally his expectation of how other people viewed him. She acknowledged the importance to him of his intellectual pursuits as a way of reassuring himself and others that he did have substance and stature in his own right. Consequently, he had overvalued work such that it had not only pulled him away from developing relationships, but also made him highly sensitive to any slight to his intellect. Marc responded to this interpretation by saying that at times he did wonder to himself what the point of life was. Bearing in mind the importance of engagement at this early stage, the therapist reflected on the sense of futility that underpinned Marc's overall presentation, but she also observed that he had nevertheless allowed himself to come for help, and that this was positive.

The therapist then elaborated further on what she had understood so far and spoke with Marc about the heavy burden of having not just to bear the meaning for him of the early loss of his father, but—perhaps even more significantly—to have to nurse his mother through her ongoing sense of loss, which he could never assuage. The therapist spoke empathically of how he seemed to feel that he had lived in the shadow of his father and brother, both of whom had managed to escape the fate of the 'clever thinkers prone to depression', leaving him feeling as if he was forever lagging behind them in some fundamental way, which nothing could change. At the same time, he was having to take care of a mother who both needed him and made him feel second best.

Marc seemed to respond positively to this formulation, but the therapist detected some hesitation. He emphasized that in the intellectual domain he had always shone, but that somehow this was never really valued, even though he had always thought that his mother, herself an academic, prized intelligence. The therapist wondered to herself whether this response might be indicative of Marc's experience of feeling in some way criticized by her, but she decided not to intervene along these lines as she did not feel she had enough evidence for this. Rather, she observed that he seemed to have always been very preoccupied with what his mother was looking for, and that he felt confused about what she valued and admired. His whole life in a way had been devoted to getting it right for his mother rather than for himself.

The therapist then wondered with him as to whether, now that they were negotiating what to work on in therapy, he might be similarly preoccupied with what he imagined *she* would prize. This appeared to resonate with Marc, who observed how anxious he had felt each time he had come for a session. He then reported a dream he had had the night before the third session in which he had been jeered at by a group of adolescents. In the dream he wanted to shout back, but no words came out.

By this stage the therapist felt confident enough to propose an IPAF (Figure 5.4). She suggested that a recurring experience for Marc in his relationships was to feel that he was small, lacking in stature, and insufficient, while the other person was more typically either explicitly humiliating and rejecting (as he had felt his boss had been recently) or more implicitly humiliating (as he felt his mother had been, leaving him feeling that he could never live

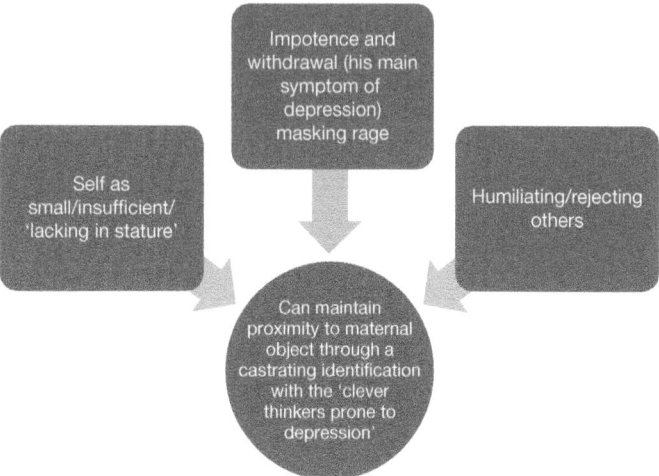

Figure 5.4 Marc's IPAF.

up to his father's/brother's stature). His only option seemed to be to follow on in the maternal family tradition of 'clever thinkers prone to depression'. Distressing though this was, the therapist suggested that this way at least Marc comforted himself with a likeness to his mother, which he felt only he shared with her. Marc was intrigued by this suggestion and told the therapist that as he was growing up what he had most enjoyed were the evenings with his mother when he used to read poetry with her. Although the therapist was moved by this image, she also sensed Marc's wish to create an intense exchange with her, which did not feel comfortable. Again, at this early stage, the therapist only made a mental note of this, and it would be interpreted only if this developed into a resistance in the course of treatment.

The therapist suggested that although Marc's overt response to the interpersonal scenario in which he felt humiliated was to feel impotent and to typically withdraw (as in the dream, he loses his voice), internally a far more angry conversation took place in which he tried to defend himself. At this stage, the therapist did not share her hypothesis that Marc also took up the position of being the humiliating, critical one in his own mind and subjected the other to harsh scrutiny, because she considered that this would be too much for him to take on board at this point and might make him feel denigrated by her. However, this would be an important theme that deserved further elaboration during the course of therapy.

REFERENCES

Kernberg, O. F. (1980). *Internal world and external reality: Object relations theory applied*. Jason Aronson.

Lear, J. (1993). An interpretation of transference. *International Journal of Psychoanalysis, 74*(4), 739–755.

6
The Middle Phase

The middle phase of dynamic interpersonal therapy (DIT) requires both the patient's and the therapist's concentrated effort to stay focused on the agreed interpersonal-affective focus (IPAF) and the goals that derive from it. The therapist works with the patient to identify and understand this dominant recurring pattern as it plays itself out in the patient's current relationships, including the relationship with the therapist, and highlights its impact on the patient's current functioning and symptoms. In this chapter, we will review in more detail the core aims and strategies that guide the middle phase (sessions 5–12).

AIMS

The overarching aim of the therapist's interventions at this stage in the therapy is to stimulate the patient's capacity to think about and understand their thoughts and feelings, and how these underpin the identified pattern of relating (and its varied behavioural manifestations) that may seem strange or self-defeating. More specifically, the therapist has several aims in mind in approaching the work of the middle phase sessions:

- To help the patient identify areas of difficulty in their relationships that pertain to the IPAF
- To support the patient's engagement in reflecting on how these difficulties relate to their current symptoms (e.g. how their feelings of panic might relate to an argument they had with a specific person during the week)
- To help the patient understand their characteristic ways of managing areas of difficulty in their relationships and

to point out the 'cost' of these strategies, that is, working actively on characteristic defences
- To help the patient reflect on their state of mind and the feelings and thoughts they attribute to others in order to highlight the activation and implications of the IPAF
- To support the patient in trying out new ways of approaching relationship difficulties.

SEQUENCE OF MOVEMENT IN MIDDLE PHASE SESSIONS

In DIT, each session may start with the patient filling in forms to provide outcome monitoring data, if required by the service setting (as has been the case in the NHS services where DIT has largely been used so far). In that sense, the therapist opens every session. The review of the forms provides a focus and entry point into discussing how the patient has been feeling in the intervening week since their previous session. The patient is invited by the therapist to reflect on how their scores relate to how they have been feeling in the week. A deterioration or improvement on the depression or anxiety scales prompts an exploration of what may have contributed to this change.

Other than this structured way of starting the sessions, there is no set agenda for the sessions as such, unlike in cognitive-behavioural therapy, for example, and yet the IPAF *is* the agenda for every session. The therapist always approaches what the patient brings with the IPAF in mind. This is important and somewhat different from the more free-floating attention characteristic of the therapist's approach in open-ended psychodynamic therapy. Having said this, in common with other psychodynamic approaches, the middle phase sessions have a more emergent quality that reflects the therapist's efforts to create a space for unconscious meanings to be elaborated and reflected upon.

Indeed, being focused, while precluding attending to all of the patient's dynamics, does not preclude listening to their unconscious communications: in DIT the therapist pays attention to the patient's imaginative life (e.g. conscious and unconscious fantasies, dreams, metaphors) and non-verbal communications (e.g. tone of voice, body posture), and uses these manifestations to deepen their understanding of the patient, and hence as the basis for a more focused interpretation related to the IPAF. Likewise, the therapist allows their own subjective associations and ideas to form in response to the patient's communications, and makes use of these to inform their understanding of the patient.

Because sessions in the middle phase are less structured, it becomes easier for the therapist to wander into more diffuse explorations of the patient's internal world. Here, it is helpful for the therapist to keep in mind the aims of DIT so as to get back to the agreed focus. At the same time, the therapist will need to tolerate a degree of uncertainty and ambiguity when trying to understand the patient's communications so as not to foreclose exploration. Balancing these dual requirements is an important skill that develops with experience of the protocol as the therapist acquires a more direct sense of what is possible to achieve within one session, and over the course of sixteen sessions, such that they can then pace themself accordingly.

The ability to pace oneself cannot be taught as such; each therapist has to find their own way of navigating through the protocol with enough room for the elaboration and exploration of the patient's experience, but with sufficient focus to ensure the patient can begin to work on an important pattern. Although sixteen sessions may strike some therapists as impossibly brief, in our experience it is often possible to help patients to make significant changes—or at least to initiate the process of change—within this time limit (Gelman et al., 2010).

The middle phase sessions are gradually structured by the five therapeutic strategies during this phase, summarized in Figure 6.1. They tend to progress from a more open-ended exploration of what is on the patient's mind at the start of the session as the symptoms and/or the preceding week's events are reviewed, and linking this to the IPAF, to a more concentrated focus on the patient's state of mind, and finally to engaging the patient in reflecting on how they might handle a problematic situation differently (Figure 6.2). This sequence describes a prototypic session in the middle phase, but it would be unhelpful to view this as set in stone: in some sessions, for example, there may be little or no possibility of engaging the patient in reflecting on alternative ways of managing how they assert their needs in a relationship, and this may not occur until the following session. It would, however, be very unusual for a middle phase session to make no reference to the IPAF: by and large, explicit reference to the

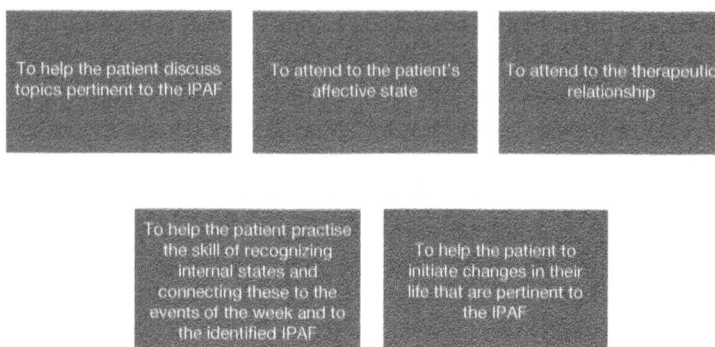

Figure 6.1 Middle phase strategies.

IPAF is frequent and consistent in every session in the absence of an acute, immediate crisis (e.g. an unexpected bereavement), which would of necessity temporarily divert both therapist and patient away from the agreed focus.

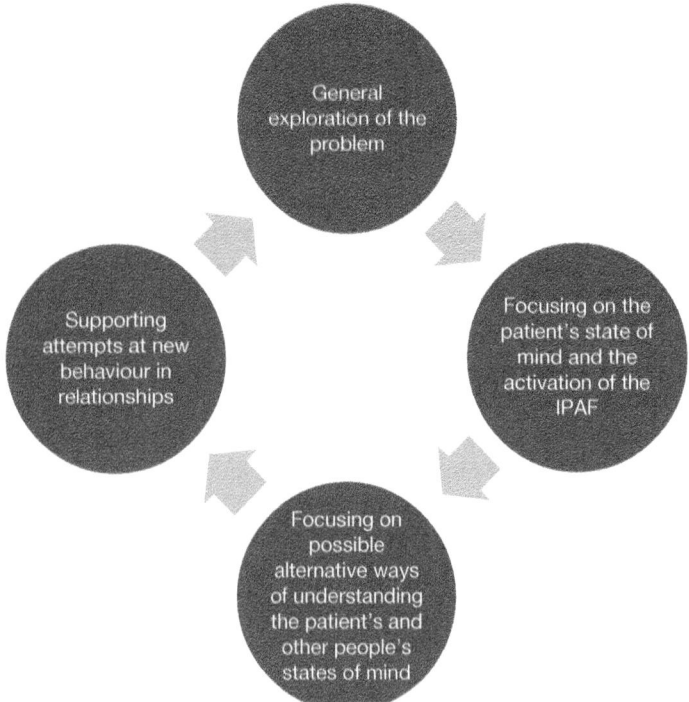

Figure 6.2 Sequence of movement in the middle phase sessions.

TRACKING THE IPAF: ELICITING INTERPERSONAL NARRATIVES TO ILLUSTRATE THE ACTIVATION OF THE IPAF

During the middle phase, a core strategy is to help the patient to explore the IPAF. This involves assiduously relating the content of interventions to the interpersonal and affective themes that the formulation has identified as the focus of the therapy. A common challenge for the novice DIT therapist is to not forget the IPAF! Here we have in mind not only actually forgetting the specifics of the IPAF (although this can and does happen) but also that *in every session* it is important to work to the agreed IPAF and towards the goals identified in the initial phase that are relevant to the IPAF. 'Working with the IPAF' means refining it progressively throughout the middle phase and right into the ending phase. It would be surprising if the IPAF agreed at the end of the initial phase did not undergo some modifications over the course of the therapy. Occasionally, the IPAF undergoes its most significant refinement in the ending phase.

One of the key interventions in this phase is to support the elaboration of interpersonal narratives (INs) because it is through these that the IPAF will become apparent. This gives the therapist an opportunity to draw the patient's attention to how a recurring and underlying pattern of interpretation and reaction—that is, the IPAF—is manifest in their current relationships and how it relates to their presenting symptoms. Connections are made, as appropriate, between current concerns and the IPAF across three interpersonal domains—the therapeutic relationship, current relationships, and past relationships—with less emphasis on the last of these.

Some patients struggle to report INs either because they have very few relationships in their current lives or because they want to avoid really thinking about their relationships, preferring instead the relative safety of discussing their problems in abstract terms. When this is the case, it will require some redirection to a more tangible interpersonal focus. For example, the therapist might say:

> You have a lot of interesting ideas about why you feel as you do, and I wonder if you could give me an example of when you felt this way with another person during the past week.

Alternatively, the therapist might consider it more helpful to take up in the transference the patient's retreat into a more cut-off, intellectual mode. Either way, the strategy is to engage the patient in reflecting on what is actually happening, now, in their relationships.

The therapist thus displays curiosity about interpersonal scenarios, asking questions and for clarifications as necessary, to bring into focus an interpersonal exchange so as to highlight a salient repetitive pattern. Whenever the patient presents an IN, as the therapist listens, they are scanning for the following information to build a picture in their mind of the patient's internal world, as summarized in Figure 6.3: who is talking/doing what to whom? Who feels what towards whom? And how does the therapist feel as they listen?

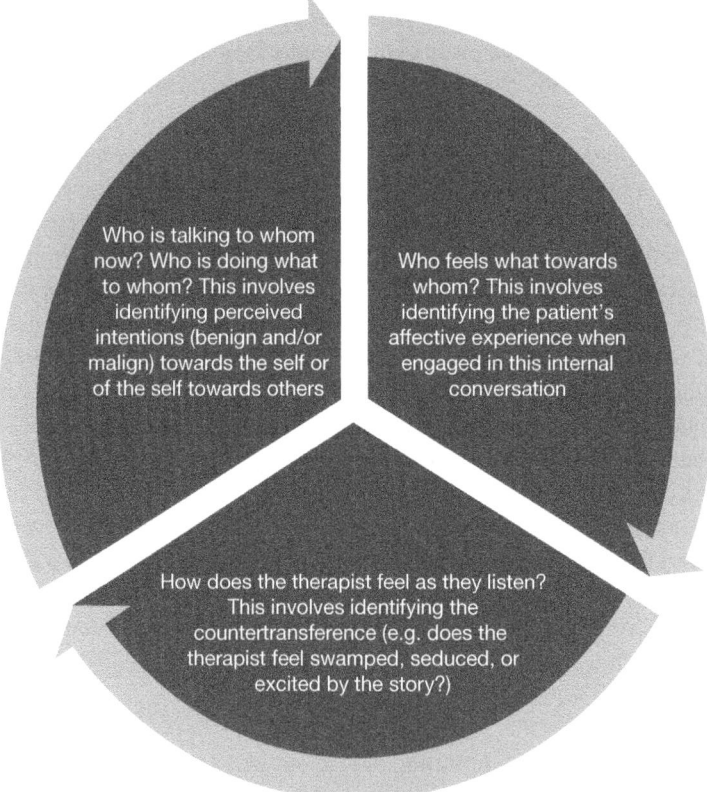

Figure 6.3 Abstracting interpersonal-affective patterns from interpersonal narratives.

Through unpacking an IN with the patient, the aim is to engage the patient in thinking about what other kinds of conversations might be possible for them, which might be helpful. This may then provide an opportunity to identify a new way of responding, which the patient can be encouraged to try out between sessions.

STAYING FOCUSED

However experienced we might be, when learning any new model, we all have to make some adjustments to our technique that will feel more or less congruent with our known and preferred way of working. Working to a specified focus can feel very difficult at first, especially for therapists who are accustomed to working long-term with open-ended contracts.

Besides the challenge of formulating rather rapidly, and hence of finding a focus for the therapy by (typically) the fourth session, the other main challenge encountered by DIT practitioners is how to stay focused on the IPAF once it has been identified (Box 6.1). Of course, we might say that *all* psychodynamic approaches have a focus insofar as the patient's unconscious mental life is what we are trying to understand. Indeed, 'maintaining a dynamic focus' describes two distinct yet related activities (Lemma et al., 2008). First, it refers to maintaining attention on the exploration of the patient's unconscious experience. Essentially, this means that all aspects of the work are approached with an analytic attitude. Second, it refers to working on a particular dynamic theme or conflict to the relative exclusion of others for the duration of the therapy. This is usually the case in time-limited therapy, as in DIT, where it is essential to negotiate with the patient a circumscribed interpersonal pattern that will provide direction and a boundary for both patient and therapist.

The IPAF is thus prioritized over other possible foci for the duration of the therapy. This is a central challenge shared by all brief approaches, but can be particularly difficult for some therapists who may feel that they are short-changing the patient by not addressing a range of unconscious processes that will be apparent to them. Here it is helpful for the therapist to remind themself of the aims of DIT, which, although more modest than the aims of longer-term

> **Box 6.1**
>
> **STAYING FOCUSED ON THE IPAF**
>
> This involves:
>
> - Helping the patient to identify relevant interpersonal and affective pattern(s) through an exploration of interpersonal narratives and (where relevant) their elaboration in the transference
> - Helping the patient to explore themes relevant to the agreed IPAF through the use of techniques such as clarification, confrontation, and interpretation (see Chapter 7)
> - Relating the content of interventions to the interpersonal and affective themes pertinent to the IPAF
> - Helping the patient to identify and explore the meaning of diversions away from the agreed focus (e.g. because it is too painful to address)

psychodynamic therapy, can nevertheless make a tangible, immediate difference to the patient's capacity to function in their day-to-day life.

Deviations from the focus will occur, however competent the therapist is. When they do, this is a cue for the therapist to think about why this may be happening: is the patient feeling the strain of working on the IPAF? Is it asking too much of the patient? Is the focus felt to be threatening the internal status quo? The task therefore becomes identifying the defensive function of the deviation from the focus.

Where the deviation from the focus occurs because the patient raises other issues that are important to them but do not pertain directly to the IPAF, the therapist sensitively acknowledges their importance but reminds the patient of the agreed focus and the brevity of the treatment, which precludes an in-depth exploration of other areas of their life. If the therapist identifies the need for further therapy, this can be discussed with the patient in the ending phase. Similarly, unexpected life events that occur during the course of the therapy should not go unacknowledged but should be responded to in some way. The therapist will need to rely on their tact and sensitivity to guide them in deciding whether the therapy can continue or whether the life event is of such magnitude that the agreed focus becomes less relevant.

Sometimes, however, the patient may keep diverging from the agreed focus simply because the wrong focus was selected. Here, as in any other situation where it becomes clear that the therapist and patient have misunderstood each other, or where there is an impasse in the therapy, the therapist approaches this openly, is receptive to the patient's experience and feedback about what they feel is not helpful, and strives to engage jointly with the patient in working out a way forward (see also Chapter 10).

A typical concern that arises for therapists applying this protocol is about becoming very repetitive because the IPAF can seem restrictive in the context of the myriad facets of any individual's internal mental life. In one sense this is true: we are explicitly selecting only one segment of the patient's functioning, and there are many others. However, the concern about repetitiveness is not one shared, on the whole, by patients, who mostly welcome this assiduous emphasis on the IPAF because it helps them to concentrate on working on something over a short period of time that can be identified and named in their current functioning and, hopefully, modified to some degree. The specificity of the IPAF is, in fact, containing for most patients. By the end of the sixteen sessions it has become internalized as something they can identify for themselves and over which they feel they have a greater degree of control, such that the activation of the self–other representation can be nipped in the bud before it takes hold in their mind and potentially distorts their experience of current relationships.

Case example

> Lara is a woman in her late thirties, referred to a male therapist because of recurrent depression and generalized anxiety disorder. Things had become particularly difficult for her following the birth of her first child two years earlier. She described recurrent periods where she would feel 'on a level' for a while but then would all of a sudden 'hit a precipice' where she would become very agitated and low.
>
> Lara recounted an uneventful early life, with no history of separation or trauma. She felt close to both of her parents until

about six years of age, when her younger brother was born. She had vivid recollections of her brother suddenly occupying all her mother's affections, and she and her sister being relegated to 'second best' at that time. She remembered in particular her mother as a critical and unsupportive person and her father as quiet and submissive. Her mother would often put her down about the way she looked, her exam results, and her dress sense. She remembered that after completing family chores, her mother would always 'inspect' what she and had her sister had done, eventually redoing the chores again to her own satisfaction. Around the age of ten, she found herself marginalized from all the other girls in her class after a rather nasty whispering campaign about her. This was deeply hurtful for her. She had always been angry that her mother did not show interest in her or support her in this situation.

Lara presented in the initial sessions as plainly dressed. She sat on the edge of the seat and nervously drank from a water bottle. She would always apologize at the beginning of sessions for being either too early or too late, and she intimated early on that she was 'relieved' that she was not seeing a female therapist. It became clear from her INs that she often felt judged, criticized, and put down by so-called successful women and mothers, and she referred to herself as 'a geek'. This had become much worse since she had become a mother—at toddlers' groups she was preoccupied with the idea that she was failing in comparison to other mothers, perceiving herself as having the worst-behaved child and being the one who coped the least well with the demands of motherhood. She would often withdraw in depression and anger, which would be sublimated and passively expressed.

The IPAF that was eventually agreed on focused on a recurrent sense of self as a 'flawed woman' and a recurrent view of the other being 'critical and superior' that triggered a conscious affect of anxiety and that appeared to defend against anger. Through the course of the middle phase, the interpersonal events of the week would invariably centre around a female friend or acquaintance by whom Lara had felt slighted or judged, and this provided a helpful opportunity for exploring the IPAF. It was apparent that she needed to revisit this pattern repeatedly, in its different guises, and never appeared to find this process unhelpfully repetitive.

Lara's repeated apologetic gestures towards her therapist were explored in the transference, revealing a constant sense that the therapist would be thinking that she was 'a geek' and 'weird', and the fantasy that the therapist was a skilled parent who had a happy marriage, a notably attractive spouse, and obedient children.

By the ending phase of the therapy, Lara had made considerable progress. She acknowledged that it was difficult to end the therapy and fantasized that the therapist would be relieved to find another patient, revealing her fear that she would be replaced in the therapist's mind. This was productively explored in the transference.

WORKING IN THE TRANSFERENCE

We will not say very much about working in the transference here because we devote the whole of Chapter 8 to this topic, but it is nevertheless important to note that interpretation of the transference is a central technique in the middle phase because it helpfully roots the therapist in working on, and through, the patient's current relationships.

In the initial phase there is some discussion about past relationships, as these inform the elaboration of the IPAF. However, in the middle phase sessions, this is less of a focus. It may, of course, be very pertinent to the IPAF for a patient to discuss past relationships. However, on the whole, during the middle phase, the therapist strives to prioritize working on *current* significant relationships that demonstrate the activation of the IPAF. The therapist thus focuses on helping the patient to explore the vicissitudes of the therapeutic relationship because for the duration of the sixteen sessions it often becomes a significant relationship in the patient's life. The therapist will make use of the experience and observation of the patient's ways of relating within the session to inform their understanding of the patient's internal world of relationships. Where appropriate, the therapist draws attention to this to highlight the enactment of the IPAF in the session. This is one of the most important uses of the transference during the middle phase. This is because the activation of the IPAF in relation to the therapist provides the most immediate and rich opportunity to examine the patient's affects and defences.

WORKING WITH DEFENCES

An important aspect of working through the IPAF involves helping the patient to identify their often unconscious 'investment' in maintaining a particular self–other representation. The patient may, for example, complain that they feel belittled by others whom they experience as haughtily superior, and yet they repeatedly allow into their world people who treat them in this way. This may be because one of the 'pay-offs' is that by doing this they remain the victim of others' criticism and they can sidestep owning their own arrogance.

As we mentioned earlier, with some patients it is only in the middle phase that the therapist will share their understanding of the defences the patient deploys and of the hidden pay-offs afforded by this defensive configuration. A core strategy in the middle phase is therefore to help the patient to explore the defences mobilized in their relationships, including the unconscious strategies they use to manage areas of difficulty in relationships. The overall aim is to help the patient to reflect on behaviours and feelings that give rise to, perpetuate, or exacerbate the core interpersonal pattern identified by the IPAF.

Any behaviour or feeling can be used defensively—or, put another way, whatever allows an alleviation of psychic pain belongs under the heading of defence. It is the psychic function of a behaviour or feeling that determines whether it is being used defensively, for example, whether it protects self-esteem.

Defences are often used to manage interpersonal anxiety generated by, for instance, a fear of being taken over or controlled by the other, or of becoming too intimate. Such object-related defences are, once again, varied. For example, some people may use distancing to protect themselves from intimacy; others may become obstinate as a way of controlling the object; and others still may become passive as a way of discharging hostility. There are also defences that destroy or attack a mental process and leave the patient bereft of their own mental capacities (e.g. attacks on thinking as a defence against understanding something painful) and defences that destroy a mental representation (e.g. splitting the representation of a significant other, reducing them to a part-object).

Defences act as the gateway to change: flexible defences that are open to challenge allow a destabilization of the psychic status quo that maintains the problems. Rigid defences instituted to protect the individual from intolerable psychic pain may prove harder to shift. A session-by-session assessment of defences is critical for determining the patient's ability to respond to an interpretation. It is thus important to assess the balance between defence and motivation alongside the strength of the therapeutic alliance in every session.

If interpretation elicits more defensive behaviour, this is suggestive of an entrenched defensive system that might well prove hard to shift in a brief intervention. If the interpretation of defences leads to regressive behaviour on the part of the patient, this would suggest the possibility of defences protecting the patient from a breakdown. For example, after the first session during which the therapist had made a trial interpretation, a patient reported going on a drinking binge that resulted in their losing consciousness. The urgent need in this patient to obliterate the session from their mind placed them at risk. In such cases it is advisable to proceed cautiously and to consider seriously the patient's suitability for a more exploratory approach. If the decision is made to continue, this would be a strong indicator of the need to strengthen the supportive aspects of the approach until there is more evidence of ego strength.

The exploration of defences is closely linked to the exploration of the patient's affect. Here we are primarily interested in helping the patient to become aware of several facets of their emotional life, namely: (a) those affects that need to be kept in check by defences, (b) those affects that function as defences, that is, affects that protect the individual from feeling other emotional states, and (c) how particular affects are managed or discharged (e.g. through self-harm or substance abuse).

Working with defences can be thought of as consisting of four interlinked strategies that build on each other: (a) the acceptance and validation of the *need* for defences, (b) the exploration of the *how* of defences (i.e. the patient's characteristic defensive strategies), (c) the exploration of the *why* of defences (i.e. the function of defences), and finally (d) the *costs* of defences (see Figure 6.4) (Greenson, 1967). Working through the defences associated with the IPAF thus begins with an

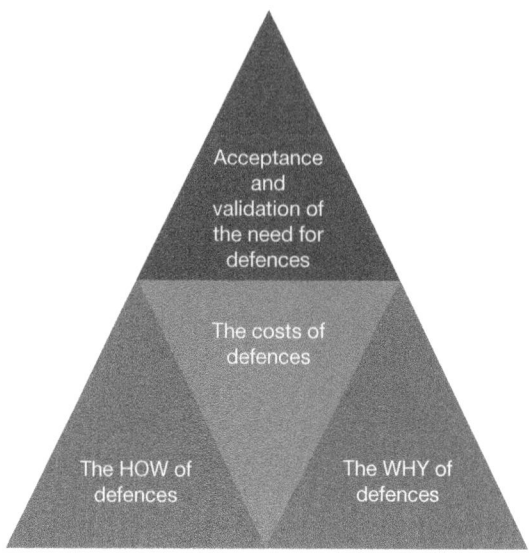

Figure 6.4 Strategies for exploring defences.

initial acceptance by the therapist of the patient's style of relating, that is, by communicating respect for the defensive needs that may underlie particular interpersonal styles. This can be facilitated through helping the patient to explore and become more aware of areas of conflict by drawing attention to feelings or states of mind that seem unacceptable or uncomfortable, without any pressure to change at this stage.

It is in this context of acceptance that the therapist can then start to focus on helping the patient to understand *how* they protect themself from particular painful feelings or states of mind, for example, by empathically pointing out how they become confused or 'unable to think'. It is important to strike the right balance between support and challenge. Challenging defences may be too demanding in the very early part of the middle phase, but we would expect some challenge of defences to occur by the mid-point of the therapy.

Using the transference can help the patient to become more aware of how they manage problematic aspects of their relationships, through an exploration of defences as they arise in relation to the therapist and significant others. This will include helping the patient to manage the anxiety generated by the live exploration of defences, which can feel very threatening to some.

Once the *how* of defences has been explored, the therapist can move on to the *why* of defences, that is, helping the patient understand why they need to protect themself from the experience of particular feelings/states of mind.

Finally, highlighting the *costs* of the defences used, by pointing out their impact on the patient's own capacities and on their relationships, is a prerequisite for engaging the patient in relinquishing defences: the costs need to outweigh the conscious and unconscious benefits if change is to occur.

SUPPORTING ATTEMPTS AT NEW BEHAVIOUR IN RELATIONSHIPS

Insight into the unconscious relational patterns that inform the patient's behaviour is a prerequisite for change, but it is often not sufficient by itself. Indeed, many patients, although grateful for the clarity that the IPAF sheds on their difficulties, might turn around and say: 'Yes, it all makes sense, but I still can't see what I can do to change.'

Psychodynamic therapists do not all subscribe to the same view of what promotes psychic change. Some believe that change will be supported through assiduous attention to the transference dynamics; others maintain that change is achieved through the provision of a 'new' relationship in the therapy; others still that it is through enhancing the patient's reflective capacity that change occurs, and different techniques are thought to facilitate this. All of these processes may well be mutative, but in the absence of active support and focus on also trying out new ways of approaching the interpersonal scenarios that activate the IPAF, it may prove very hard for the patient to leave the brief period of therapy with some confidence that they can actually respond differently in their current relationships.

Working in the transference provides a valuable opportunity for practising, as it were, two of the key 'skills' that we hope to impart to the patient during a course of DIT: noticing the activation of a relational pattern and the associated affect, and using this enhanced self-reflective capacity to create the possibility of a different response. Practising these skills in the transference is important, but the therapeutic relationship is often (although not always, of course) also experienced as a relatively safe place within which to take interpersonal risks. Consequently, it may be more difficult for the patient to generalize this learning to other relationships.

Moreover, although with some patients the therapeutic relationship very rapidly becomes the focus of their imaginative life and feelings, with others the transference is not always sufficiently emotionally live to provide adequate opportunities to work on these dynamics over sixteen sessions, and hence the patient's external relationships may carry greater affectivity and relevance and will help to consolidate change. From the patient's point of view, exposure of a dynamic in the transference therefore needs to be reinforced with attempts at novel behaviour in their current relationships outside the therapy.

The new interpersonal behaviours that the patient is encouraged to try out will be informed by the goals that were agreed at the end of the initial phase. Like the IPAF, the goals will also be refined as the therapy unfolds in light of the new insights that emerge. The patient is actively invited to review the early goals so that these can be adapted if required. The exploration with the therapist of the success or failure of the patient's attempt at change offers yet more opportunity to understand the interpersonal and affective processes that inhibit change. Anticipating with the patient what may prove difficult is an integral part of the process of supporting change. Often this involves helping the patient to understand the link between the anxieties mobilized by the prospect of change and the defences brought into play to deal with them. For example, a patient who dreads conflict and wants to try to be more direct about what they need from others might revert to appeasing the other instead of communicating what they feel unhappy about in the relationship. Examining the outcomes of these attempts at new ways of being in a relationship is an important part of the work of the middle phase.

We emphasize that the therapist actively supports the patient to try out different ways of responding. The timing of this will, however, vary depending on the patient and how they are progressing during the middle phase. The total absence of any overt attempts to engage the patient in trying out different ways of relating to others would, nevertheless, suggest that the therapist is not 'on model' in practising DIT.

Some patients display marked resistance at the level of implementing interpersonal change despite the insight they have gained about recurrent relational patterns. In these patients, this relative inflexibility generates what we refer to as 'relationship-interfering behaviours', which maintain the problematic relational constellation. DIT for complex care (DITCC; see Chapter 13), with its extended number of sessions, allows the therapist more time to help the patient to work on these defensive constellations.

REFERENCES

Gelman, T., McKay, A., & Marks, L. (2010). Dynamic Interpersonal Therapy (DIT): Providing a focus for time-limited psychodynamic work in the National Health Service. *Psychoanalytic Psychotherapy*, *24*(4), 347–361. https://doi.org/10.1080/02668734.2010.513556

Greenson, R. R. (1967). *The technique and practice of psychoanalysis.* International Universities Press.

Lemma, A., Roth, A. D., & Pilling, S. (2008). *The competences required to deliver effective psychoanalytic/psychodynamic therapy.* Research Department of Clinical, Educational and Health Psychology, University College London. https://www.ucl.ac.uk/pals/sites/pals/files/ppc_clinicians_background_paper.pdf

7
Techniques

A key intervention in dynamic interpersonal therapy (DIT), as we described in Chapter 5, is to help the patient to stay focused on the agreed interpersonal-affective focus (IPAF). All the techniques deployed in DIT support this core aim, that is, of helping the patient to better understand what is happening for them, in their mind, when things go wrong in their relationships. This will include, as we have seen, how the IPAF is enacted in the therapeutic relationship. To this end, DIT draws on expressive/exploratory, supportive, mentalizing, and directive techniques, which we will discuss in this chapter.

LISTENING WITH AN ANALYTIC EAR

Before we can intervene, we have to listen. Tuning into unconscious communication is not a passive process. It involves actively being with the patient, moment by moment, and tracking the changes in the patient's states of mind, which indicate shifting identifications and projections. These changes are imperceptible to the untrained ear.

Listening to unconscious communication is demanding. It requires patience because unconscious meaning is seldom immediately obvious. Not only can an aspect of the environment, or its image, be used metaphorically, but also the people the patient refers to may represent—stand in for, as it were—other people. Sometimes they may represent the patient themself as a whole or as a part.

In the evolving conscious and unconscious dialogue between patient and therapist, the patient gives voice to complex schemata of self and other that indicate the activation of different states of mind, contemporaneously or in sequence. For example, an experience of the self as a child raging at a punitive parent may give way to an experience of the self as a child yearning for an absent parent. Within the same session the patient may then oscillate between feeling the subject of angry impulses and, at other times, feeling like the object of someone else's neglect. These shifts are seldom conveyed directly through language, but we can infer them from the stories patients recount and, importantly, how they recount them.

There are numerous vehicles for unconscious communication that are non-verbal, for example, posture, gesture, movement, facial expression, tone, syntax, rhythm of speech, pauses, and silences. Gestures, including bodily postures and movements, always accompany the speech process. The power of gestural messages rests precisely in the concealment that they afford and so they become ideal vehicles for the communication of unconscious mental contents (Fónagy & Fonagy, 1995).

The patient's 'idiolect' (Lear, 1993)—that is, their use of language that is unique to them—endows the conscious narrative with unconscious resonances. Patients' preconscious attitudes are often expressed at the paralinguistic level, preceding their emergence in the patients' verbal utterances. Meaning and unconscious phantasies may be expressed through the way the patient speaks rather than in what they say: a harsh tone, a soft, barely audible voice, or a fast-paced delivery can convey far more about the patient's psychic position at a given point in time than the words themselves.

The 'how' of the patient's narrative also alerts us to the importance of its structure. The attachment research by Main and colleagues draws our attention to the meaning that is inherent in the organization of language itself (Main et al., 2008). The coding system developed by Main and Goldwyn (1998) was a major landmark in the study and classification of attachment narratives, with an explicit and operationalized distinction between coherent and incoherent narratives. Main et al. (2008) distinguished between language that is collaborative and coherent and language that is incoherent, distorted, or vague. Incoherent narratives make it necessary for the listener to infer linkages of which the speaker may be unconscious so as to create organization and to deduce the real or underlying meaning in the story that is being told. This distinction encourages us to listen closely to moment-to-moment changes in linguistic fluency and to shifts in voice, lapses in meaning and coherence, absence of memories or flooding by memories, and fragmentation of the narrative, all of which have been found in research studies to be indicators of attachment insecurity in adult speech (see e.g. Main et al., 2008).

Listening to the structure of the patient's narrative sensitizes us to the quality of the patient's early experiences of attachment (Slade, 2000) and how this might be translated into the patient's current relationships. Secure or reflective patterns of language and thought indicate the presence of an internalized other who can contemplate or contain the breadth and complexity of the child's needs and feelings (Fonagy, 2001). In this sense, the breaks, incoherencies, and contradictions observed in the narratives of insecurely attached adults are said to imply a break in the caregiver's capacity to respond to the child's need for care and comfort. So-called *earned security*, that is, a coherence and/or mentalizing even about distressing or traumatic experiences, can be shown where a person has had support in processing very difficult memories and/or struggled with anxiety or depression in childhood or adult life (see Roisman et al., 2002). In the 23-year longitudinal study by Roisman et al. (2002), for instance, adults within a high-risk sample classified as 'earned secure' on the Adult Attachment Interview were found to have experienced particularly good maternal care.

Analytic listening, unlike ordinary listening, therefore takes place simultaneously on multiple levels and in reference to multiple contexts. This kind of layered listening acknowledges the complexity of the patient's communications and the hidden agendas. It not only underscores the central importance of the therapist's receptivity to the patient's conscious and unconscious communications, but also points to a key aspect of analytic listening, namely that it is impossible to listen without involving ourselves. This confronts us with a paradox:

> It is necessary for the analyst to feel close enough to the patient to feel able to empathize with the most intimate details of his emotional life: yet he must be able to become distant enough for dispassionate understanding. This is one of the most difficult requirements of psychoanalytic work—the alternation between the temporary and partial identification of empathy and the return to the distant position of the observer. (Greenson, 1967, p. 279)

Bollas (1996) approaches this dual demand on the therapist by distinguishing two types of listening, which he refers to respectively as the 'maternal mode' and the 'paternal mode'. The terms used by Bollas inevitably evoke restrictive gendered assumptions about what is 'maternal' and what is 'paternal'. We retain Bollas's original terms because these are his words, but we regard these terms as denoting different functions, not restricted to a particular sex, reflecting qualitatively distinct modes of listening. The maternal mode denotes a more receptive, 'holding' therapeutic stance, whereas the paternal mode reflects a more active and interpretative therapeutic stance. Bollas argues that both modes play complementary roles in the analytic process, and this is certainly the case in DIT, which calls for different stances at different stages of the therapy and sometimes even within the same session. For example, if a patient is very distressed this may require the therapist to operate in a more 'maternal' mode than during times when the patient can withstand a more challenging exploration of the IPAF. Neither stance is better than the other; rather, they complement each other. This takes us back to the importance of the therapist's ability to implement DIT in a flexible way so as to respond to the patient's changing needs.

Monitoring multiple levels of discourse simultaneously is essential. Communication, however, would fail if we did not take the first level of implication of what the patient says to us at face value. An overemphasis on what the patient is not explicitly saying to the exclusion of what they *are* saying does not contribute to the development of a good therapeutic alliance. In DIT, the therapist's interventions ideally convey an acknowledgement of both the manifest content of what the patient communicates and the possible latent content. Patients are less likely to feel misunderstood, bemused, or angered by our interpretation of unconscious meaning if we acknowledge first what they have actually said before making a link to its possible unconscious meaning (Figure 7.1).

EMERGENCE VERSUS STRUCTURE IN THE SESSIONS

A range of techniques support DIT's organizing principles and aims, namely to intervene so as to generate, clarify, and elaborate interpersonally relevant information and to encourage the patient's curiosity to reflect on what happens in their mind. All techniques 'structure',

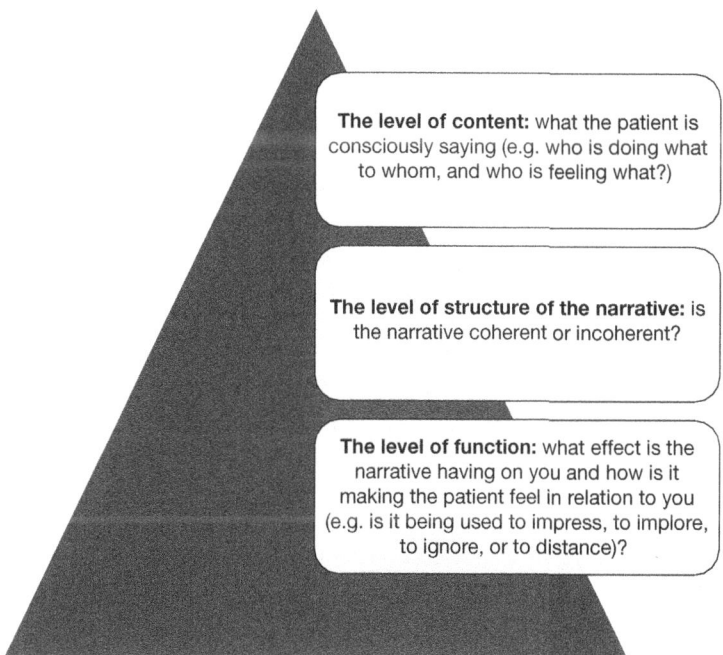

Figure 7.1 Levels of listening.

to an extent, a session, insofar as whatever we do, or do not do, has a structuring impact on the therapeutic interaction. Obviously, some techniques impose far more structure than others.

One of the delicate balancing acts for the DIT therapist is between allowing space, and hence silences, within which the unconscious aspects of the patient's experience can be elaborated, as we have been describing, and the necessary requirement to be more active and focused, which inevitably introduces a degree of structure into the sessions that may well, at first, feel rather alien. Listening to a DIT session nevertheless feels very different from listening to, for example, a cognitive-behavioural therapy (CBT) session because of the more emergent quality of the patient–therapist dialogue that is characteristic of DIT.

The more questions we ask, the more we structure the dialogue. Although clarificatory questions are encouraged in DIT, as we will explain later in this chapter, equally we are interested in what emerges more spontaneously in the patient's mind, and for this to happen we need to allow the patient some silent space. At times silence indicates a quiet, reflective mood, which is beneficial or even necessary to allow the emergence of latent affect. At other times it can be a sign of resistance or an attack. The pregnant pauses may also feel like a pressure to relieve the patient from their own introspection or the responsibility of thinking for themself. No matter how difficult silences may feel, we caution against premature impingement and pressurizing the patient to overcome them. We, too, of course, may use silence as a way of discharging our own hostility towards a patient. Therefore, it is important to monitor our own silence and ensure it does not veer into withholding or neglect and perpetuate a misalliance. Having said all this, given the time-limited nature of DIT, its focus, and its aim to help the patient to effect some changes in their life, frequent or protracted silences would be very unusual in a DIT session.

EXPRESSIVE/EXPLORATORY TECHNIQUES

Once they have tuned into listening with an analytic ear, the therapist makes use of expressive/exploratory techniques to engage the patient in reflecting on what is being communicated. These techniques used in DIT, namely confrontation, clarification, and interpretation, will be familiar to all psychodynamically trained clinicians. This technical constellation has a long history and can be traced back to Greenson's (1967) classic text on psychoanalytic technique. In our view it provides a helpful reminder to the therapist of a sequence of interventions, underlining that interpretation is a process (see 'Features of helpful interpretations', below)—that is, we gradually put in place the steps building up towards an interpretation. At its best this process means that the patient can be helped to arrive at their own interpretation.

Confrontation

The first stage in helping the patient to work through the IPAF is to create a shared 'marker' of the issue that requires further clarification so as to gather the information we need to formulate an eventual interpretation. In other words, the therapist brings to the patient's attention the ostensible problem (e.g. lateness for sessions) to engage them in recognizing that there is something to be understood—that is, the therapist confronts the patient with this 'fact' as something meaningful and interesting.

For example, one patient arrived very late for one of her sessions, which had followed a cancellation by the therapist the previous week. As the patient sat down, she looked very low and said she had been feeling more depressed than usual—a deterioration that was also reflected in her depression questionnaire scores. The therapist had a very clear idea in her mind about the lateness because it had followed her own cancellation, and she thought this was of significance to this patient given the IPAF. She hypothesized that the patient might be sensitized to cancellations in a particular way since the IPAF identified a self-representation as 'insignificant' and an other-representation as 'neglectful'. Despite the therapist's conviction about the meaning of the lateness, in DIT she would be discouraged from jumping in with an interpretation without first ensuring that the patient recognized that her lateness was important.

Let us now follow the progressive efforts the therapist made before sharing an interpretation. The therapist began by straightforwardly confronting the patient with the fact of her lateness. The deterioration in the patient's symptomatic depression scores, along with her self-report of lowered mood at the start of the session, were also important signs and deserved acknowledgement:

> T: I can see from your scores and what you have said to me that you have been feeling more depressed than usual. And today you also arrived unusually very late—what do you make of this?
> P: I haven't been good at all... don't know why really... it goes in cycles... don't know about the lateness... I know you said it was important to have all the sessions and all that, but I just didn't get my act together this morning...

The therapist at this stage is factual, but immediately engages the patient in reflecting on the *meaning* behind her scores and her behaviour (i.e. the lateness): 'What do you make of this?' The patient does not elaborate at all in her response, but she nevertheless reveals that she knows getting to her sessions on time is important and that it is what the therapist has encouraged her to do. She does not dismiss the lateness as insignificant; she simply says she does 'not know' about it.

The therapist takes this as a cue for *clarifying* the interpersonal scenario that has arisen in the here-and-now.

Clarification

Clarificatory questions or statements allow the therapist to engage the patient in exploring the problem that is now openly acknowledged: 'I have been arriving late and this is getting in the way of making use of the therapy.' Clarificatory interventions serve to bring this problem into focus. They are apparently simple yet underrated techniques.

Questions, traditionally, have been discouraged in psychodynamic practice, typically out of a concern that they introduce too much direction or they avoid the elaboration of painful affect. There is some truth in this, some of the time, with some patients. For example, asking questions may be used to fill in uncomfortable silences, but this is not an intrinsic quality of therapist-initiated questions. Some of the turning points in DIT are heralded not by the interpretation of transference but by asking the kinds of questions that engage the patient in thinking deeply about what is happening in their mind, or that draw their attention to a detail that speaks volumes but that they had ignored.

An appropriately timed question that invites the patient to pause and reflect can be mutative, and has the added advantage that it does not present the patient with the therapist's more completely formed formulation (as an interpretation); rather, it invites the patient to actively engage with their mind. This is why we encourage therapists to ask questions in order to clarify the patient's experience in their relationships and to help the patient to elaborate their mental states. Particular emphasis is placed on using clarificatory prompts to help the patient to reflect on unverbalized feelings. Here, as elsewhere in DIT, the therapist makes use of their own emotional reactions to the patient as a basis for facilitating this type of exploration.

Let us return to the patient who is very late for her session.

> T: I think it would be helpful to try to make some sense of what's been happening in your mind over the past two weeks because I am concerned that you are feeling worse. And although we don't yet know what made you late today, perhaps

this is not irrelevant, and may help us to better understand how you have been feeling.

P: I don't really know why I am late . . . I got up on time, and had set plenty of time aside to get here for ten o'clock and then I ended up tidying up the house and by the time I looked at my watch I realized I was running fifteen minutes late. I don't know why I did that because then I felt anxious about being late.

T: OK, so it sounds like you clearly had the session in mind when you got up this morning. And then something else started to happen in your mind . . . can you recall what went on? [silence]

P: I was listening to the radio over breakfast and it was some discussion about soft sentencing for child abusers. Some woman was banging on about how the perpetrators are *victims* [the patient said this word in a dismissive way and carried on expressing her outrage at this, shaking her head] . . . I don't know what this has got to do with being late here though . . .

T: You feel outraged and very angry with this woman because you felt she was ignoring the plight of the victims . . . [patient interrupts]

P: Well, it's all very well being sympathetic to the abuser. I'm sure they've had a tough time and all that, but what about their victims—who's got *them* in mind?

T: There is something in this radio interview that is so important to you and relevant to what we have been working on here: someone neglecting the needs of others who deserve and need care but who are somehow not kept in mind, who are insignificant . . .

P: Yes, that really gets to me—there are so many invisible people in the world. Take the homeless on the streets . . . [patient continues in this vein]

In this example we can see how the therapist gradually draws in the patient to elaborate on the events of the morning that preceded her late arrival for her session. The radio interview is recounted with very live affect and strikes the therapist as especially relevant. The therapist speculated that her cancellation of the patient's session the previous week had activated the patient's IPAF, casting the patient back into the familiar experience of feeling 'insignificant' to the object and casting the therapist as the 'neglectful other'. The process of clarification was important not only because it substantiated the therapist's hypothesis through the narrative about the woman on the radio who was neglecting the invisible victims, but also because it engaged the patient in a process of reflection that would be bypassed if the therapist had just delivered her 'expert' interpretation. Indeed, the patient arrives at the important realization that she reacts to situations where people are treated as 'invisible', even though this important insight is immediately diluted by the patient's digression into a discussion about global poverty. This term 'invisible' struck the therapist as even more emotionally accurate as the self-representation descriptor than 'insignificant'.

Clarificatory questions also provide an important corrective because it is all too easy for us to be seduced by the assumption of shared meaning. Words carry with them a personal and uniquely individual meaning. In order to understand what our patients are trying to communicate, we need to check what they are intending. We can do so only by gently questioning something that appears to make sense but may in fact conceal a great deal that is new for the therapist.

Interpretation

Once the matter of the patient's lateness and its context has been sufficiently elaborated through clarification, the therapist uses interpretation to address the dimension of the IPAF that is closest to the patient's current awareness and that has a bearing on the lateness. Where appropriate, the therapist makes a linking interpretation between the IPAF and the symptoms to help the patient to identify the relationship between symptoms and the activation of the IPAF. Given the brief nature of the intervention, the focus of interpretation is primarily (but not exclusively) on pre-conscious material rather than more deeply unconscious or distal events.

Let us return to our case example.

> T: You used just now an important word: 'invisible'. And it made me think that perhaps it captures even more closely the position you often find yourself in: that *you* become invisible to

others, that your needs are not recognized, and this makes you feel very angry and then you withdraw.
p: I had not really thought about that, but yes, invisible actually is what it feels like . . . invisible . . . with no voice . . . sometimes I feel like screaming but nothing comes out.
t: Yes, this does make sense because feeling you have no voice is part of the problem, which then makes it hard for you to tackle what is distressing you in a relationship. For example, here I have been wondering whether it has been hard for you to find a voice today to tell me how you really feel about me cancelling your session the other week. You haven't directly mentioned this, but I think that when I cancelled the session, this left you feeling that I was neglecting you, not 'seeing' you and your needs. We know from the work we have been doing together here that when you feel 'invisible' in this way this leads you to withdraw, which is perhaps why you were late today. I wonder if this is what may have led you to feel even more depressed over the past few weeks. Does this make any sense to you?

An interpretation is a hypothesis. It invites the patient to comment on it, if they wish to, or to ignore it. This is why an interpretation is ideally couched as a tentative statement, question, or formulation that conveys to the patient, 'This might be one way of understanding what you are saying. What do you think?' An interpretation is not a statement of truth where we tell the patient what they are really thinking even if they do not yet know it; rather, it is an invitation to consider another perspective, which may or may not fit.

Interpretations in DIT can focus on a wide range of thoughts, feelings, or behaviours:

- They can draw attention to contradictory 'versions' of people, including the therapist, and the anxieties that lie behind the construction of such contradictory representations.
- They can address specific defensive manoeuvres that compromise the patient's self-awareness and connection to the therapist in the session, that is, transference interpretations.
- They can be directed at the patient's self and other representations, helping the patient to explore positive and negative attributes.

- They can centre on the identification of patterns in the patient's actions, thoughts, and feelings, especially as they relate to the IPAF.

It is important to remember that the process of interpretation aims not only to capture the patient's conscious and unconscious experience, but also to introduce a new perspective on their experience provided by the therapist's view of things. This is best achieved in an open-minded and questioning rather than dogmatic way, modelling exploration and adding meaning in a flexible way, thus stimulating the patient's confidence in, and use of, their own self-reflective capacities (Box 7.1).

Finally, when interpreting we always need to keep in mind that even though an interpretation is a hypothesis, it can nevertheless be experienced by the patient as an action, that is, as the therapist doing something to the patient. For example, an interpretation of the unconscious motivation that may lie behind the patient's investment in the IPAF could be experienced as the therapist making a critical comment. Knowing when and what to interpret thus relies on our ongoing assessment of the patient's shifting states of mind, within a given session, and over time, which will determine how the patient hears an interpretation. It also requires that we are attuned to the patient's experience of an interpretation and can respond to this with empathy and curiosity.

Box 7.1

CHARACTERISTICS OF HELPFUL QUESTIONS

Helpful questions:

- Are relevant to the agreed IPAF and support its elaboration
- Encourage reflection on and elaboration of mental states, underlying interpersonal experiences and the patient's moods, including the active consideration of alternative assumptions and perspectives
- Encourage the patient to consider alternative ways of behaving in response to their interpersonal difficulties.

Features of helpful interpretations

A good interpretation is simple, to the point, and transparent. By 'transparent' we mean that the interpretation shows the patient how we have arrived at our particular understanding. This is especially important in the early stages of DIT, when the patient might be unaccustomed to working with the unconscious and may therefore experience an interpretation as 'plucked out of the blue' unless it is grounded in the context of what they have been talking about in the session.

The therapist works collaboratively with the patient to facilitate their active involvement in the process of self-understanding. Questions and observations that stimulate the patient's own self-reflective process are prioritized over interpretations of deep unconscious content that may contribute to the patient's experience of being the passive recipient of the therapist's understanding.

A core aim of interpretation in DIT is to stimulate the generation of multiple perspectives on the patient's predicament. The therapist takes the many opportunities provided by the patient's description of real-life interpersonal incidents to help the patient to exercise flexible understanding of the possible feelings and thoughts of the different individuals involved, getting the patient to elaborate on different internal scenarios perhaps underlying these incidents, and questioning habitual assumptions.

In considering the task of interpretation we thus need to think about two aspects: the *process* of interpreting and the *content* of interpretations. As we have already suggested, interpretation in DIT is best seen as a process (i.e. based on a series of interventions over time, rather than on a single comment). The therapist draws on the use of clarification and confrontation to gradually bring feelings, fantasies, and behaviours to the patient's attention and as the basis for eventually making an interpretation (Box 7.2). This involves a number of related strategies:

- Helping the patient to explore and become more aware of painful conflicts by pointing out unacceptable or uncomfortable feelings that are otherwise managed by being kept out of the patient's conscious awareness
- Drawing the patient's attention to communication that is unclear, vague, puzzling, or contradictory, with the aim of encouraging the patient to elaborate on these elements

> **Box 7.2**
>
> **CHARACTERISTICS OF HELPFUL INTERPRETATIONS**
>
> - *Clear* (i.e. succinct enough for the patient to be able to take in what is being said)
> - *Appropriately timed* (a) in relation to an assessment of what the patient can bear to think about at any given point and (b) relative to the amount of time left in a session (i.e. not introducing new topics that may be unsettling to the patient too close to the end of a session)
> - *Of appropriate depth* (i.e. moving gradually from preconscious content to more unconscious content)
> - *Pertinent* to the interpersonal-affective focus of the session
> - Framed in a *tentative* way, such that the patient is invited to discuss rather than necessarily agree with the therapist's view.

- Helping the patient become aware of incongruent elements in their communication by pointing out and giving meaning to discrepancies and incongruities in what is being communicated through different 'channels' (e.g. a contrast between verbal and non-verbal communication)
- Identifying and pointing out to the patient unverbalized affect when it is manifested in the session.

Focusing on affect

The IPAF contains an important affective dimension, and throughout DIT we are closely attentive to the patient's emotional experience. We listen not only to the affect present in the content of what the patient says, but also to the affect that is communicated through the process of the joint interaction in the room.

Our aim is to facilitate the expression of unexpressed or unconscious feelings by communicating to the patient that their feelings can be tolerated and thought about by us (i.e. through the therapist's understanding, empathic stance) and by responding to the patient's non-verbal cues and linking these to unexpressed or unconscious feelings.

The therapist enquires into the subjective meaning of the patient's use of particular words, dreams, fantasies, or non-verbal behaviours to help to focus the exploration on the patient's affective experience, drawing attention to the internal and interpersonal obstacles to the awareness and expression of particular feelings (especially in the context of the relationship with the therapist).

Many of our interventions throughout DIT essentially aim to help the patient to:

- Identify what they feel, and stay with a current feeling as it emerges in the session
- Communicate what they feel more effectively
- Build greater facility in connecting their feelings, thoughts, and actions, and how these relate to others' internal states and behaviour.

The affective dimension of the IPAF is integral to the working through of the IPAF. The therapist thus strives to help the patient to identify the way in which their feelings are guided by the particular self and other representation that is activated in a given relationship. The patient's conscious affect, although important given that this is what the patient feels troubled by, may conceal latent affect that may be even more disturbing to the patient.

SUPPORTIVE TECHNIQUES

No therapy can occur without some supportive techniques. Support and empathy are necessary components of all therapies. Because DIT is brief, is used with patients with moderately severe problems, and aims to engage the patient very quickly, supportive interventions are an integral part of the approach. In practice this means that it is important to start with a basic supportive stance and to work towards making more demands on the patient's capacity for self-reflection over time. The therapeutic skills of reflective listening and accurate empathy are a fundamental aspect of DIT. This does not mean that we agree with everything the patient says: confrontation and challenge are equally important aspects of DIT.

Because DIT is used with patients whose depression and/or anxiety may be comorbid with personality disorders or other conditions such as intellectual disability, in addition to language, cultural, or developmental differences, the therapist needs to titrate the level of supportive interventions offered to a given patient. The less impaired patient with a higher level of premorbid interpersonal functioning is more likely to make greater use of expressive/exploratory techniques without requiring more supportive interventions to bolster defences and support day-to-day functioning. The ability to apply the model flexibly and to balance supportive and expressive techniques is therefore essential.

MENTALIZING INTERVENTIONS

Mentalizing-focused interventions in DIT aim to support a therapeutic process in which the mind of the patient is central. As we have emphasized, the objective is for the patient to find out more about how (not just what) they think and feel about themself and others, how that dictates their responses, and how distortions in understanding themself and others lead to (unhelpful) actions in an attempt to retain stability and to make sense of incomprehensible feelings.

How to identify failures of mentalizing

The process of addressing problems with mentalizing begins with the therapist identifying a break in mentalizing. How does a therapist know when such a break has occurred? This obviously takes some practice and experience, but being familiar with the smooth and coherent discourse of a mentalizing narrative is a helpful start. Box 7.3 lists some of the features of good mentalizing. It is helpful to note that many of the features, such as awareness that we cannot know what someone else thinks or feels, are something that we normally take for granted in daily conversations—not just in therapeutic contexts.

> **Box 7.3**
>
> **WHAT DOES GOOD MENTALIZING LOOK LIKE IN RELATION TO OTHER PEOPLE'S THOUGHTS AND FEELINGS?**
>
> - Acknowledgement of opaqueness
> - Absence of paranoia
> - Contemplation and reflection
> - Perspective-taking
> - Genuine interest
> - Openness to discovery
> - Understanding and forgiveness of others
> - Predictability
> - Perception of own mental functioning
> - Appreciation of changeability
> - Developmental perspective
> - Realistic scepticism
> - Acknowledgement of preconscious function
> - Awareness of impact of affect
> - Self-presentation, e.g. autobiographical continuity
> - General values and attitudes, e.g. tentativeness and moderation.

In the context of psychotherapy, we typically encounter at least two common types of discourse in which mentalizing is restricted. These are rooted in two different modes of experiencing subjectivity that are normal in early childhood, but in adulthood would be expected to be moderated, as needed, by mentalizing (these modes were first introduced in a series of papers entitled 'Playing with Reality', most notably Fonagy & Target, 1996, 2000; Target & Fonagy, 1996). The most common is what we refer to as *psychic equivalence*. In theoretical terms this refers to patients treating mental reality as if it were the same as outer reality, thus assuming that how they see a situation is how it *is*. Although this type of egocentric perception would be normal among preschool children, when it arises between adults it leads to significant conflict. The patient cannot respect (or even recognize) alternative perspectives. When there is a difference, finding fault in the other replaces self-reflection. Indeed, the patient expresses uncanny certainty about the thoughts or feelings of others, so that any other point of view might be treated as deceit (e.g. 'He stared at me so he was obviously planning to attack me; if he says not, that just proves he's a liar as well'). The cost of this is not only interpersonal; negative thoughts about oneself in psychic equivalence can also feel frighteningly real ('I feel bad; that shows I really am evil'), and inescapable because doubt has been lost.

In psychic equivalence, mental states are often not described, because they are assumed to be obvious from the events: for example, 'She didn't call me after the row, so it's obviously over.' The patient appears not to think much about the feelings of self or others, or about the relationships between thoughts, feelings, and actions. When relating interpersonal narratives (INs), the patient may provide great detail about the events that occurred, but not about their own or the other's intentions. Particularly in patients needing complex care (see Chapter 13), patients may also focus excessively on external or social factors, such as the motives of institutions (e.g. the hospital or the local council being 'against them'). When these individuals do note mental states, they typically concentrate on descriptions of behaviour or personality (e.g. lazy, depressive, has a short fuse) rather than an actual state (angry, scared).

Another type of constrained mentalizing is known as the *pretend mode* of subjectivity. It is named after a normal state of mind for a young child, or an adult pretending, in which one is absorbed in an 'as if' world, like a child immersed in play, or an adult actor. In this mode of subjectivity, the patient's ideas do not bridge inner experience to outer reality; instead, they superimpose their mental world on to external reality, disposing of its constraints. Just as a child can play freely within their game, the patient might talk about thoughts and feelings very freely, as though they are in charge of what everyone is doing and why they are doing it. The patient's affect can come across as false because it is connected to a phantasy situation. The term *pseudomentalizing* has been used to describe this type of discourse in a session: it might sound like mentalizing at first because thoughts and feelings are central, but its unconscious aim is to paint a picture that justifies a felt position (e.g. being rejected, having a 'mad' family). Without specific and plausible examples, the position asserts a subjective scenario that is presented as an external reality.

How to use mentalizing interventions

It is not the content but the process of understanding, feeling, and experiencing that is at the heart of this component of the intervention. From this perspective, therefore, it is not for the therapist to 'tell' the patient about how the patient feels or thinks, or what the underlying reasons are, conscious or unconscious, for their difficulties. Instead, the therapist 'models' interest in what is experienced by the patient to jointly arrive at a tentative understanding.

The mentalizing component of DIT underlies the therapist's enquiring or 'not-knowing' stance. It conveys that mental states are opaque and that the therapist cannot magically know what is in the patient's mind; they need to communicate about and clarify this together. When we say that the therapist adopts a 'not-knowing' stance, this does not mean having no knowledge. Formulating the IPAF represents the therapist's understanding—albeit tentative—of what is troubling the patient. The enquiring, open stance implies that the therapist does not assume they know what the patient is thinking, but would like to understand.

When the therapist shares the IPAF or an interpretation, and this may involve taking a different perspective from that of the patient, this should be verbalized and explored in relation to the patient's alternative perspective, without making assumptions about whose viewpoint has greater validity. The task is to determine the feelings and thoughts that have led to alternative viewpoints and to consider each perspective in relation to the other, accepting that diverse outlooks are possible, and sometimes inevitable.

The focus of mentalizing interventions includes affect. Such interventions are simple, always focusing on the mind more than behaviour, and as much as possible on current (in-session) affect and experience. The therapist provides a mentalizing model, and is required to own up to their own non-mentalizing errors, such as making an assumption; these are treated as opportunities to learn more about feelings and experiences (e.g. 'I think I misunderstood that; when I said depressed I meant mainly sad, I didn't realize you meant depression mainly as anger. Depression includes both, and it is really helpful you cleared that up.'). The therapist articulates what has happened in order to demonstrate that they are also noticing what goes on in their own mind, and are willing to question it without being defensive: 'When I linked your lateness to my cancellation, I did not have in mind what you had told me, that you had been very worried about going for a scan later. Both of those things might have come into it, but I can understand how worried you must be about being ill. I not only missed a session, but missed this important worry. Perhaps you felt really invisible.'

The principal aims are always the same: to be aware of the loss of mentalizing, particularly when the patient is upset, for example, while talking about an intensely conflictual attachment relationship, and then to work to reinstate mentalizing (see Box 7.4). This is achieved by 'rewinding'—going back with the patient to the point in the narrative where mentalizing was lost. The temptation is to try to help the patient to 'understand' offline mentalizing: for example, the patient's belief, based on a glance, that a friend hates them. The impression that a friend, who has been loyal and supportive, suddenly turned against the patient represents rigid mentalizing; in a psychoanalytic framework one might say that the unconscious conflict and motivation cannot be elicited just by reasoning about it. Exploring it in a rational way usually gets the therapeutic dyad into a pretend mentalizing process where the patient is coming up with thoughts and feelings that they do not truly have but think might be what the therapist wants to hear. In such instances it is often more productive to take the patient

---

Box 7.4

STEPS IN MAKING AN INTERVENTION

- Identify a break in mentalizing
- Rewind to a moment before the break in subjective continuity
- Explore the current emotional context in the session by identifying the momentary affective state between patient and therapist
- Explicitly identify and own up to the therapist's contribution to the break in mentalizing
- Seek to understand the mental states implicit in the current state of the patient–therapist relationship (mentalize the transference).

back to the moments before they had this feeling. For example, the patient may remember thinking that they felt frustrated by the friend's anxiousness to please, or was angry about some minor infraction of the friendship. Contextualizing the experience in this way, and linking it to actual experience, makes it far more likely that a meaningful understanding of the experience will emerge.

The therapeutic aim in such situations is to help the patient to stabilize their mentalizing in the context of attachment relationships. By painstakingly working through the example above, the patient might become more able to understand what happened in their mind that time. Then, they may be able to notice how they often switch off their thinking and start attending to clues of limited relevance and significance ('go down a rabbit hole'), which can profoundly disturb their experience in relationships, for example, by leading them to distrust friends and distance themself after small misunderstandings. This is of great generic value. It can be 'marked as important' (usually by agreeing a shared memory handle for the experience—e.g. 'that irritation thing') and used later in the same session or in later sessions as something to go back to. In general, the therapist aims to help the patient to find such clues or signals to mentalizing failure that might alert the patient that the feelings and thoughts that follow such signals may be unreliable, poor mentalizing that makes things more difficult for them.

Of course, mentalizing others can be helpful too. Identifying restricted mentalizing that explains others' actions often meets with far less resistance in the patient than applying this in relation to themself. The therapist might therefore choose, strategically, to formulate with the patient an example of failed mentalizing by someone other than the patient (usually an attachment figure) and only slowly encourage the patient to see this as something that might often happen in them too.

The mentalizing therapeutic stance includes: (a) humility deriving from a sense of 'not knowing'; (b) whenever possible, taking time to identify differences in perspectives; (c) legitimizing and accepting different perspectives; (d) active questioning of the patient in relation to their experience, focusing initially not on 'why?' but on 'what?'; and (e) not feeling obliged to understand (particularly, to pretend to understand the non-understandable).

It should be remembered that in the course of a treatment, particularly with a patient who shows features of a personality disorder or whose mentalizing is mostly offline, the therapist may lose their own capacity to mentalize. This may lead to an enactment, for example, 'correcting' the patient about what they are feeling. This is an expected crack in the therapeutic alliance, something that has to be acknowledged and reflected upon. As with other instances of breaks in mentalizing, the process is 'rewound' and explored (see also Chapter 13).

Communication analysis

Communication analysis is another intervention, which is not specific to DIT because it is also used in interpersonal therapy (and other psychotherapeutic approaches). We use it in DIT because it supports the enhancement of mentalizing, which is a basic process in all psychotherapy. Communication analysis helps the patient to reflect on their communication with others, to identify ways in which they express (or deny) strong affects, and to identify alternative strategies for managing interpersonal conflicts.

This approach is especially helpful when the patient reports a difficult interpersonal exchange. It is a simple but powerful technique that involves the therapist listening to a particular IN and then inviting the patient to pause and reflect on it in great detail. The emphasis here is on the 'movie script' level of detail that is gathered (e.g. 'So when you said that, what did you feel? Do you think you conveyed to him how angry you felt? When he responded by walking off, what went through your mind?'). Through the questions the therapist asks, the interpersonal exchange is magnified in as live a manner as possible, with particular attention given to the patient's emotions and other mental states. Identifying unhelpful communication patterns often involves listening for the assumptions that the patient makes about another person's thoughts or feelings and what the patient feels about themself as they relate to the other person. The overall aim is to help the patient communicate more effectively.

DIRECTIVE INTERVENTIONS

Once the link to the IPAF has been established, the therapist can use more directive interventions to support the translation of the patient's understanding of the IPAF into change in their current relationships. As we have noted before, the therapist enlists the patient as a collaborative participant from the outset, engaging them actively in finding and working on the pattern encapsulated by the IPAF. Doing this within a time limit requires the judicious use of more directive interventions.

The most 'directive' intervention in DIT is the focus on the IPAF, which requires tracking the focus and actively redirecting the patient to it where necessary. However, the therapist's higher level of activity, compared with psychodynamic therapy in general, also includes interventions such as some use of psychoeducation or actively helping the patient to solve interpersonal dilemmas. More active interventions like these may well be less familiar to psychodynamic therapists trained in long-term work, since they are generally proscribed in that approach. In DIT, however, interventions such as active encouragement to try out different ways of approaching a conflict with another person are considered to have a subtle structuring impact on the patient's ways of thinking about their experience.

Let us look more closely at some of these more directive interventions and what they are *not*, given that providing direct advice and suggestions is discouraged. (The therapist might, however, exceptionally do so; for example, if a patient has been having suicidal thoughts, the therapist might make a plan with the patient about how to manage them if they arise outside the session.)

Unlike CBT, where the patient might be asked to do specific 'homework' or keep a diary that is then reviewed in the next session, in DIT the therapist employs non-specific directives. These directives allow the therapist to signal that action is needed and engage the patient in reflecting on what might stand in the way of progress. After having explored a problematic interpersonal scenario with a patient—say, a difficult exchange with a partner, during which the patient felt they could not express what they were feeling—the therapist might say:

> You feel very stuck and you are clearly telling me this is causing you a lot of distress. The more you avoid talking with your partner about what's on your mind, the more you withdraw into yourself, and then the more depressed you seem to feel. If you could replay this exchange what do you think you might do differently?

The therapist would then closely track what the patient says they might wish they could do differently and help them to identify the interpersonal 'steps' that are required. Close attention is paid to the areas of vulnerability linked to the IPAF that stand in the way of change. Once this is clarified, the therapist would straightforwardly ask the patient what they imagine might happen if they did try to put into practice a different way of engaging with their partner, so as to anticipate some of the obstacles the patient might encounter.

Sometimes the patient will spontaneously report a scenario where they have tried out a different way of relating. It can be very helpful to extrapolate from a situation where the patient has found a constructive and novel solution, articulating the significance of this, to support some generalization of a more constructive way of managing relationships. But, of course, things do also go wrong, and the therapist needs to be alert to this possibility and receptive to the patient's negative feelings about the therapy—and the therapist—when this happens.

Psychoeducation is used very sparingly, but it can be helpful for some patients, especially in the initial phase, to orient them to DIT's relational frame of reference and its focus on mental states. In other words, we do not educate the patient about their symptoms per se, but about a way of understanding their symptoms. For example, we might say to a patient who gets angry easily but who is unconvinced by the therapist's focus on their mind:

> I can appreciate that it might well be difficult at this stage to see how this might help, but what goes on in our minds—what we feel, think, imagine to be happening—all this actually informs how we relate to others, what we expect from them, and what we imagine they expect from us. So if we can get a better picture of what is going on in your mind when you lose your temper, for example, this might actually help you to not be pulled in that direction all the time, which is so distressing to you.

The use of directive techniques in DIT is always framed in the context of a good understanding of the meaning that the therapist's more directive stance may acquire for the patient in light of the IPAF. For example, an anxious patient for whom separation is felt to be terrifying may well be very compliant with the therapist's direction because non-compliance is felt to pose a threat to the relationship. Yet, in spite of the therapist's support and encouragement, little change occurs for this patient. In such a situation, the DIT therapist would be very attuned to the unconscious meaning that may be latent in the patient's wish to please the therapist and would actively take this up with the patient, linking it to the identified IPAF and the lack of progress in the therapy.

REFERENCES

Bollas, C. (1996). Figures and their functions: On the oedipal structure of a psychoanalysis. *Psychoanalytic Quarterly*, 65(1), 1–20. https://doi.org/10.1080/21674086.1996.11927480

Fónagy, I., & Fonagy, P. (1995). Communication with pretend actions in language, literature and psychoanalysis. *Psychoanalysis and Contemporary Thought*, 18(3), 363–418.

Fonagy, P. (2001). *Attachment theory and psychoanalysis*. Other Press.

Fonagy, P., & Target, M. (1996). Playing with reality: I. Theory of mind and the normal development of psychic reality. *International Journal of Psychoanalysis*, 77(2), 217–233.

Fonagy, P., & Target, M. (2000). Playing with reality: III. The persistence of dual psychic reality in borderline patients. *International Journal of Psychoanalysis*, 81(5), 853–873. https://doi.org/10.1516/0020757001600165

Greenson, R. R. (1967). *The technique and practice of psychoanalysis*. International Universities Press.

Lear, J. (1993). An interpretation of transference. *International Journal of Psychoanalysis*, 74(4), 739–755.

Main, M., & Goldwyn, R. (1998). *Adult attachment scoring and classification system*. Unpublished manuscript. University of California at Berkeley.

Main, M., Hesse, E., & Goldwyn, R. (2008). Studying differences in language usage in recounting attachment history: An introduction to the AAI. In H. Steele & M. Steele (Eds.), *Clinical applications of the Adult Attachment Interview* (pp. 31–68). Guilford Press.

Roisman, G. L., Padrón, E., Sroufe, L. A., & Egeland, B. (2002). Earned-secure attachment status in retrospect and prospect. *Child Development*, 73(4), 1204–1219. https://doi.org/10.1111/1467-8624.00467

Slade, A. (2000). The development and organization of attachment: Implications for psychoanalysis. *Journal of the American Psychoanalytic Association, 48*(4), 1147–1174. https://doi.org/10.1177/00030651000480042301

Target, M., & Fonagy, P. (1996). Playing with reality: II. The development of psychic reality from a theoretical perspective. *International Journal of Psychoanalysis, 77*(3), 459–479.

8
Working in the Transference

Working in the transference is one of the cornerstones of psychodynamic technique, and transference interpretation is held by many to be the 'royal road' to psychic change. As we saw in Chapter 7, a range of techniques is deployed in dynamic interpersonal therapy (DIT), but we consider that working in the transference is a fundamental intervention that facilitates the exploration of the interpersonal-affective focus (IPAF). In DIT, the therapist makes systematic use of the transference—that is, the therapist monitors their experience of the transference and of their own countertransference in order to inform their understanding of the patient's state of mind and hence how to intervene. In practice, this may entail not making a verbal interpretation. In our view, we should always 'use' the transference as a compass to orient us in relation to the unfolding of the therapeutic process (Lemma, 2012), but we need to consider carefully how its interpretation furthers the therapeutic aims at any given point in time and whether the patient can tolerate it. In this chapter, we will therefore outline how to formulate a transference interpretation and the rationale for doing so in DIT.

USING THE TRANSFERENCE TO EXPLORE THE IPAF

As deployed in DIT, a transference interpretation is an intervention that uses the 'here and now' of the therapeutic interaction to bring to the patient's attention the activation in their mind of a specific representation of self in relation to an other—that is, the IPAF.

The transference can take many forms, for example, positive, idealized, negative, or sexualized. A transference interpretation makes explicit reference to the patient–therapist relationship and its particular quality at a given point in time. Working in the transference relies primarily on interpreting the current relationship between therapist and patient (i.e. as opposed to interpreting the childhood origins of the patient's current interpersonal patterns). In DIT we share this focus on the here-and-now, but we also make links and draw parallels between the patient's subjective experience with the therapist and that with current others outside the therapy (and vice versa) to illustrate the relevance of the IPAF across different interpersonal contexts and temporal dimensions.

Whereas some patients become very quickly and consciously preoccupied in their own minds with the therapist, others do not, and may find links to the therapeutic relationship irrelevant or even odd. Others might be quite consciously preoccupied with the therapist, but they do not find it easy to report on the therapeutic relationship. In order to support the elaboration of the IPAF, the therapist actively encourages the patient to discuss and explore their perceptions of, and feelings about, the therapist and how they think the therapist may feel or think about them. Working in the transference thus rests on our receptivity to the patient's view of us—however distorted this may be—so as to allow a particular experience of the patient's self in relationship to us to emerge in the session. This requires an ability to recognize the patient's need to 'test' the relationship with us in the transference and to communicate this understanding to the patient, who may be worried, for example, about our anticipated rejection.

There are a number of ways in which a transference interpretation can support the exploration and working through of the IPAF:

- Transference dynamics are live and more immediate, and hence more verifiable in the here-and-now than the patient's report of past experiences or relationships outside the therapy. What the patient tells us has happened to them is subject to the distortions of memory. So, although this is a valuable source of information about what is troubling the patient and how they manage their life, the information is inevitably at one remove. Because the events are in the past and the therapist has only the patient's memory to go on, it is hard to look at it afresh. By contrast, the relationship that develops between patient and therapist provides a more immediate experience of some of the patient's interpersonal

dynamics that occur outside the therapeutic relationship. It allows the therapist to make these conflicts explicit to the patient as they are happening in the room, thus providing raw material to reflect on with the patient.
- Some patients are very adept at telling stories, but they struggle with expressing affect. The transference interpretation allows the therapist to make use of the emotional immediacy of the therapeutic relationship to counter intellectual resistances. The immediacy of the interventions based on this more direct source of information can have a very profound, and often moving, effect on the patient.
- The transference interpretation facilitates an increase in interpersonal intimacy by allowing the therapist to demonstrate attunement to the patient's current experience. A well-timed and accurate transference interpretation is perhaps one of the most powerful expressions of the therapist's empathy, as it shows the patient that they have been heard at various levels, not only in terms of what has happened, but also in terms of what *is* happening. For those patients who have not had the experience of being with another person who reflects back to them what is only indirectly implied in their communications, a transference interpretation can be experienced as containing and transformative.
- The transference interpretation allows the therapist to address the patient's defences against intimacy as they emerge in the therapeutic relationship, and so contributes to a strengthening of the alliance. We all recognize that patients turn up for their sessions but this does not necessarily mean that they want to be there. The transference interpretation squarely focuses on the reasons why the patient might want to avoid the therapeutic relationship by trying to reflect on the anxieties it generates. At its best, this kind of interpretation helps the patient to move on from a resistance.
- Through a transference interpretation, the therapist models a way of handling negative perceptions and interpersonal conflict. Many transference interpretations highlight the patient's negative perception and experience of the therapist.

In making an interpretation that acknowledges these, the therapist implicitly conveys to the patient that it is possible to reflect on such feelings without catastrophic consequences.
- Transference interpretations enhance the patient's capacity to recognize and think about their states of mind. Because they usually pull together strong but confusing feelings and unconscious, distorted thoughts and behaviour, they help the patient to see the relevance and helpfulness of taking a new perspective, and understanding what is happening between them and an important other person.

For all the reasons just listed, a transference interpretation is a powerful intervention. This is why it is also important to evaluate its impact. As with any intervention we make, it is essential to note and respond to the emotional impact of transference interpretations on the patient so that their use is 'titrated' in a manner that reflects the patient's capacity to receive them. In a more general sense, we work to understand and help the patient to manage the emotional impact on them of the transference relationship, where appropriate, because the patient might experience an increase in their feelings towards us—whether positive or negative—as confusing or frightening. To this end it is helpful to consider:

- The patient's conscious and unconscious response to the interpretation (e.g. what associations/understandings follow an interpretation)
- The therapist's evaluation of the quality of the working alliance following an interpretation (i.e. a strengthening or weakening of the alliance)
- The patient's level of distress following an interpretation (however 'correct' our interpretation might be, if the patient feels too persecuted by it, it is of no use to them).

FORMULATING A TRANSFERENCE INTERPRETATION

Let us now look more closely at the components of a transference interpretation. For an interpretation to be useful to the patient, as we suggested in Chapter 7, it needs to make some sense rather than being experienced as coming out of the blue, apparently unconnected to what the patient has been saying. It is therefore helpful to start from the patient's conscious experience of what is transpiring between them and the therapist. In other words, such interpretations begin by describing the patient's experience, as in the following example of work with a patient whose IPAF identified a self-representation as 'unlovable' and an other representation as 'cruel', with rage as the linking affect. Early on in this patient's thirteenth session, the therapist reminded the patient that they were now approaching the ending of therapy. The therapist had been mindful of this patient's difficulty with endings throughout the therapy, but even so, the patient responded to this reminder in a striking manner.

T: We have three more sessions left after today . . .
P: [The patient interrupts, stiffens in her posture, and looks taken aback.] What do you mean?
T: You seem to be taken aback by my reference to the end of our work together as if I have just broken the news to you for the first time.
[Silence]
P: [Dismissively] You must have mentioned it . . . but I have had more worrying things on my mind . . . I probably didn't take it in. It doesn't matter . . . [At this stage the therapist has responded only to the patient's manifest communication. The therapist then tries to engage the patient in clarifying and exploring the feelings that have been evoked, in order to elaborate the experience.]
T: I have the strong feeling that it does actually matter to you even though I can see that it might feel easier to just ignore what you really feel about this . . .
P: What's the point of talking about it . . . it won't change the facts . . . it's not like you will offer me any more sessions . . . anyway it's fine . . .
T: We are on familiar territory here: you feel upset and you push me away because you anticipate that I'm not interested in your experience . . . [Silence]
P: I need to detach, otherwise it's too painful . . . [Long silence and then patient becomes tearful]
T: Something does feel very painful . . .

P: I hate saying goodbye ... my life has been littered with goodbyes or people turning their backs on me. I can't face another one here. I'd rather just get up and leave now—be done with it.

T: I can understand why that might seem like the least painful solution right now. And it would also be you turning your back on me rather than me doing this cruel thing to you, which, I think, is how it felt when I reminded you of the three sessions we have left...

P: [The patient sounds very brittle and angry] What is it to you anyway? You're a therapist and it's your job—nothing wrong with that, but at the end of the day it's just another ending for your notes. You won't even remember my name in a few weeks' time...

At this point the therapist has elicited enough information to make a link to the IPAF, that is, the therapist can abstract the relational pattern that has been activated in the patient's mind by the ending of the therapy and its interpersonal implications.

T: There seems to be room for only one script here: I'm a ruthless therapist who won't even remember your name and I'm abandoning you. You now feel like 'just another patient', someone I can easily disregard, not someone I have grown to know well over the past few months and whose feelings about the ending are very important. But if we get stuck in this particular conversation we can't think together about how the ending feels for you, and this only makes you feel more alone and abandoned by me.

How we share with the patient our understanding of the transference deserves some consideration. Of course, we each have our own particular therapeutic style that influences how we present our interpretations to the patient and there is no 'right' way of doing it because every patient is different and, to an extent, we always adapt our style accordingly. We have found that with some patients—especially those who are not acculturated to a psychological approach to their problems—it is helpful to present the transference dynamic as a kind of 'internal conversation'. For example, we formulate that at a given point in a session the patient feels criticized by us and that their way of managing this is to become contemptuous of our interventions. In this scenario, we might share our formulation in the following way:

> I think that when you experience me as critical in your mind you are no longer talking with someone who is on your side, but with someone who is attacking you. The only way you feel you can then protect yourself is by putting me down as if you are saying to me, 'I don't need you any more. What you have to offer me is worthless.'

If the patient finds this way of thinking congenial, the work of therapy can then be framed as aiming to help them to have different kinds of 'internal conversations', which, in turn, can expand the range of the actual conversations they can have in their external relationships.

CRITERIA FOR INTERPRETING THE TRANSFERENCE IN DIT

As we mentioned earlier, DIT makes active use of the here-and-now therapeutic interaction. However, this should not be taken to mean that all that is discussed is what transpires between therapist and patient—transference interpretations are used in a more circumscribed manner in DIT than they are in longer-term psychodynamic therapies.

Moreover, the aim of a transference interpretation in DIT is not only, or even primarily, to arrive at an insight; the equally important goal is to engage the patient in the process of making sense of how their mind works. Using what happens in the transference often provides the most immediate way of doing this, but there may also be other interpersonal experiences outside the therapy that carry a strong affective charge and could be equally useful to this end.

There are several cues for interpreting the transference in DIT (see Box 8.1):

1. The main rationale for interpreting the transference in DIT is *to enhance the exploration of the IPAF.* This means that the therapist is monitoring the extent to which the interpersonal narratives (INs) the patient brings carry

> **Box 8.1**
>
> CRITERIA FOR INTERPRETING THE TRANSFERENCE IN DYNAMIC INTERPERSONAL THERAPY
>
> - When it enhances the exploration of the interpersonal-affective focus (IPAF)
> - When making a link between the transference and an external relationship adds immediacy and validity to the work
> - When the patient finds it difficult to report interpersonal narratives (or is very isolated), and hence what transpires between the patient and therapist is the most 'live' material available to work with
> - When the therapist considers that the interpersonal narrative reported by the patient is being used to create emotional distance from the IPAF and a transference interpretation about what is going on in the here-and-now serves to refocus the patient
> - When there is a resistance to the work of therapy.

sufficient emotional immediacy to support the exploration of the IPAF or whether the IPAF can be discerned more clearly, and with greater immediacy, within the context of the therapeutic dyad.

2. There may be occasions when the therapist deems that making a link between the transference and an external relationship *adds immediacy and validity to the work* or demonstrates the IPAF's relevance across several interpersonal domains.
3. Working in the transference is essential *when the patient finds it difficult to report INs*, or is very isolated, and hence what transpires between the patient and therapist is effectively the most 'live' material available to work with.
4. Taking up the transference can also be used to *reinforce the working alliance* when this is threatened by the activation in the patient's mind of negative feelings or unsettling fantasies

about the therapist (e.g. if there seems to be a danger that the patient will drop out of therapy because the patient believes that the therapist wants to get rid of them). These feelings or fantasies may or may not be part of the chosen IPAF but should be attended to nevertheless as they pose a risk to continuation of the therapy.
5. When the therapist considers that the INs reported by the patient are being used to create emotional distance from the IPAF (e.g. the pattern is something happening 'out there'), a transference interpretation about what is going on in the here-and-now helps *to refocus the patient on their more immediate experience and the IPAF.*

Case example

Graham was in his mid-forties. He presented to his general practitioner (GP) requesting help with his increasing unhappiness, low self-esteem, and self-doubt. His personal and professional life was becoming difficult. He felt 'old' and 'fragile'. The GP noted that he had experienced anxiety and depression for the past year, he was finding social situations difficult, and his libido had decreased.

On meeting Graham for the first time, the therapist was struck by his physical appearance. He was very tall and seemed to tower over her in the waiting room. She had an immediate experience of feeling small. He was also thin and appeared awkward in his body, stooping in an attempt to reduce his height. He looked pale and slightly dishevelled, and seemed young, dressed like a teenager. Also striking was his beaming smile, which conveyed hope and expectation. This smile became familiar to the therapist as Graham showed it at the beginning and end of every session.

In the first four sessions, the therapist explored Graham's relationships, past and present. Graham was the middle of three siblings. He had one sister two years older than him and another three years younger. His sisters did not feature much at all in his account of family life. His father was in banking, 'not happy or successful'. Work-related stress permeated family life. Graham described his father as 'objective' and as his harshest critic, displaying no physical affection or emotional support. He had felt like a constant disappointment to him. He reported that his father made attempts to hide his disappointment and displeasure by 'objectivity', but Graham felt that he could easily 'see through' this. His relationship with his mother was different, he said. They were very close; there was nothing to hide. He felt that he knew her so well he could anticipate her emotional state, especially when she was stressed and upset. Overall, he felt that he had been experienced as a demanding and needy child. His grandfather had told him he would often make his mother cry because he was so demanding.

The therapist was interested to note that she did not experience Graham as demanding—quite the opposite. He was clearly anxious but did not challenge or question her. However, he did seem somewhat brittle and guarded, which had an impact on the therapist; she felt anxious about intruding too much. She also felt that he was hiding the extent of his distress from her.

In this initial phase of the therapy Graham was very preoccupied with his body. Because of his height and thin physique he had always felt different from others and lacking in physical strength. He described this as feeling 'wonky'. He felt embarrassed by his body and mostly kept it covered up, even in hot weather. Sports activities as a child had been a cruel reminder of his 'wonkiness', and as an adult he tried hard to avoid any kind of exercise. In his mind it became apparent that the trigger for his help-seeking had been his perception of his 'failing' body. The cracks were showing for all to see, he felt. He was experiencing aches and pains, which he saw as a confirmation of his ageing body. He said that he 'hated feeling old'.

Graham's interpersonal world was quite impoverished. He mentioned two or three important friends from the past, but no current ones. The most important relationship was with his partner. As Graham spoke about these relationships, the therapist was able to see a clear pattern emerging: Graham was often left feeling very judged and criticized by the other person, just as he had felt by his father. This was beginning to emerge in the transference, too. The therapist's countertransference was of note: she was beginning to feel that *she* needed to keep herself free of criticism from *him*, and often felt a pressure to 'get things right'. She monitored her use of words and her facial expression, as if alert to the possibility of criticizing him. She was able to explore this in the transference, illustrating to Graham how their relationship was suffused with his expectation that she would be critical and crushing of him and that his need for help was simply confirmation of his 'wonkiness'.

Through his narrative and her understanding of the evolving transference–countertransference, the therapist developed the following IPAF: Graham had a long-standing experience of a critical and unaffectionate father who was unable to disguise his disappointment in him. He had grown up with the family 'story' that his neediness made his mother cry. As a young child, he began to anticipate his mother's moods. Importantly, he began to develop a view of himself as demanding, inferior, and 'wonky'. His awkward body was a visual representation of his wonky self. He began to experience and expect others to be critical of this wonky self and to have no capacity to respond to his neediness, ultimately disappointing him. The IPAF that was agreed on focused on a 'critical, judging' other representation and Graham's self-representation as 'wonky and inferior', which triggered a feeling of depression and loneliness, as he then invariably withdrew from others.

Graham seemed to accept the IPAF. He responded to it by giving an example from his primary school days that helped the therapist to further fine-tune the IPAF: he was trying to make a prop for the school play and was intent on making it the best in his class. He wasn't content with second best. His mother, seeing him struggle, offered to help. Graham said he had felt irritated and angry. He knew how he wanted it to be. It emerged that what had made him so angry was his belief that his mother would succeed only in making the prop the 'same as everybody else's': ordinary. This was unbearable for two reasons: his need for help had been uncovered, and there was an intention, so he felt, to reduce him to something ordinary and not special.

This story was explored in the transference. There was evidence that Graham had been anxious to know if he was the therapist's only patient, and she had increasingly experienced him as needing to be in a one-up position when he was beginning to feel vulnerable or criticized by her. She was reminded of her first meeting with him and her feeling of smallness. The therapist therefore took up in her eventual interpretation how Graham feared exposure of his need for her. Importantly, the therapist began to understand that alongside Graham's view of himself as wonky and inferior, and hence his anticipation that the other might criticize him, there was another self-representation as someone special and superior.

Graham also described ways in which he avoided knowing about the ordinary aspects of his relationships and how he had a secret contempt for the prosaic. He often sabotaged experiences by reducing them to a cliché. As a teenager he had looked for something profound and special in his relationships. He also began to explore how his work as an academic had kept him in an elevated position. As a student he had been in a special place, as he had been taken under the wing of a prominent professor. This had been an effective way of preserving his self-esteem until younger, more successful students came along to challenge his view of himself and left him feeling old.

The middle phase of therapy was spent looking at the loss and pain involved for Graham in facing his ordinariness, his neediness, the limitations of his ageing, and the implications of all this for his work. The elevated, superior part of him needed help to accept that there might be things in life that he would never achieve, and to free himself from the internal critical father figure that he had spent so much of his life relating to. The therapy also explored the consequences of keeping others at a distance. He was able to see that he was missing out on a lot of pleasure in his life. Graham was tempted to reduce the IPAF to a cliché—a 'midlife crisis', but he managed not to, and worked hard at challenging his familiar ways of being in relationships.

The therapist was able to anticipate that the ending would be difficult for Graham. It meant giving up on the idea of a 'special' therapy, just for him. Exploring this in the transference was very important. It helped Graham to acknowledge his need for help, revealing more of his fragile and wonky self, which lay him open to feeling exposed.

THE BRIDGE TO CHANGE

In longer-term psychotherapy, the emphasis remains more firmly placed on work in the transference, and links to other current relationships are generally discouraged. In DIT, as we have been suggesting, the transference is actively used to help the patient to observe the manifestation of the IPAF in other current relationships so that it can be used as a 'bridge' to supporting change. While it would be clearly unhelpful to be prescriptive about the timing for this, in DIT there is a more explicit effort to help the patient to eventually extrapolate from the transference to their external world of relationships so as to support attempts at new ways of relating.

Case example

Sara—a young woman experiencing debilitating anxiety—struggled with therapy from the outset. This was largely because of the fact that Sara felt she had to rely entirely on herself. This emerged as an expectation that had taken root early on in her life when she felt that her parents were emotionally unavailable to her. In her eighth session, Sara's anxiety scores revealed a further deterioration in her anxiety, which had in fact been worsening over several weeks.

The therapist invited Sara to tell her what she made of this. Sara discussed difficulties with her husband: she found it very hard to communicate to him what she needed from their relationship. She then talked generally about the bleakness of the future, how nothing could really change things, that her marriage was stuck, and that she was dreading raising with her husband the fact that she did not want to visit her in-laws over the forthcoming holidays. She wished she could just 'magically disappear' so as to avoid this confrontation.

The therapist felt that Sara sounded distant and disconnected as she spoke. She experienced Sara as hopeless about the therapy, and thought to herself that Sara might not come back for her session the following week—that she might 'disappear' so as to avoid a more direct discussion about the therapy. The therapist eventually said:

T: I think it would be helpful if we pause for a minute to look at what has just been happening here between us, because it seems to me that you are feeling rather despairing and hopeless about whether coming here can be of any help to you, and your anxiety does seem to be getting worse, and yet you are not communicating this directly to me. Instead, I feel you withdrawing. We know how difficult it is for you to be in the position of feeling that you are on your own with a problem and that the other person cannot help you with it. This often leaves you feeling angry, but instead of expressing what you feel, you shut down communication. This is so similar to what happens with your husband when you get into a conflict with him, just as you were describing to me earlier on in the session.

P: I know. I do that. I don't feel able to change this. I don't seem able to communicate normally with others. It must be frustrating for you...

T: What is difficult here is that you pull away instead of us being able to think together about how you are feeling worse and how you feel the therapy is not helping. The risk then is that you might just not come back, that you might disappear...

P: [Sounds taken aback] I have been thinking about whether it's worth continuing with this... I hadn't wanted to tell you, though, in case you thought I was being difficult.

T: So it's safer not to tell me, but this also then means that there is no possibility for us to work out a way forward.

The therapist and patient were then able to unpack this impasse further, making it eventually also possible for the therapist to invite the patient to reflect on how she might approach the unspoken tension between her and her husband in relation to the dreaded stay with the in-laws. The therapist actively encouraged the patient to try to speak to her husband about it, just as she had managed to speak to her in the session.

If we unpack the therapist's first intervention, it reveals several components. The first step is to 'mark a moment' in the interpersonal exchange in the here-and-now and invite the patient to pause to reflect on it:

I think it would be helpful if we pause for a minute to look at what has just been happening here between us...

The second step involves exploring the uncomfortable feelings that are not directly communicated:

> It seems to me that you are feeling rather despairing and hopeless about whether coming here can be of any help to you, and your anxiety does seem to be getting worse, and yet you are not communicating this directly to me.

The third step involves empathizing with and beginning to explore around the edges of the self–other representation that is being activated (i.e. the IPAF), which may reflect a particular defensive function:

> Instead, I feel you withdrawing. We know how difficult it is for you to be in the position of feeling that you are on your own with a problem and that the other person cannot help you with it. This often leaves you feeling angry, but instead of expressing what you feel you shut down communication.

The fourth step involves linking the transference pattern to other current interpersonal contexts that are being focused on in the therapy:

> This is so similar to what happens with your husband when you get into a conflict with him, just as you were describing to me earlier on in the session.

The final step marks the invitation to work on a current interpersonal issue, as the therapist and patient went on to do in this case.

REFERENCE

Lemma, A. (2012). Some reflections on the 'teaching attitude' and its application to teaching about the use of the transference: A British view. *British Journal of Psychotherapy*, *28*(4), 454–473. https://doi.org/10.1111/j.1752-0118.2012.01302.x

9
The Ending Phase

The focus on the importance of attachments means that in dynamic interpersonal therapy (DIT) the separation from the therapist is regarded as an important event. The last four sessions are therefore devoted to an exploration of the conscious and unconscious meaning for the patient of ending the therapy, reflecting on the work that has been achieved and anticipating future challenges. In this chapter, we will review the aims and strategies of the ending phase.

THE PATIENT'S RESPONSE TO ENDINGS

At the core of psychodynamic accounts about the significance of ending therapy lies the assumption that endings re-stimulate other salient experiences of separation, such as bereavements, transitions (e.g. leaving home), or the ending of other significant relationships.

Each patient reacts differently but, generally speaking, ending therapy elicits feelings of loss as well as provoking anxiety about separation. These feelings are not always expressed directly. One of our tasks in the ending phase is to help the patient to articulate their feelings about ending. This requires us to closely monitor and respond to the patient's experience, to minimize the likelihood of a premature ending or other 'acting out' during this phase, which is typically associated with a difficulty in processing the experience of ending.

For many patients, endings force upon them the reality of separateness—an awareness that can be especially challenging for some. In one sense the end of every session is a separation, which is why the end of sessions often provides an opportunity for acting out (e.g. the patient who seemingly ignores that the therapist has called time). The end of each session can feel like an unwelcome reminder that the therapist and patient are two separate beings. As the therapist calls time, the patient hears and feels different things, depending on their own experiences: they may feel rejected, abandoned, or humiliated. For those patients who experience separation in this manner, the final ending of therapy serves only to accentuate further their feelings and phantasies associated with loss.

For some patients, the briefness of DIT may 'dull' some of the feelings that longer-term and more intensive therapy typically accentuates when the therapist becomes a very central attachment figure over a long period of time. Yet, clinical experience frequently illustrates that even over a period of sixteen sessions, many patients develop intense feelings towards the therapist. For example, for some patients, the briefness of the encounter itself may mobilize an intense transference in which the therapist is experienced as tantalizingly seductive and cruel, inviting them into an intimacy only to then leave them. Moreover, precisely because of the brevity of the therapy, such feelings can emerge in a more intense manner because the patient cannot 'push to one side' in their own mind the experience of separation, as it is clearly present from the outset.

How the patient is able to end the therapy encapsulates their level of psychological functioning at the time and, in many cases, is a good indicator of how the patient has progressed in therapy. This is because ending 'well' (i.e. in a way that allows the expression of disappointment, loss, and/or gratitude) involves a number of related processes:

- *Ending entails mourning.* The work of mourning requires of the patient that they can relate to the therapist as a whole object with imperfections without this overshadowing the strengths or qualities that will also be missed. Ending requires accepting the separateness of the therapist and the pain that this can give rise to. Working through this loss promotes internalization of the therapeutic relationship. This then allows the patient to establish the therapeutic process as a structure within their mind: that is, the patient becomes self-reflective. This internalization can occur only once the patient has accepted the therapist's separateness and mourned the loss.
- *Ending involves re-owning projections.* Over the course of therapy the therapist often becomes the container of the

patient's projections—a repository for the split-off aspects of the self. Ending involves relinquishing this container as the patient has to re-own what belongs to them and learn to bear it within themself.

- *Ending requires relinquishing sole possession of the therapist.* It involves coming to terms with being replaced by the next patient. This requires that the patient manages the feelings of envy and rivalry this may arouse without recourse to destructive attacks that devalue the therapeutic experience in the patient's mind, thereby allowing them defensively to come to terms with its loss.

PREPARING FOR ENDING

As with any brief therapy, in practice, the ending is not a discrete phase, even if we set it out as such here for the sake of clarity. Rather, endings are worked on from the start, as the patient is reminded regularly of the brevity of the treatment. The therapist will be attuned, from the outset, to direct and indirect references to termination/separations. Throughout, the therapist will keep in mind, and help the patient to reflect on, the meaning of the time frame of therapy. This will be more or less relevant depending on the patient. In other words, the patient's history of loss and separation, which will invariably emerge as we sketch out the interpersonal map, will alert us to whether ending is likely to be challenging, and in what way. It is not so for all patients, however. We also need to recognize that, for those patients for whom separation is not a major psychological challenge, we do not need a sledgehammer to crack a nut: that is, we may not need to do the same kind of work around endings with all patients.

There are two core strategies for preparing the patient for ending and these are actively used from the start (Box 9.1). From a purely practical point of view, as we described in Chapter 4, we contract with the patient a set number of sessions at the start, and we frequently refer to the number of sessions that are left. This need not necessarily happen every week, but once the middle phase work is underway, it is helpful to refer to the number of sessions left every few weeks. We also prepare the patient by drawing their attention to their subjective

> **Box 9.1**
>
> **ENDING PHASE STRATEGIES**
>
> - Encourage the patient to express affect related to ending.
> - Normalize the experience of anger, sadness, and loss if the patient is struggling to express their feelings.
> - Interpret the defensive aspects of denigrating or idealizing the therapy and the therapist as the ending nears.
> - Systematically draw attention to, and address, the patient's feelings, phantasies, and anxieties about the ending of therapy.
> - Respond to indications of regression near the end of treatment (e.g. symptomatic deterioration) by linking these to the feelings and phantasies associated with endings.
> - Help the patient review the therapy as a whole (e.g. whether they have achieved their aims, whether the attachment style descriptions the patient had selected in the initial phase have changed).
> - Offer a 'goodbye' letter, which reviews the original agreed formulation and outlines what progress has been made in working on the issues identified at the outset.
> - Help the patient express gratitude and/or disappointment, as appropriate.

experience of separations as they occur in the context of the therapy and in their life in general.

For those patients for whom endings are difficult, we may be put under pressure to extend the therapy (and hence avoid facing the ending). In these situations, the therapist needs to maintain the boundary created by the time-limited nature of the therapy and help the patient to explore what the ending means to them. This exploration may well start before session 13 if we consider that the patient will find the ending especially challenging. As always, we are guided by what the patient as an individual brings rather than following the manual to the letter.

Although the ending will therefore always be in our mind, it is only in the last four sessions that there is an increasing specific focus on the experience of ending. We will be especially alert to the opportunity during the ending phase of treatment to revisit the IPAF that has been worked on in the therapy. Not infrequently it sheds helpful light on why the patient might find the ending difficult.

INTERPRETING THE UNCONSCIOUS MEANING OF ENDINGS

The particular emotional colouring that the ending assumes will vary considerably between patients depending on their unique developmental histories. The fact that the patient knows about the ending from the outset does little to avert the phantasies that are often activated as the ending approaches. No matter how amenable or even positive the patient's conscious response to the ending is, it is best not to be seduced by it. It will always be closer to the truth to anticipate a mixed response, even when the work has gone well and the patient has made gains.

Some patients become very preoccupied in their own minds with the end. In these cases, an important strategy in the ending phase is therefore to identify the phantasy that the patient has about why the therapy is coming to an end (Box 9.2). These phantasies mostly concern the patient's view of the therapist's mind and the therapist's perceived intentions in relation to the patient. In other words, they

---

Box 9.2

PREPARING FOR ENDING

- Make contracts clear and specific at the outset.
- Work with the ending from the start—keep referring to it in each session, if necessary, as a reminder from the middle phase onwards, and explore the patient's reactions to this systematically.
- Think about whether there are particular features of the patient's background and experiences that might make the patient especially sensitive to endings.

reflect the patient's experience of themselves in relation to their object. Broadly speaking, the phantasies fall into two kinds, each respectively linked to more or less borderline/psychotic or neurotic levels of personality organization (this list should not be considered as exhaustive).

Paranoid and manic phantasies

- *Paranoid phantasies* reveal how the therapist is experienced as malevolently or ruthlessly leaving the patient behind because they no longer want to see the patient. In these cases, the patient's own hostility about ending is projected into the therapist, who is then experienced as the one who is harming the patient by leaving. (This goes beyond what may be a reality—that the therapist has imposed the time limit and the patient would like, or would benefit from, more sessions. The feeling is one of being treated cruelly or hatefully.)
- *Manic phantasies* reflect the operation of primitive defensive manoeuvres to manage the ending (a) by attributing to the therapist a sense of failure and incompetence (e.g. the patient who views the ending as proof of the therapist's inability to manage them), (b) by retreating into an omnipotent denial of the therapist's significance in the patient's life (e.g. the patient who denies any feelings of loss and diminishes or devalues the therapist's helpfulness in their own mind), or (c) by manically praising the therapist (gratitude that has a false and controlling quality), creating the phantasy that the therapist is the patient's own creation.

Neurotic phantasies

Neurotic phantasies can be classified into two kinds:

- *Depressed phantasies* reveal the patient's preoccupation about their impact on the therapist, for example, a phantasy that the therapist is ending the work—or at the very least not

discouraging the patient from ending—because they find the patient boring or too demanding.
- *Oedipal phantasies* reveal the patient's preoccupation with who else is occupying the therapist's mind and is experienced as more lovable, interesting, or exciting than the patient is. Two qualitatively different phantasies have an oedipal flavour. In one version, the therapist is thought to be ending the therapy because they have a more special patient in mind. In the second version, the therapist is ending the therapy because there is another patient who needs them more (e.g. 'I understand that we have to stop. There are more needy people than me'). The second phantasy reflects a defensive approach to the existence of the rival—it is a defensive 'giving up' of one's space to an 'other', which usually masks resentment.

PREMATURE AND PROLONGED ENDINGS

We offer sixteen sessions in standard DIT (twenty-six in DITCC; see Chapter 13) but the patient may well decide to have fewer sessions. Such decisions always deserve exploration in order to identify the conscious and unconscious factors that may be influencing them. Although a premature ending may reflect the patient's way of managing the anticipated ending, or it represents an enactment of the IPAF, or it simply expresses the patient's difficulty in staying with the IPAF, we cannot assume that this is always the case. It is also important to explore non-defensively the possibility that the patient does not feel that DIT and/or the therapist's style are helpful. Equally, some patients may not require sixteen sessions, and we need to be open to this possibility too.

At the other end of the spectrum we will encounter the patient who struggles to end and tries to prolong the therapy, for example, through repeated cancellations. This is one reason why we advise therapists to make it clear at the outset that the therapy is sixteen sessions long, to offer a clear outline of the schedule of sessions with planned breaks, and to explain that sessions are not automatically replaced. These are only guidelines and each therapist, partly depending on the service context and the protocols in place for missed sessions, may need to modify these guidelines. The main point is to ensure that there are some structures in place that help the therapist to stick to offering DIT over sixteen weekly sessions in close succession rather than over a protracted period of time. This is important because when working briefly the momentum of the work is maintained partly through the continuity of sessions. The focus on change can easily be diluted by irregular sessions.

THE THERAPIST'S PERSPECTIVE ON ENDING

Endings pose a challenge not only to the patient but also to the therapist. Just as our patients make an investment in us, and develop an attachment to us, we have an emotional investment in the therapeutic process and in the patient's life.

Endings are a time when, as well as the patient reviewing their progress, we as therapists assess our helpfulness or otherwise. If the patient has improved, we vicariously partake in this achievement and we experience satisfaction in our work. Some patients will leave us feeling that we have done a good job, whereas others leave us feeling as if we have failed and should start looking for an alternative career. Sometimes the sense of failure we experience can be understood as an attack by the patient, that is, their defence against loss: we become in the patient's mind a failed, useless object whose loss becomes trivial, thus easing the pain of separation.

In some cases we have to recognize that, unfortunately, we do fail our patients. This can be uncomfortable to bear. Some so-called failures are avoidable, but here we also have in mind the more ordinary failures that are unavoidable because no matter how good we are as therapists, we can never be more than 'good enough'. Moreover, therapy can never hope to 'correct' the deprivations some of our patients have suffered. It can offer understanding of the past, but it can never undo it. What we recognize rationally to be the limits of therapy can nevertheless be experienced by some patients as our personal failure towards them.

Because endings are infused with ambivalence, at the risk of sounding ungrateful, it is important to approach the patient's gratitude at the end of therapy with curiosity to begin with rather than take it at face value. Hopefully, most of our patients are genuinely grateful to us for the help they have received. Gratitude is rooted in a realistic appraisal that therapy has not been a magic cure and that we are not all-wonderful but the patient still feels that we have offered something helpful. With some patients, however, the conscious expression of gratitude is excessive: we are talked about as 'saviours' or as the parent they never had. As we approach endings we need to beware the seduction of idealization as much as the danger of denigration. Neither position will help our patients to deal with the infinitely more difficult psychic task of saying goodbye to a therapist who is both loved for what they have offered and hated for what they could not put right.

THE GOODBYE LETTER

A central organizing strategy in the ending phase involves the therapist writing a goodbye letter to the patient. This is an important feature of cognitive analytic therapy (CAT) (Ryle, 2004; Ryle et al., 1990) and we have directly borrowed from this model the idea of including a goodbye letter as part of the DIT protocol. We have done so because it is, in our view, a very helpful intervention that assists the work of ending the therapy and may even be beneficial in preventing relapse (the latter is a hypothesis that requires testing). Unlike in CAT, however, the DIT therapist does not write a reformulation letter in the early stages of the treatment, but only at the end.

Why do we provide a letter? There are a number of reasons why we consider this to be an important adjunct. From a practical point of view, a 'goodbye letter' provides a helpful way of punctuating the beginning of the ending phase and provides a tangible focus for the joint evaluation of the therapy. In a brief therapy, where the pace and rate of learning for the patient are inevitably faster than in longer-term psychodynamic therapy, the scope for consolidating gains is correspondingly more limited. The letter provides a record of the therapeutic work that the patient can refer to and reconsider once the therapy is over.

For many patients, as Ryle (2004) recognized, the letter is also important because it has the quality of permanence (Hamill et al., 2008). The letter may have symbolic value where the patient's own narrative is characterized by the impermanence of their attachments. The letter may thus be said to provide some kind of reassurance at the point of separation—a type of transitional object that may contribute to the internalization of a benign attachment figure (Ingrassia, 2003). It gives the patient something to take away as a memento of the work and to remind them of the understanding they have gained if they have difficult periods later, or simply miss the relationship with the therapist.

It is, of course, legitimate and important to raise the possibility that such letters bypass the working through of the pain of separation. Instead of facing loss, the patient and therapist could be seen to work together on a letter that somehow avoids the more immediate experience of separation. We would suggest, however, that while this possibility needs to be borne in mind and taken up in the transference with the patient where appropriate, in our experience, if the patient's affective experience of ending is addressed directly, as is advocated in DIT, the letter aids the working through of separation rather than avoiding it.

Moreover, the repeated clinical experience is that these letters provoke strong affects and are often experienced by patients as supportive and challenging in equal measure. The letter squarely focuses the patient on a realistic appraisal of the therapy, on what they have gained and also on what has not been possible to achieve; that is, it does not sidestep the reality of disappointment. For the therapist, too, the act of writing the letter can be very powerful and challenging, especially where the work may not have been as successful as they had hoped for.

The discipline of reflecting on the work to arrive at a succinct yet affectively meaningful account of the therapy and its impact on the patient can sometimes alert the therapist to countertransference experiences that they can then take back to the therapy and explore with the patient.

The goodbye letter in practice

In practice we draft a letter, which functions as both a summary formulation and a 'progress report', written in words familiar and accessible to the patient and referring clearly to the IPAF that has been the focus of the work. The letter is a 'realistic' account of the work and therefore includes reference to what has been difficult or challenging for the patient, linking this to a reminder of how the patient managed to overcome these difficulties. Striking the right balance between reminding the patient of their resilience and their ongoing vulnerability is part of the skill in writing these letters, which are typically felt to be challenging and time-consuming by therapists who are new to this part of the work.

The letter is offered to the patient in session 13 or 14, to allow time for them to make suggestions, to discuss it, and to change it. It is typically announced in session 12 so that the patient is prepared for its arrival. The letter acts as a helpful signal that the therapy is moving towards its conclusion and invites the patient to reflect on what they have achieved—and what has not been achieved. The acknowledgement of disappointment is just as important as the gains.

The writing of the letter is intended to be a collaborative process. Even though it is initiated by the therapist, the final draft should reflect the patient's feedback. When the first draft of the letter is presented to the patient, they are invited to choose whether they want to read it and, if so, how they want to approach this. The way the patient relates to the letter is in itself often very interesting. One patient, for example, did not want to read the letter in the session; they took it away and re-presented it the following week, retyped and edited, which left the therapist feeling that the patient had taken it over, leaving the therapist as the abandoned and incompetent one. We are as interested in how the patient negotiates the presentation of the letter as we are in how they feel having read it. In other words, and just as we do when we introduce the relationship questionnaire or outcome monitoring tools (see Chapter 4), we remain attuned to the interpersonal and affective process that unfolds when these events take place in the therapy.

The letter should be about one and a half pages long, two at most. There is often the temptation to make the letter over-inclusive and long. This is not necessary; capturing the IPAF, the patient's characteristic defences or self-defeating patterns, as well providing an outline of what has changed and what might need more attention in the future, are the most important components.

The language should be jargon-free with an emphasis on putting things, as far as possible, in the patient's words, or using live examples that have been worked on during the course of therapy and that may have become 'landmarks' of sorts in the work. The letter is intended to reflect the fact that it is a product of a shared therapeutic process and, as such, it should not read purely like an impersonal summary of the work or like the kind of letter we might send back to a referrer. To this extent, the letter has a more personal feel, even though it remains a formal document that will be included in the patient's notes.

It is important to devote some time to reflecting with the patient on what they will do with the final letter. There may be anxieties about where it is stored, for example, or the patient might want to share it with their partner but is concerned about the partner's potential reaction. Sometimes there may be a wish that the letter is 'accidentally' stumbled across by someone significant in the patient's life so as to communicate indirectly about the issues that are important to the patient. In other words, part of the work of ending involves exploring the meaning of the letter in the context of the therapeutic relationship as well as its potential 'use' in the patient's other relationships.

When constructing the letter, it is helpful to bear in mind the following questions (see Box 9.3):

- Does the content capture the IPAF?
- Does it communicate clearly and supportively to the patient what change(s) has taken place?
- Does it convey a balanced appraisal of the process of the therapy?

Box 9.3

GUIDELINES FOR WRITING THE GOODBYE LETTER

The letter should cover the following aspects, with an emphasis on the collaborative nature of the work (i.e. the 'we-ness' of the experience):

- What has been worked on (i.e. the IPAF)
- What problems/challenges have been encountered
- What has been achieved (i.e. what has been helpful in managing the challenges)
- What remains outstanding.

- Does it address what has not been possible to achieve and future goals where relevant?
- Does the tone convey to the patient a sense of the therapist's involvement in the process?

Examples of goodbye letters

Here are some examples of goodbye letters. There are some individual variations in style as they have been written by different therapists, but they also share common characteristics that reflect some of the key principles we have outlined (see Box 9.3).

This was the letter Timothy's therapist wrote (see Chapter 5 for the case example):

Dear Timothy,
As our sessions are coming to an end, I have written down my thoughts about the work we have done together. This letter is for you to take away as a reminder of the work and the changes you have made, as well as an acknowledgement of some of the things you may continue to struggle with and work on.

You initially came to your GP wanting help with feelings of depression. At the beginning of your sessions with me, you talked about how easily and how often you feel like 'a loser' in relation to other people whom you expect to treat you badly and to humiliate you in some way. This leaves you feeling humiliated and angry and wanting revenge. In your description of growing up in your family, I could understand how these feelings about yourself and others may have come to be. During our work together, we discovered how much of an effort you put into trying to resolve this situation and how these things actually might make things worse for you and contribute to your depression.

One of the things we talked about was how, rather than risk being treated badly and feeling like a loser, you keep other people at arm's length ('DTA'—'don't trust anybody'). You do this by, in a sense, 'being on the run' from really being known by other people, and by yourself. We realized how sometimes you do this by being 'speedy', sometimes by trying to be the favourite or most special, and sometimes by not being honest with yourself or others about yourself (the 'false' Timothy that we got to know a bit). We looked at how this makes you feel, at times, that you don't know who you are. By always being on the run from others, in case they treat you badly or see you as 'a loser', you find yourself feeling very lonely, and this makes you feel sad.

We also noticed together that sometimes you get yourself into trouble by doing things that appear, at first, to reverse the situation and make someone else into a loser (like the Japanese tourists or the guy in the loading bay at work) and put you in the position of being the one who humiliates someone or treats them badly. What we realized, though, is that this doesn't actually make you feel any better, at least not in the long term. What it actually does is that it keeps you feeling like a loser because you lose jobs and make enemies. It also stops other people (most of all your family) from getting to know the 'real' Timothy.

As our sessions together progressed, you experimented with doing things a bit differently. You tried to be more 'real' with others (and we struggled together to allow you to be more 'real' with me), to be less 'speedy' at work, and to not always have to be the 'golden boy'. This was not always easy, and I know that you are still struggling with allowing the 'real' Timothy, who may not always be the 'golden boy' or 'Jack the lad', but is not a 'honey monster' either, to have a voice. It would not be helpful to think that this is something that will happen quickly or easily. I think that sometimes you believe that you can achieve this by going somewhere else, or leaving without telling anyone where you are going.

I know that you are still struggling with feeling depressed at times, and I think that we have to acknowledge that you have started a journey rather than completed it. You have been really courageous, though, in making changes in your life outside and in the therapy with me. I hope this letter is useful in highlighting the insights you have gained and that you can use it to help you to continue to allow the 'real' Timothy to be more present.

With best wishes

This was the letter Graham's therapist wrote (see Chapter 8 for the case example):

Dear Graham,
As our sessions are coming to an end I have written down my thoughts about the work we have done together. This letter is for you to take away as a reminder of the work and the changes you have made.

You initially came to your GP wanting help with feelings of depression and 'melancholia'. At the beginning of your sessions with me you were preoccupied with bodily aches and pains, and felt 'old and fragile'. We quickly began to see how your sense of yourself in relation to others was clearly linked to these feelings of depression. You have been able to show me your 'wonky' self and how you easily expect to feel criticized, even humiliated, by others, leaving you feeling even more 'wonky', irritable, lonely, and anxious. We were able to explore together how you understandably want to protect yourself from this by working hard to keep yourself in a 'one up', 'special', and superior position. You talked about how your work has played a large part in keeping you in a 'special' position, and that this had been a motivating force and to a certain extent 'kept you going'.

As the sessions progressed, however, we have seen how this familiar way of relating has been more limiting, particularly in friendships and more intimate relationships. We have explored your anxiety about getting close to others and difficulty with asking for and accepting help. You have been worried about someone 'taking the whole hand'. We have seen clear examples of this, particularly in your relationship with your partner, when she has invited you to be close and you have felt yourself 'closing down'. You very helpfully have identified your tendency to spoil and sabotage experiences when you feel threatened.

It would be unhelpful to think that these discoveries have been easy and uncomplicated. I have been impressed by your willingness to tackle these difficult issues head on and the many changes you have made in a relatively short space of time. Given your initial anxiety about me being yet another person who would humiliate you or simply see your problems as boring, it must have been difficult to let me know what has really been on your mind. It has been helpful to see the relationship with me as a testing ground for other relationships. By doing this you have been able to experience quite a different way of being with somebody. You have been able to open up and show a more vulnerable side of yourself and not immediately feel embarrassed or humiliated. This has allowed you at times to begin to behave differently towards your partner and, in turn, you have experienced her differently. You have identified your greater awareness of these interpersonal dynamics and that you are less ready to 'close off' when she invites you to be close or needs your help. You have also been able to stick with the more ordinary 'domestic' aspects of a relationship such as going to the supermarket together—which previously you might have reduced to a cliché.

We all need to continue working at our relationships, and it would be unrealistic to think that sixteen sessions could have resolved all of the interpersonal difficulties for you. However, you have shown a real capacity for change and we should not underestimate this. I hope this letter is helpful in highlighting this and in motivating you to continue with the valuable work you have started.

With best wishes

This is the letter that Lara's therapist wrote (see Chapter 6 for the case example):

Dear Lara,
As our sessions are coming to an end, I have written down my thoughts about the work we have done together. The letter is for you to take away as a reminder of what you have achieved in the sessions as well as an acknowledgement of some of the things you may still continue to find challenging and might want to continue to work on.

When we first met, you told me that you had been struggling with anxiety and depression most of your life. You mentioned that things had become worse since the birth of your first child. You noticed that you would be OK in relationships for a while but that sooner or later you would hit a 'cliff edge' and feel that you 'went over', and would become anxious and depressed.

When we looked at this, it seemed to be related to powerful negative feelings you had about yourself, especially in relation to other women whom you described jokingly as 'the cool kids to be with'. On that note, I was struck by the fact that you viewed yourself as the 'geek'. You seemed time and time again to see yourself as a failure and different from others, especially other women. When we looked at this more closely we agreed that you felt a constant sense of failure as a woman and mother, and that others could seem harsh and critical of you in this regard or, even more painful, appear so much more 'together' and 'sorted'. This created a lot of anxiety for you in social situations with other mums and eventually you would become down ('go over the cliff'). You also felt this way with women whom you considered 'more successful' and 'more attractive'. To deal with the anxiety you felt, you would often push your feelings down and just withdraw or, alternatively, find a way to show your anger and envy in more civilized ways, in veiled criticisms in e-mails or passing comments. Sometimes the emotions would get so overwhelming that you would just 'lose the plot'—as you once described when out socializing one evening.

As we moved on in the sessions, we noticed this pattern happening in several situations in your life, especially with key women you considered to be the ideal. I noticed that in our sessions you would often say 'Oh dear, I'm really sorry'. We have understood that this was more than likely related to your sense that you may have felt flawed in comparison to me and that you just assumed that I was always right and, moreover, the man who was a 'model father' with the 'perfect kids and family life'. This highlighted, even between us, how you often feel flawed and you anticipate that others will be critical of you or humiliate you given the chance.

I know that you still struggle with anxiety and feeling depressed at times. We need to acknowledge that it is unrealistic for sixteen sessions of therapy to completely resolve all ongoing struggles. In a way we have only started a journey rather than completed it. In saying this, I want to really acknowledge and commend you for working hard at looking at painful feelings in our work together.

With best wishes

REVISITING THE ATTACHMENT DESCRIPTORS

In session 14 or 15 it is helpful to revisit the attachment statements the patient had rated at the beginning of therapy when completing the relationship questionnaire (see Chapter 4). The patient is asked to rate themselves again on the same statements. In a similar fashion to when the relationship questionnaire is first introduced in the initial phase, we use its review in the ending phase to stimulate discussion about the patient's perception of what has changed and what they might wish to change in future.

It is very unusual to observe significant shifts in the patient's scores because attachment patterns are unlikely to change over such a short period of time. However, it might be possible to note changes in the patient's more realistic appraisal of what they find difficult or in their wished-for changes in this respect. The questionnaire is thus used primarily as a prompt for this kind of evaluative reflection rather than for assessing outcome in any formal sense. It is important to make this clear to the patient, who may otherwise be left with the feeling that they, or the therapy, have failed.

WORKING WITH RESISTANCES IN THE ENDING PHASE

When ending stirs a lot of ambivalence it is unsurprising to find that, as the therapy approaches termination, this phase is ripe for acting out. Strictly speaking, acting out refers to the bypassing of a secondary representation of a feeling (e.g. being able to think about a feeling, or even know that it is one, as opposed to, for instance, construing it as a physical symptom, or boredom, etc.), which is instead expressed indirectly through action. Let us now review some of the most common forms of acting out in the ending phase.

- The *patient misses sessions* (especially the last one). This is one way in which the patient turns what may feel like the passive experience of being left into an active one whereby they are doing the leaving.
- The *patient has nothing to talk about* in the last few sessions. This is often the patient's way of discharging aggression,

leaving the therapist feeling impotent and redundant and that they are the one who has to work hard to reach the patient.
- The *patient's symptoms reappear or deteriorate*. Patients often repeat old patterns in the termination phase and in so doing express a wish to begin treatment again. Sometimes the deterioration reflects the anxiety generated by the anticipation of leaving the therapist. The return of symptoms may also be used to undermine the therapist, showing them what a bad job they have done as the symptoms have not been 'cured'.
- The *patient displaces hostility on to other figures in their life*. The wish to have a 'good' ending can militate against the free expression of ambivalent feelings towards the therapist.
- The *patient avoids ending by replacing the therapist* with another therapist or helping figure, thereby reversing the patient's own anticipated experience of being supplanted in the therapist's attentions once the therapy has come to an end. The seamless transition from one therapist to another is another way of denying the pain of separation and loss.

THERAPEUTIC STANCE IN THE ENDING PHASE

Unlike longer-term psychodynamic therapies that encourage a degree of regression, DIT aims to foster throughout the development of a therapeutic relationship that is more attuned to reality. As we have seen, however, transference distortions will occur and are explored with the patient as the therapy unfolds. One of the tasks of ending involves helping the patient to consolidate a more realistic relationship to the therapist. This is a natural and desirable by-product of the patient's increasing awareness of their projections.

As the ending approaches, we support this more reality-attuned relationship by engaging in a review of the therapy, allying ourselves with the patient's reflecting ego. The experience of two adults taking stock of the work of therapy and thinking about what has changed, and what might yet have to change, is a form of collaborative activity that reinforces the patient's adult, more realistic self.

In the final sessions it is helpful to give some realistic appraisal of how the therapy has proceeded and to share with the patient in their achievements, without shying away from acknowledging what could not be achieved. Bearing the imperfections of the therapy together is an important part of ending and of helping the patient to develop a realistic relationship with us.

REFERENCES

Hamill, M., Ried, M., & Reynolds, S. (2008). Letters in cognitive analytic therapy: The patient's experience. *Psychotherapy Research*, *18*(5), 573–583. https://doi.org/10.1080/10503300802074505

Ingrassia, A. (2003). The use of letters in NHS psychotherapy: A tool to help with engagement, missed sessions and endings. *British Journal of Psychotherapy*, *19*(3), 355–366. https://doi.org/10.1111/j.1752-0118.2003.tb00089.x

Ryle, A. (2004). Writing by patients and therapists in cognitive analytic therapy. In G. Bolton, S. Howlett, C. Lago, & J. K. Wright (Eds.), *Writing cures: An introductory handbook of writing, counselling and therapy* (pp. 59–71). Brunner-Routledge.

Ryle, A., Poynton, A. M., & Brockman, B. J. (1990). *Cognitive-analytic therapy: Active participation in change. A new integration in brief psychotherapy*. John Wiley & Sons.

10

When Things Go Wrong

MANAGING DIFFICULTIES IN THE THERAPEUTIC RELATIONSHIP

No matter how well trained or how much personal therapy we have undertaken, some of the time, we all get it wrong. This 'getting it wrong' may have different sources and meanings. It may indicate a momentary lapse in attentiveness, for example, which says more about our state of mind than being the result of the patient's projections. There are also those occasions when things go 'wrong' because we are drawn into an enactment, responding to unconscious pressure from the patient to behave in particular ways that resonate with their interpersonal-affective focus (IPAF).

Some patients need to 'test' the relationship with the therapist in the transference. For example, we may need to stand the test of the patient's hostility or mistrust. Sometimes, we will find ourselves behaving towards the patient just as they anticipated. Such experiences, however difficult for us, require careful processing, rather than being 'batted back' through a premature interpretation, which might leave the patient feeling that we cannot tolerate their feelings towards us.

A classical analytic position presumed the analyst's capacity for objectivity, and so neutrality, with privileged knowledge, and skills to discover a hidden 'truth' about the patient. The therapist might, at the extreme, have been seen as an objective presence interpreting to a subjectively self-deceiving patient. Increasingly, however, therapists across schools of psychoanalysis recognize that, for the most part, unconscious processes govern the patient–therapist interaction. Notions of neutrality then become problematic and, together with abstinence and anonymity—the classical triad emblematic of the analytic stance—appear antithetical to the unavoidable mutual interaction at work in the patient–therapist dyad.

Despite theoretical and technical differences, there is a fair degree of consensus that some enactments by the therapist are unavoidable because the therapist is a participant in the analytic process and also has an unconscious mind (see e.g. Steiner, 2000). In dynamic interpersonal therapy (DIT), we pay particular attention to the way the IPAF becomes actualized in the transference so that we can step back and understand how the pattern has been activated.

Reflective practice: monitoring the countertransference

At their best, the patient and therapist strive together to be observers of the states of mind that emerge during the course of a therapy so that they can be reflected upon, but since we are frequently pulled away from an analytic stance by factors in both the patient and in ourselves, the work of therapy relies on our capacity to re-establish this reflective stance.

Working in the transference involves recognizing our countertransference and making use of it to add to the formulation of the transference, moment by moment. We attend to the specific quality of the feelings, thoughts, flow of associations, and phantasies that are evoked in us during the exchanges with the patient in order to hypothesize about what the patient may be expressing indirectly. We underline, once again, that it is a hypothesis, not necessarily a fact, because it is easy to equate our own emotional experience (e.g. 'I felt so angry as I listened to the patient and I think this is what she cannot bear to know in herself') with the patient's state of mind. The countertransference is an important source of information, as rich in the insights it can facilitate as it is in the possibilities it also offers us for misattributing states of mind to the patient that, in fact, belong to us. This is because the countertransference is a complex phenomenon and consequently it can be misused: in this sense the countertransference is the best of servants, but the worst of masters (Segal, 1993).

As we define it here, the countertransference consists of three dimensions: (a) the therapist's ordinary emotional response to the patient's predicament; (b) the therapist's own transference to the patient; and (c) the patient's projections into the therapist, which give rise to emotional responses in the therapist. All three dimensions need to be borne in mind when trying to understand the therapist's feelings or fantasies, so that it becomes part of routine practice to consider critically the meaning of the therapist's emotional reactions to the patient. This way we can minimize the risk of unsubstantiated speculation ('wild psycho-analysis'; Freud, 1910) or of misattributing to the patient feelings that belong to us.

In order to use our responses to the patient as the basis for interpretation, we have to reflect on our involvement in the therapeutic process in the context of the rapid shifts that can occur in the patient's states of mind (and that sometimes recruit us into taking up highly specified roles in relation to the patient). The therapeutic process relies on our ability to be open to experiencing transitory identifications with the patient's projections through allowing the patient to view us in a manner that is incongruent with our own self-perception, so as to understand the meaning of this for the patient (i.e. not interpreting this prematurely).

Maintaining an 'observing distance' from the part of us that is involved in the process is best facilitated through regular discussion of cases with peers or supervisors. This is especially important when learning a new way of doing things: the anxiety normally associated with demonstrating competence in the new model not uncommonly results in clinicians becoming so preoccupied with 'doing it right' that in the process they neglect basic therapeutic skills with which they are familiar and experienced. In other words, in these circumstances, the potential for enactments is enhanced.

Enactments, as we have been suggesting, are not only inevitable, but also potentially helpful as long as we can process their meaning and use the understanding gleaned to further the therapy. Being drawn into an enactment gives us first-hand experience of what happens in the patient's relationships. However, some enactments can lead to the violation of boundaries that damage the work and the patient, and hence we need to be vigilant and monitor ourselves. We can never justify an enactment that breaches ethical boundaries, even if it is on account of the interactional pressures placed on the therapist by the patient. Patients may well want to transform us into all kinds of different objects, but we always remain, in reality, a therapist who must practise within professional boundaries.

Therapeutic stance when managing misunderstandings and misattunements in the therapist–patient relationship

Like any relationship, the therapeutic relationship can suffer the strains of misunderstandings and misattunements. When these do occur, we approach them with an 'open to correction' stance that signals to the patient that we are prepared to examine what may have gone wrong in a non-defensive manner. The critical part of the process is to slow the discourse down so that the misunderstanding can be explored fully and carefully. Approaching these difficulties with interest in the patient's experience of the therapist, and being committed to identifying and taking responsibility for the respective roles of patient and therapist in contributing to the problem that has arisen, implicitly models a mentalizing stance. Where appropriate, we recognize and acknowledge our contribution to the patient's response. For example, a therapist yawned and the patient reacted with anger. In exploring this, the therapist acknowledged yawning and that this had been felt to be provocative by the patient, inviting them to think about the particular meaning of the yawn to them.

If we have somehow contributed to the patient's experience through an enactment, this needs exploration too. This is important because a major aspect of working in the transference is to model a capacity for reflecting on what happens in relationships, which involves acknowledging mistakes or misunderstandings. Notwithstanding this, acknowledging our 'mistake' does not require explaining why we made the mistake: this is the patient's therapy, not ours. It is crucial to acknowledge that we did something that, ideally, we should not have done, that this had an impact on the patient, and that we are keen to understand that impact. The patient's conscious and unconscious fantasies, for example, about the cause of a therapist's temporary lapse in attentiveness would then become the focus of joint exploration of the patient's conviction that this was owing to how boring they are. It is important for the therapist to be open about the way their own mind works while at the same time not making personal disclosures and losing the analytic frame. This engenders curiosity as well as creating motivation for adopting alternative perspectives. This stance is important for several reasons. The acknowledgement of an error models honesty and courage, as well as that everybody can fall short. Taking responsibility for the 'error' or a behaviour that was felt by the patient to be provocative in some way also tends to lower the patient's arousal. Finally, it offers an opportunity to revisit how such scenarios arise out of mistaken assumptions about opaque mental states and how misunderstanding can lead to aversive experiences.

The therapeutic relationship is strengthened by the experience of difficulties that can be openly discussed and resolved. Misunderstandings and ruptures in the therapeutic relationship allow the therapist to model how to manage interpersonal conflict, and how to disentangle the intentions and attitudes of those involved.

Case example

Ms A, a rather brittle young woman, had always felt herself to be in the shadow of her older and seemingly more successful sister. She had comforted herself with being the 'good daughter' who had stayed close to her parents and taken care of them in their old age.

The IPAF that was agreed on centred on her recurring experience of feeling herself to be 'undesirable' relating to an object that was felt to be 'preoccupied and unavailable' to her. This invariably gave rise to a despairing affect that paralysed her. Her recent depression had followed the sudden death of her mother and she had then struggled to manage taking care of her father, whose grief and pining for his wife left Ms A feeling that her care and attention were 'insufficient'. She spoke about her mother as a very engaging, funny woman whom her father loved and admired. It felt to the therapist that Ms A had hoped that she could somehow replace her mother in her father's affections, and that she could finally be the one who was desired. The father's seemingly entrenched grief, however, was interpreted by Ms A as the painful, if all too familiar, confirmation that she was simply not desirable enough. The object, as far as she was concerned, always had a more desirable 'other' in mind.

In session 7, the therapist and patient agreed to change the time of the next session at the therapist's request. The following week, the patient turned up at the correct 'new' time, but the therapist was not there—she had, in fact, got confused and was expecting the patient the following day. When she later realized her mistake, the therapist wrote to the patient to apologize for the confusion.

When they finally met again, Ms A was late, and the therapist felt her to be hostile. Even before the therapist could say anything about the previous week's events, the patient began to speak in a very pressured manner. The therapist thought that Ms A was desperately suppressing her rage. The patient spoke about her disappointment with the therapy and with the therapist:

P: It's not as though I had high expectations . . . that would have been unreasonable, and no one knows how this verbal therapy works . . . perhaps medication is better, I read that somewhere . . . I don't know . . . I wish I had not embarked on this . . . you said it was important to attend all sessions . . . the importance of not losing momentum . . . at the very least I had expected I would be treated with respect, not treated like a second-class citizen who can't even rely on being seen at the right time . . . It was so embarrassing being in the reception in front of other patients and being told 'your therapist is not here' . . . they were all looking at me . . . glaring as if there was something odd about me.

T: It was entirely my confusion that led to you being left stranded without a session last week and exposed to the harsh glare of the other patients, and, as I said in my letter, I am sorry about this. It is understandable that you should feel upset about it and unsettled, especially since I have been so emphatic about the importance of attending sessions.

The patient visibly calmed down at this point. The therapist then went on, trying to link the 'event' in the therapy to the IPAF:

T: I think that it would nevertheless be helpful to think together about what has made my mistake feel so upsetting in this very particular kind of way, because what strikes me about your experience in the reception area is how you felt harshly scrutinized by the other patients. It wasn't only that I was not there, but that you then felt that my absence exposed something unappealing about you.

P: [The patient nodded] It felt just awful . . .
T: Awful . . .
P: I mean, ashamed, like I wanted to dig a hole and disappear and then also angry, furious, like I was about to explode . . . incensed . . . that's what I felt—I could both believe that this was happening to me—because these things *always* happen to me—and at the same time I felt incensed.
T: I think that your connection with the feelings of shame followed by outrage is important. My not being here for you last week cast you right back into that painful familiar role of being the undesirable, insufficient one who is not kept in mind—instead someone else gets the attention you so desperately feel you need and is due to you—and I think this is what you imagined the other patients could see. And you sway from feeling ashamed to then feeling outraged, that it's unfair . . .
P: When I was told by the receptionist that you were not here, I felt at first that I was to blame—I always feel that even though I knew I had the right time in my diary. Still, I thought the receptionist must have got it wrong . . .
T: So, at that moment you were still holding on to some hope that this could not be happening, that you had got it right and that I would also get it right and appear, as I should have done.
P: Yes, exactly, but as time passed and you didn't turn up, I started to feel really angry towards you. It was like a wave of rage, which I still felt as I got here today . . .
T: Rage towards me for not being here . . . where did you think I was?
P: I was convinced that another patient had called in, someone with more important, interesting issues than the crap I repeat every week, and that you just offered to see them instead of me.
T: So, the rage you felt then and are still feeling today has something to do with me becoming in your experience someone who actively neglects you because you are not as interesting as the patient you think I chose to see instead of you . . .

The patient's elaboration of her fantasy about the reason for the therapist forgetting her session provided an immediate opportunity to help the patient observe the activation of the IPAF in the transference.

Irrespective of what motivated the therapist's confusion in the first place, this incident became an important landmark in the work, which gave Ms A greater confidence in her therapist's ability to tolerate her rage and reinforced the relevance of the IPAF. The therapist's ordinary openness about her error was an important precondition for this development because it modelled a way of taking responsibility for something that had gone wrong and for how conflict can be resolved.

It is easier for patients to give voice to negative feelings if they trust that the therapist can tolerate the expression of these feelings without retaliating or trying to minimize their significance. As was the case with Ms A, responding to such feelings requires that the therapist can scrutinize critically their own contribution to any difficulties or impasses in the relationship.

FORMS OF RESISTANCE

In the therapeutic situation, defences manifest themselves as resistances, which undermine the conscious contract both therapist and patient have signed up to. The term 'resistance' essentially means *opposition*. Resistance can take many forms. It refers to any defensive manoeuvre, as deployed in the therapeutic situation, which impedes the therapeutic work. It signals an avoidance of unsettling feelings or thoughts by the patient that is subjectively experienced by the therapist as being somehow drawn away from the agreed focus. Resistances can be 'obvious', for example, when the patient arrives late, or they can be 'unobtrusive' (Glover, 1955), such as when the patient appears compliant but the compliance masks hostility to the process.

Because resistance occurs in the context of the therapeutic relationship, it is incumbent on us to acknowledge the 'external' triggers that may compound a resistance, for example, cancellations by the therapist, as shown in the case example of Ms A. It is also very important to differentiate resistances from the patient's disagreement with us: the patient's 'No' sometimes does mean just that.

Starting therapy always represents a threat to the patient's emotional status quo. The early stages of DIT are thus ripe for resistances of various sorts because the patient's anxiety about beginning therapy will be very active and has not yet been sufficiently reflected upon with the therapist for that process to provide sufficient containment.

To understand resistance, we need to think about the different—and all too often conflicting—motivations that lie beneath the patient's resolve to seek help. In other words, we need to consider the patient's relationship to help and its internal meaning. Suffering often, but not invariably, acts as a spur to seeking help. For every wish to be helped, we often find the converse wish—within the same patient—to maintain the status quo, owing, for example, to the threat of therapy to the patient's self-esteem or the patient's need to keep the pain alive (i.e. secondary gain). Often, the patient wants to both get better and stay the same. Some patients are more fundamentally 'against understanding' (Joseph, 1983, p. 139) and these patients are highly unlikely to benefit from DIT.

The patient's relationship to help is organized around expectations and habitual patterns of reacting in the context of care that have probably been set in early childhood. Such procedures will be activated when beginning therapy, and will become known to us in the transference. This is what we often aim to capture when we listen to 'cautionary tales' (see Chapter 4). Enquiring at the assessment stage about the patient's previous experiences of therapy or relationships with other health care professionals, friends, and family will enrich our formulation and help us to anticipate particular difficulties for the patient in engaging with the therapeutic process.

It is beyond the scope of this book to cover all possible forms of resistance. This section is therefore restricted to describing common scenarios that are encountered especially, but not exclusively, in the initial stages of DIT, and which may act as a form of resistance.

Requests for information about DIT

It is important for the patient to have information about DIT in order to give meaningful agreement to entering treatment. Answering some of the patient's questions about this form of therapy is therefore part of good clinical practice. For some patients, however, these questions are imbued with meaning (e.g. wanting to discuss the reason for the exact number of sessions compared with a cognitive-behavioural therapy programme the patient has heard of) that goes well beyond the need for informed consent. In such a scenario, the therapist might say:

> Beginning psychotherapy can make people feel anxious because it is frightening and painful to confront certain aspects of ourselves. I'm wondering if asking me a lot of practical questions is perhaps your way of letting me know that you are worried about what you are letting yourself in for?

In the vast majority of cases, picking up on the anxiety behind the question is enough to ease the patient into therapy.

Personal questions about the therapist

Many therapists struggle with how to manage requests by patients for information about themselves (e.g. the therapist's age, culture, or family circumstances). On the face of it, some of these questions might seem reasonable, and the therapist may fear that choosing not to answer the question will create awkwardness in the interaction.

There is, of course, natural curiosity about the kind of person the therapist is, but this apparent curiosity is often multilayered and may serve a range of defensive functions that require understanding. For this reason, in DIT therapists are discouraged from disclosing personal information about themselves. It is more productive to approach these requests by acknowledging the importance of the question to the patient and then inviting them to be curious about 'what else' they might be trying to communicate or ask for.

Having said this, when these questions arise in the first sessions, we need to balance exploration with engaging the patient in the therapy. For those patients who are not acculturated to a psychodynamic mode of working, our declining to answer such questions may seem odd. We need to ensure that in remaining true to our 'model', we do not shame or alienate the patient. In a response to a question, for example, about whether the therapist has children, the therapist might preface the invitation to explore what lies behind the question by saying something like:

> I appreciate that this is an important question for you and that my not answering it may seem odd to you, but I am interested to understand the difference it might make to you if you knew whether I have children or not?

Now, if this question about children was posed by a patient who had been unable to conceive, we might hypothesize that the question is emotionally loaded given the patient's history and would have a particular poignancy. The therapist might then say:

> I can imagine that this is a really important question for you given what you have been struggling with in your own life. You may well be wondering how I could understand your loss if I don't have children . . .

Requests for direction or advice

Generally speaking, giving direct advice is proscribed in DIT (except, for example, if the patient is suicidal and action needs to be taken to ensure their safety, or if the patient might require a referral on to another professional). Requests for advice are not uncommon, however, in the early stages of DIT, especially from patients who know little about how psychotherapy works and who consequently base their expectations on the model with which they are most familiar with, that is, the medical model, where advice is given liberally. The patient's cultural background may also be relevant in this respect: in cultures where psychotherapy is not common and where the expectation is that the 'doctor' gives pills or instructions, requests for advice are best addressed first by explaining the nature of psychotherapy and then exploring how the patient feels about this. For example, the therapist might say:

> I can see that in coming here you expected me to give you advice and practical suggestions to help you with your difficulties. I wonder what it feels like to discover that I am a different kind of therapist from the one you had expected.

In some cases, the request for advice may betray the patient's wish for an idealized therapist who is omnipotent and will cure them of their ills, or it may reveal the patient's characteristic passive stance in relation to their problems. Here, it will be important to take this up with the patient and to articulate the possible meaning.

Challenging the boundaries of the therapeutic relationship

Patients can use the therapeutic frame as the focus of their resistance, for example, by coming late or trying to extend sessions. Requests for contact between sessions may represent another means of challenging the boundaries of the therapeutic frame. The particular meanings that such behaviour might have will be specific to each patient, but often such challenges to the therapeutic frame are a call to the therapist to take these up in the transference—for example, giving more time or unscheduled contact may mean to the patient being treated as the special child by a caring parent.

The IPAF as an intellectual defence against feeling

Patients come into therapy in search of answers. Some patients, however, convey an urgent need to be relieved of their symptoms and the uncertainty resulting from this state of 'not knowing'. This anxiety may be managed by a retreat into a search for certainty. For such patients, the IPAF may provide the kind of certainty they are seeking, and the formulation is therefore enthusiastically welcomed, but soon the therapist is left feeling that no real contact can be made with the patient, that the links to the IPAF are superficial and nothing changes. Here, the use that is made of the IPAF becomes the focus of exploration.

The compliant patient

It is not uncommon for patients to project their own critical superegos into us so that we are then experienced as judgemental or punitive (often, playing out the IPAF in the transference). When this occurs, the patient may retreat into compliance and will try to say or do the right thing to avoid our disapproval. The patient may agree with the IPAF, dutifully bringing examples each week that confirm it, and the therapist may be pleased with their ostensible progress. And yet, there is little change in the patient's life. In so doing, the patient is resisting the process because they are not able to examine this dynamic, something that might, in turn, expose them to their own more critical, hostile feelings towards the therapist. The problem for the therapist in these cases is that it is all too easy to fall into the comfortable trap of being in therapy with the patient who is always nice, appreciative, and interested, but who simply does not change because we collude with their defence.

Difficulty in being the patient

One way of avoiding exploring oneself and denying feelings of vulnerability or dependency is to defend against being a patient. Rationalizing, intellectualizing, or acting seductively may all be deployed as a means of avoiding vulnerability. Patients who use this type of defence may be very adept at drawing us into intellectual discussions. These can be stimulating, but serve the hidden function of abolishing differences between the therapist and the patient so that their vulnerability is avoided, and the purpose of the relationship—to help the patient change and reduce their suffering—is bypassed and implicitly denied.

Idealizing the therapist

The DIT therapist makes the most of the positive transference, when it is accessible, in order to engage the patient and drive the therapy forwards. The therapist does so mindful that this will likely give way to the negative transference some of the time. A positive transference is, however, quite different from an idealized one that reliably gives way to denigration.

Given our own narcissistic needs, it may be difficult to resist the pull of the patient who thinks we are wonderful (although it helps to remind ourselves that we will invariably find ourselves knocked off that pedestal!). The patient may need to think we are brilliant because any other thoughts and feelings might be too threatening. If we become too identified with being a 'wonderful' or 'brilliant' therapist, we will not be able to stand back and help the patient think about what their idealization defends against.

Sexualized behaviour

Sexualization of the therapeutic relationship is often used as a means of resisting feelings of vulnerability or powerlessness. Seduction can be quite explicitly erotized, or it may be more subtle and therefore more difficult to grasp. A subtle form of seduction, for example, can be observed in the way some patients disclose information: some patients tell their story enigmatically or very colourfully and we find ourselves gripped by the story, wanting to hear more. Often this reflects the patient's attempt to draw us out of our interpretive function through seducing us. Again, this is a call for the therapist's self-reflection.

The therapist's resistance to time-limited work

It is not just the patient who may engage half-heartedly in the therapy. Therapists, too, can bring into play their own resistances. We have in mind here specifically the resistance to time-limited work.

In order to work in any therapeutic modality, therapists need to feel that they are delivering a therapy that has integrity and is felt to be potentially beneficial to the patient. DIT is no exception, but its delivery may pose particular problems for practitioners who are very committed to long-term, open-ended therapy and who may consequently feel that they are somehow short-changing the patient if they offer sixteen sessions.

In our experience it is not uncommon for these therapists to present what they are offering the patient in exactly these terms: 'We will meet for *only* sixteen sessions.' Our prejudices about brief therapy may well leak through in this way and convey to the patient our belief that what we are offering them falls short of what they need. Of course, with some patients, this will indeed be the case, and it will be important to help the patient to express their own experience of disappointment as well as the therapist's recognition that further help will be needed. Another way in which this resistance plays out is in selecting very challenging, highly defended, and complex patients for DIT, including those with several failed attempts at therapy under their belts.

Notwithstanding this, for a therapist who is trained in long-term therapy, it may also be difficult to imagine that sixteen sessions could be enough to help a patient to make some important changes, or that for some patients this may be all that they can manage at a given point in time. It is therefore incumbent on all of us to examine our own belief systems in this respect so as to be freed of unhelpful assumptions that might set up the therapeutic encounter to fail.

WORKING WITH RESISTANCE

The first stage of working with resistance requires a formulation of the patient's relationship to help: that is, we strive to make sense of what internal object relationship is activated when the patient experiences themselves as needy and vulnerable in relation to us as the helper. This may or may not be relevant to the IPAF, but if the patient is resistant to being helped, then this becomes the therapeutic priority.

As we mentioned earlier, many resistances emerge specifically in relation to the anticipation of receiving help. For example, a patient whose experience of being vulnerable had become equated early on with being humiliated found it intolerable to take in anything the therapist offered them, because the patient experienced their own need and 'not-knowing' (which they equated with being a weak and needy person) as deeply humiliating. The patient therefore met all the therapist's interpretations with contempt, making the therapist feel like the 'stupid' one who always got it wrong. This internalized object relationship got in the way of the patient being able to derive help from the therapy, and hence had to be addressed. This could be a very useful opportunity to point out to the patient a 'reverse IPAF'. The IPAF may have been something like 'self: weak; other: dismissive; affect: hopeless and sad'. The defensive function of this IPAF may have been formulated by the therapist so as to relieve the patient from knowing about their own dismissiveness and contempt, which could (and might well already have) led to the patient spoiling relationships through subtly putting down others. That pattern could lead to the patient being not only rejected but disliked or even hated, which is worse than being seen as weak. This could lead to depressed feelings of sadness and despair, with the patient unconsciously maintaining the status quo of the IPAF. This hidden dynamic and fear would therefore be unconscious at the beginning of therapy, but would probably come into some interpersonal narratives. The superior and dismissive behaviour emerging in the transference gives the therapist a valuable opportunity to help the patient to see this other side, a reversal of their usual self-image, giving rise to greater fears and reinforcing the conscious IPAF as an unconsciously preferable alternative.

Once we have grasped the quality of the patient's relationship to help, we can begin to reflect on whether they 'won't'—or 'can't'—accept help. This distinction relates to the important consideration of whether the resistance results from an internal conflict or from a deficit. The greater the degree of personality integration typically associated with a neurotic personality structure, the more likely it will be that the resistance arises from a conflict between a part of the patient that wants help and another that finds some substitute satisfaction or safety in maintaining the symptoms.

The less integrated patient may, by contrast, be resisting help because to allow another person into their world is simply experienced as too dangerous. This is the kind of patient who feels that they cannot afford to take the risk of allowing the therapist to know about them. In such histories, we often encounter developmental deficits. Our task here is to find ways of communicating that we understand what the experience of being in therapy might feel like for the patient. This patient, for instance, may have a template for being helped that involves an abusive other masquerading as a helper. In such instances, the therapist strives to convey respect for the defensive structure that has protected the patient and names the feared risks of letting the therapist into their life.

Working with resistance is approached in the same way as we suggest approaching defences (see Chapter 7), that is, gradually and through building up to an interpretation once the patient has first been helped to acknowledge that they are not allowing themself to be helped (Greenson, 1967) (see Figure 10.1). For example, say the patient has been arriving late for a few sessions and that this is occurring in the latter part of the middle phase, that is, as the therapy is inching

When Things Go Wrong

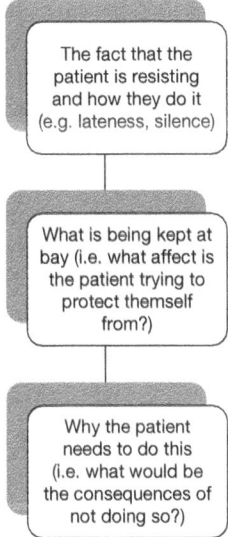

Figure 10.1 Steps for interpreting resistance in the therapeutic relationship.

closer to the end. The therapist would go through the following steps before making an interpretation:

- The therapist begins by pointing out to the patient that they are resisting, using unambiguous examples of why the therapist thinks this: 'This is the third time you have arrived late this month, and I think this is perhaps not just accidental.'
- The therapist then invites the patient to be curious about the meaning of their behaviour before making an interpretation: 'Do you have any thoughts about this?'
- The patient may or may not provide any response to this. Either way, the therapist tries to develop an understanding through what the patient says and/or what they unconsciously convey. In particular, the therapist formulates the affects the patient needs to protect themself from before interpreting the content of the resistance: 'You seem to feel quite anxious in the sessions of late. I wonder if when you arrive so late, at least you feel in control of what happens here between us?'

- The final step is to make a fuller interpretation that takes into account the unconscious meaning of the resistance and links it to the IPAF where relevant: 'It seems as though, since I brought up the ending a few weeks ago, you have found it very hard to arrive on time. I am wondering if my reminder felt like me pushing you away. We know from the work we have been doing that when you feel this way in your relationships you withdraw and can actually start to do the rejecting. I think this may be what has been happening here: you come late and I am the one waiting here, the one who is left out, not knowing whether I have a patient or not.'

WHEN THINGS GO WRONG FOR THE DIT THERAPIST WHEN LEARNING THIS MODEL

Up to now, we have largely focused on the way things can go wrong for the patient. We will now highlight some of the areas where new DIT therapists can become derailed in their practice, based on our experience of supervising in this model over many years.

Working in a new model requires us to be mindful of our preferred practices, so that we can make conscious choices about the interventions we make in DIT. The DIT therapist has to strike the right balance between being active versus sitting back, between being supportive and using psychoeducation judiciously versus using interpretations to bring difficult experiences to the patient's attention, including challenging the patient where appropriate. We want to ensure that the psychoanalytic stance that informs DIT, together with the emergent quality of sessions, is preserved, notwithstanding the structure of using sessional outcome measures (if they are required by the service context), encouraging change, and working with a focus. DIT therapists can run into difficulties if we find ourselves avoiding exploring the transference, particularly negative transference, in favour of being more supportive, or by becoming overly cognitive and directive. Some DIT therapists find working with questionnaires and outcome measures uncomfortable, and tend to ignore them rather than finding ways of working with them from a psychodynamic perspective and integrating the relationship questionnaire into the formulation (see Chapter 4). Similarly, using mentalizing techniques can be an area with which DIT therapists are less familiar, and they may stay away from this important tool in our repertoire of interventions. They might find it hard to integrate with an interpretive stance; that is, the mentalizing therapist does not tell the patient what they—as 'expert'—can see is in the patient's mind. However, it is entirely possible, and in fact familiar to many psychodynamic therapists, to introduce tentativeness to an interpretation; it is a suggestion rather than an assertion. For example, where a patient wants to have contact between sessions, or prolong their time, the therapist might say: 'I wonder whether you have any thoughts about why you want to have more time? I have imagined it might make you feel more cared about, like having a close family member on call, or maybe being given more time makes you feel that I really understand you?'

Another area of difficulty in sustaining a psychodynamic approach can occur where DIT therapists operate in busy primary care settings, where there are pressures to discharge patients after they drop below 'caseness' (i.e. their outcome scores indicate recovery) or when a session is missed. It is important to hold the analytic frame in brief work, where a break in treatment holds conscious and unconscious significance for patient and therapist. This may require adopting a slightly different approach to the primary care service, where, for example, cancellations may be permitted or patients are discharged after a missed session or two.

We find that the evaluation side of DIT accreditation causes anxiety that tends to find particular focus in session recordings. Supervisees are required to share recordings of key sessions for evaluation by DIT supervisors against a set of competences for the model (see Appendix 3). This is often the first time that supervisees have had a supervisor listen to their clinical work. While this is a rich source of information for both self-supervision and feedback on the progress the supervisee is making, we have found that things often go wrong with the recording process for a session that is being evaluated. Technology can express therapists' resistance to their understandable anxiety at being evaluated and often feeling deskilled when undertaking further professional training. They may also sometimes be reassured by listening to the recording on their own (or watching, where a video recording is available) and observing that it is better than they might have feared; they might also themselves notice some areas for improvement, which they can take to supervision. We encourage DIT therapists to test out their recording equipment well in advance and to trial sending the material—in an agreed safe and confidential way—to their supervisor.

Initial phase difficulties

Some of the common difficulties that emerge in the initial phase include not gathering enough interpersonal narratives, meaning that there is insufficient material to establish a robust enough IPAF. There can be a tendency to allow the patient to tell their story, with the result that we end up with a well-rehearsed narrative that does not allow us to elicit the components of self, other, and affect that make up the IPAF. Brief work inevitably requires us to be more active and metaphorically to lean in towards the patient, asking more questions than we would otherwise in open-ended, longer-term psychodynamic work. The IPAF should link with early relationship patterns as well as current relationships across several different domains.

Therapists can struggle to settle on an IPAF, sometimes getting confused between the different parts of the pattern, using an idealized, defensive view of the self (e.g. a hardworking or caring self-representation) instead of the underlying problematic view of self, and thereby avoiding taking up a more unsettling and honest self-view. Being unable to find a focus for the work, even with supervision, can be a sign of patient complexity that may suggest brief focused work is contraindicated.

When it comes to negotiating the IPAF (typically in session 4), the DIT therapist has to hold the pattern in mind, without drawing it up beforehand in a way that would fix the IPAF before getting the patient's input and adjusting it as required. This is a challenging stage in the DIT model, arguably the most taxing part of the model. Some therapists fail to establish the rationale for this session upfront, so that they do not link the pattern to the reasons the person came for therapy ('why now?'). They can also present the pattern in a condensed way, without allowing time for the patient to reflect on the descriptors and/or narrow down the best word or image to capture their self- or other-representation and the affect linking the two. The dynamic aspect of the formulation can be lost, with the therapist not presenting the way the self-representation responds to the other-representation and then gives rise to the affect. Some therapists end up with a multiplicity of descriptors for the IPAF, suggesting difficulty in arriving at a clear formulation. This muddies the work, and it can lead to a vague pattern that neither therapist nor patient has grasped clearly. We encourage therapists to get agreement on the one—or at most two—key descriptors that capture the sense of self and other, with the conscious and unconscious affects that flow from this interpersonal pattern.

The therapist has to titrate the IPAF so that the patient can reach a shared understanding around the formulation. When the wording that is chosen for the IPAF is not the patient's own imagery and language, it can make the IPAF feel less personal to the patient, as if it has been taken 'off the shelf'. We are aware that while we are all unique, there are shared experiences among us when it comes to IPAFs. We are aware there are some 'off-the-shelf' IPAFs that most patients would feel are relevant to themselves, such as the 'not good enough' self with a critical other. We would encourage DIT therapists to make the IPAF as ideographic as possible for the patient.

There are IPAFs that are not generalizable to more than one relationship, which results in too much specificity. There are also self-representations that confuse the self with a defensive, false self-representation such as 'pleasing' or 'hard-working'. Here, it is best to get hold of the underlying difficulties the patient is having, as prompted by the following questions: 'What would happen if you didn't work so hard to please others? What would you feel about yourself then?' We would encourage therapists to avoid conceding a more powerful descriptor in the face of something more palatable like 'not good enough', which may veer away from something more compelling like 'worthless' or 'useless'. Some therapists can confuse the self- or other-representations with affect and vice versa, for example, using 'angry' or 'sad' as self-representations.

We are also aware that there can often be confusion between the defensive function of the IPAF and the patient's use of defences to cope in the face of the painful affects generated by the pattern. When negotiating the IPAF, it is important to suggest to the patient the reason we think they keep this unhelpful pattern going. We have stressed that this is a dynamic model whereby the self is often projecting unwanted parts into the other in a defensive manner. One of the goals of DIT is to start to take back these unwanted projections. This involves becoming aware of the reverse IPAF—the way the patient will often step into the shoes of the other—thereby giving the other an experience of how they are feeling. This can happen in the transference, where we can be left feeling stupid, inadequate, or helpless as therapists in our countertransference; in this way, we are being given an experience that the patient often suffers.

Finally, therapists often dodge asking patients to agree some goals for change over the course of treatment once they have established the IPAF. This may highlight difficulties in working in a more focused way. In our experience, therapy can run adrift in the middle phase of the work without having some agreement from the patient regarding areas they wish to improve. We do want to encourage a positive attitude towards change, and a patient's unwillingness to set any goals is suggestive of their resistance to the work and possible scepticism about the impact of therapy. This should be acknowledged and addressed by the therapist.

Middle phase difficulties

As we move into the middle phase, new challenges are encountered. Even where goals have been agreed, there can be a tendency to stay with describing the IPAF rather than moving into helping patients translate insights into action by making changes in their interpersonal behaviours.

Earlier, we described the way the patient can treat the IPAF in a concrete manner. Similarly, the DIT therapist can become wedded to the pattern that they worked hard to establish, and it becomes solidified. The IPAF should be seen as a starting point, rather than the holy grail of DIT. We would expect the IPAF to be continually refined during the middle phase, with some adjustments made to the descriptors or a shift in the focus as the work deepens. The other direction that some DIT therapists veer towards is forgetting the IPAF altogether. We would expect the pattern to be referenced several times during a middle phase session. It is the focus of the work; without holding to a focus, we run the risk of the middle phase slipping into 'work as usual', whether that is more psychodynamic or analytic at one end of the spectrum, or more cognitive or supportive at the other. Other challenges in the middle phase include not paying enough attention to the affect in the IPAF, as well as staying away from the way the IPAF plays out in the transference.

Ending phase difficulties

The ending phase is heralded with the goodbye letter. A draft letter is usually shared with the supervisor ahead of the session in which the letter is shared with the patient. Writing a letter to patients can be another aspect of the DIT model that feels very unfamiliar to some therapists. Common pitfalls in this stage of therapy include forgetting to give the patient advance notice that the letter is on its way. There should be time to consider with the patient their potential anxieties and hopes around receiving the letter. With some patients, the letter may activate their IPAF, and it can be experienced as a bad school report or work appraisal in those patients with a judgemental, critical other in the IPAF.

The therapist may write an overly lengthy letter that is too much for the patient to take in. The goodbye letter should not include surprises and new observations from the therapist that take the patient aback. It is best to discuss these in the context of the letter and then produce a revised draft of the letter for the next session. Some therapists fix the letter at the start of the ending phase; rather, it should be treated as a living document that is worked on until the last session. If there are changes to be made, then the letter can be sent to the patient after the work has ended. The letter can be introduced too rigidly, without allowing the patient some choice as to how they want to go through it in the session. We encourage the therapist and patient to go through the letter paragraph by paragraph so that it can be discussed in bite-sized chunks.

Both therapist and patient can avoid facing the ending and yet a quarter of the sessions in DIT are dedicated to this purpose. If a therapist is resistant to brief psychotherapy, this can find expression in the ending phase of the work, with a tendency to keep going as usual. Therapists do not always shift gear at the ending stage, where we are focused on evaluating the work we have done together, taking up the achievements alongside the disappointments, considering the challenges on the horizon, and thinking about our patients' future needs for support and how to access it if required. Part of this evaluation process includes repeating the relationship questionnaire (discussed in Chapter 4) and comparing the scores with those on the questionnaire they completed at the start of therapy. Although attachment styles are not expected to change radically, we do find meaningful shifts in patient scores that indicate greater awareness of their attachment vulnerabilities and the way this connects with the IPAF, as well as more acknowledgement of interpersonal anxiety. Therapists who find the relationship questionnaire challenging often forget to repeat it in the ending phase. We also find that therapists struggle to explore the unconscious meaning of the ending with their patients, perhaps linked to difficulties in taking up the transference with their patients during this stage of work.

SUMMARY

In this chapter, we have reviewed the different kinds of therapeutic challenges that may arise in the course of the therapeutic encounter from the point of view of both the patient and the DIT therapist. We hope that we have conveyed that exploring what happens in the transference is very important when there is a need to explore difficulties in the therapy, but, as we saw in Chapter 8, its use is more circumscribed than is the case in other psychodynamic models, as it is informed by the main strategies of DIT: exploring the IPAF; helping the patient to better understand their mental states; and encouraging change. The transference is also taken up early in DIT in relation to the 'cautionary tale' in order to address negative feelings and deepen the therapeutic alliance. We hope that in flagging up areas of the DIT model where therapists can go 'off-model' we can help to better understand our own points of vulnerability in relation to working with this model so that these can be anticipated and addressed.

REFERENCES

Freud, S. (1910). 'Wild' psycho-analysis. In J. Strachey (Ed.), *The standard edition of the complete psychological works of Sigmund Freud* (Vol. 11, pp. 219–228). Hogarth Press, 1957.

Glover, T. (1955). *Technique of psychoanalysis*. International Universities Press.

Greenson, R. R. (1967). *The technique and practice of psychoanalysis*. International Universities Press.

Joseph, B. (1983). On understanding and not understanding: Some technical issues. *International Journal of Psychoanalysis, 64*(3), 291–298.

Segal, H. (1993). Countertransference. In A. Alexandris, & G. Vaslamatzis (Eds.), *Countertransference: Theory, technique, teaching* (pp. 13–20). Karnac Books.

Steiner, J. (2000). Containment, enactment and communication. *International Journal of Psychoanalysis, 81*(2), 245–255. https://doi.org/10.1516/0020757001599735

11
Frequently Asked Questions

HOW DOES DIT DIFFER FROM INTERPERSONAL PSYCHOTHERAPY?

Dynamic interpersonal therapy (DIT) is significantly different from interpersonal psychotherapy (IPT). For a start, IPT is not a psychodynamic approach. However, both approaches share a clearly identified interpersonal focus and aim to help the patient to address current interpersonal problems, although they use very different strategies to do so. The IPT therapist achieves this primarily through formulating the patient's symptoms in the context of four predetermined focal areas, each with its specific strategies and goals. By contrast, DIT adopts a very idiographic approach to formulation, selecting a core unconscious pattern of interaction that is meaningfully connected to the patient's symptoms/difficulties. Distinctively, whereas DIT deploys the transference relationship as one of the ways of helping the patient work through the identified focus, in IPT the therapist does not work in the transference.

The differences between the two models are clearly reflected in the different competences required to deliver DIT and IPT (see Lemma et al., 2008; Lemma et al., 2010).

HOW DOES DIT DIFFER FROM OTHER BRIEF PSYCHODYNAMIC THERAPIES?

DIT explicitly draws on the manuals reviewed as part of the competence framework for the effective delivery of psychodynamic therapy (Lemma et al., 2008). To this extent we expect many colleagues who have developed other brief psychodynamic models to find features of their model reflected in DIT. One of the most interesting outcomes of the work on the competences was to bring to light the significant areas of technical overlap between models drawing on different theoretical traditions in psychoanalysis. All that DIT does is to systematically integrate into one protocol shared psychodynamic principles and techniques, grounded in the extant evidence base and required to deliver a time-limited intervention with depressed and/or anxious patients. This may be why DIT appears to be acceptable to therapists trained in a variety of psychodynamic traditions.

IS DIT A SUPPORTIVE PSYCHOTHERAPY?

If all brief psychodynamic models were to be placed on a continuum, ranging from the most expressive/exploratory to the most supportive, then without doubt DIT would be situated at the more supportive end of the spectrum. In this respect it is more explicitly supportive and strengthening of the patient's ego than intensive short-term dynamic psychotherapy, for example, which is more challenging of the patient's defensive structure. However, the supportive components of DIT sit alongside a systematic focus on a segment of the patient's interpersonal functioning, which is typically experienced by the patient as very challenging. The emphasis on helping the patient to try out new ways of managing their relationships, not just on developing insight, also challenges the patient's investment in the status quo. DIT therefore does require of the patient some capacity to withstand being challenged in this way. For this reason it would be contraindicated for patients who had no interest in and/or capacity to reflect on some of their own contribution to perpetuating unhelpful dynamics in their relationships.

IS DIT AN ADAPTATION OF MENTALIZATION-BASED TREATMENT FOR MOOD DISORDERS?

We believe that all psychotherapeutic approaches that are helpful to patients more or less explicitly support psychic change through facilitating the patient's capacity to reflect on their states of mind and those of others. The techniques used to this end differ between approaches, but the process they facilitate is probably shared. In other words, we see a focus on mentalizing as being a core feature of effective interventions with patients across a range of clinical presentations. Maintaining a focus on the patient's mind is core to DIT—but this is not the same as saying that DIT is a form of mentalization-based treatment (MBT).

MBT was originally developed for the treatment of patients with borderline personality disorder (BPD), who typically show significant deficits in their capacity to mentalize; hence the assiduous focus on mentalizing, which is the hallmark of MBT, along with a range of other interventions targeting the needs of this particular patient group (Bateman & Fonagy, 2016). However, not all depressed or anxious patients share with BPD patients this more characteristic primary mentalizing deficit, at least not to the same degree. Of course, we all experience some failures of mentalizing on a daily basis, and when we feel depressed and/or anxious our capacity to mentalize is undermined to an even greater degree, but these failures are not invariably the central deficit in an individual's mood disorder. Thus, in the DIT protocol we do make use of mentalizing techniques when the patient's capacity for reflection is weak. However, unlike in MBT, this is not the central focus; DIT is rooted in a psychodynamic approach suited to neurotic patients, with a greater emphasis on the interpretation of transference and of the patient's defensive manoeuvres. In the DIT for complex care (DITCC) adaptation for secondary care patients with histories of personality disorder and trauma, we use mentalizing techniques more regularly, and the work is more closely aligned to MBT approaches (see Chapter 13).

HOW CENTRAL IS WORKING IN THE TRANSFERENCE IN DIT?

It is very central to the therapist's understanding, but it is not a predominant or even a primary technique. That is, understanding of transference is central to the therapist's model, but is not always referred to by the therapist in interpretations to the patient. Any negative transference is taken up early in therapy in relation to the 'cautionary tale' (see Chapter 4), to strengthen the therapeutic alliance. DIT draws on a range of other interventions, such as more supportive interventions, mentalizing interventions, and, more sparingly, some directive interventions.

In DIT, the therapist approaches the clinical situation with three main therapeutic priorities in mind: (a) to help the patient to explore the interpersonal-affective focus (IPAF), (b) to help the patient to reflect on their states of mind, and (c) to make some changes in relation to the problematic relational pattern. The choice of techniques is determined by these priorities; hence, the transference is used when and if it supports these strategies, which in practice is often, but not always.

WHAT TRAINING DO I NEED TO PRACTISE DIT?

DIT was explicitly developed to support psychodynamically trained therapists and counsellors to hone their existing skills and experience in order to deliver a brief psychodynamic intervention for the treatment of mood disorders. Entry into the standard training therefore requires a diploma-level or equivalent qualification in psychodynamic therapy or counselling, followed by a five-day course and two supervised cases, which are audio (or ideally video) recorded and rated for adherence to the protocol. This is not a protocol that can be implemented without prior demonstrable competence in working psychodynamically, but it does not require prior training in intensive (i.e. more than once weekly) psychodynamic therapy. The DIT training and supervision protocol is set out in Appendix 5.

More recently, we have developed a twenty-day DIT training programme, which was designed for clinicians without prior psychodynamic training. In this extended programme, we introduced video recording as a requirement because we felt that it was necessary in order to assess and support the therapist's ability to focus on holding an analytic stance, the frame and setting, alongside learning the specific DIT interventions. Where possible, we recommend video recording sessions for training and supervision, but, apart from in the twenty-day format, it is not a requirement.

DOES THE DIT THERAPIST WORK WITH DREAMS AND UNCONSCIOUS PHANTASIES?

Yes, definitely. However, as we have emphasized throughout this book, the primary strategy in DIT is to support the working through of the selected IPAF. In other words, dreams and unconscious phantasies may be interpreted if they serve the function of illustrating to the patient the activation of the IPAF in their current life and interpersonal context. Of course, the function of a patient's use of sessions is always important to monitor. If a patient mostly brings dreams to their DIT sessions, we would be curious about what might be avoided by focusing on their dream life (e.g. intense dreams might be a welcome distraction from coming back to the IPAF), and in some cases a patient might be trying to please the therapist by reporting dreams (which they might assume all therapists want).

DOES THE DIT THERAPIST USE THE COUNTERTRANSFERENCE AS THE BASIS FOR INTERVENING?

Yes. Using the countertransference to inform the therapist's understanding of what is transpiring between themselves and the patient is central to DIT. Without consideration of the impact the patient has on the therapist we cannot see how therapists could arrive at a comprehensive understanding of the patient, or how they can effectively manage difficulties in the therapeutic relationship. Again, this is something the therapist can think about privately and with a supervisor, rather than speaking to the patient about their reactions.

DOES DIT FOCUS ON THE PATIENT'S PAST?

Yes and no. DIT is underpinned by an understanding of developmental theory, which contextualizes the patient's current functioning in light of developmental models of 'self-in-relation-to-an-other', which have been internalized on the basis of early experience with significant attachment figures. Although such an understanding of the early origins of internalized object relationships is important, the focus of the therapist's efforts is to help the patient understand the way in which the pattern itself is active in their current life and relationships. We would also be interested in the timing of when a patient moves to speak about their past, and consider whether this is a defensive manoeuvre away from the heat of here-and-now relationships.

The focus in DIT on the activation in the present of internalized object relationships is consistent with most contemporary psychodynamic models, where reconstruction of the past is no longer regarded as the primary intervention leading to psychic change. Having said this, given DIT's brevity and the importance of formulation within this protocol, there is a place for helping the patient to contextualize their difficulties with reference to significant experiences in their life that may feel especially salient for them or that may have been unhelpfully neglected. The formulation arrived at in early sessions of DIT therefore draws on an understanding of the early origins of the problems, to provide the patient with a narrative that will orient them to the task in hand and is focused on working on their current relationships.

WHAT SHOULD I EXPECT IF I CHOOSE TO TRAIN IN DIT?

The first thing to say is that it is always harder (not least on one's narcissism!) to learn an adaptation of an already acquired model. This is partly because learning to deliver an adaptation, such as DIT, will expose you to ideas and techniques that are familiar (and hence ones that you will most likely feel competent in) but are nevertheless integrated in ways that will feel more or less unfamiliar, and this may leave you feeling somehow wrong-footed and incompetent. It might possibly also feel in conflict with a training superego that proscribes some of the techniques that are actively encouraged in this protocol.

In our experience, the steepest learning curve is in the requirement to explicitly formulate and then work assiduously to a focus (the IPAF). This involves tolerating what often feels like 'ignoring' fascinating aspects of the patient's varied and complex mental life. Therapists regularly feel that this is even more challenging than integrating outcome monitoring into every session, where that is a requirement of the service in which they are working.

REFERENCES

Bateman, A., & Fonagy, P. (2016). *Mentalization-based treatment for personality disorders: A practical guide* (2nd edn). Oxford University Press.

Lemma, A., Roth, A. D., & Pilling, S. (2008). *The competences required to deliver effective psychoanalytic/psychodynamic therapy*. Research Department of Clinical, Educational and Health Psychology, University College London. https://www.ucl.ac.uk/pals/sites/pals/files/ppc_clinicians_background_paper.pdf

Lemma, A., Target, M., & Fonagy, P. (2010). The development of a brief psychodynamic protocol for depression: Dynamic interpersonal therapy (DIT). *Psychoanalytic Psychotherapy, 24*(4), 329–346. https://doi.org/10.1080/02668734.2010.513547

12

Research on Psychotherapy Outcomes, Fidelity and Mechanisms of Change in Dynamic Interpersonal Therapy

The evidence base of dynamic interpersonal therapy (DIT), as for most interventions for depression, depends less on the outcome of randomized controlled trials (RCTs) of DIT itself and more on the general strength of empirical support for short-term psychodynamic interventions for depression. There are two reasons for this.

First, national guidelines for the treatment of depression tend to take large-scale reviews of the major categories of psychological interventions as their data source (e.g. National Institute for Health and Care Excellence, 2019; National Institute for Health and Care Excellence, 2022). Such reviews tend to ignore differences between specific implementations of major categories of therapy. Instead, psychological therapies are classified into modalities or types (e.g. interpersonal psychotherapy). DIT is an example of a brief psychodynamic psychotherapy, and its credibility is highly influenced by findings about the effectiveness of this larger group of psychoanalytically rooted interventions relative to other available therapies.

Second, whether the therapy is implemented in a particular context depends on evidence beyond RCTs, as well as other contextual factors. Evidence from RCTs might be considered necessary, but it is not sufficient. The validity of the psychological model that explains pathology (symptoms) as well as therapeutic benefit is increasingly regarded as crucial evidence (Kazdin, 2009). Practice-based evidence (i.e. how well the treatment is working for patients seen in clinical practice) is critical (Cartwright & Munro, 2010). Patient preferences are important, particularly if outcomes do not differ greatly between available alternative therapies. There are also pragmatic considerations, such as the breadth and prevalence of conditions encountered in the service, the availability of trained clinicians, the availability and cost of training for clinicians who wish to train, and, of course, the therapy's compatibility with the culture of the health service provider.

THE META-ANALYTIC EVIDENCE BASE OF PSYCHODYNAMIC THERAPY FOR DEPRESSION

Clinically meaningful exploration of the available scientific information about psychotherapy is surprisingly complicated. Narrative reviews that summarize and synthesize a body of research rely on the statistical significance of a study. This is determined by many issues of internal and external validity, including the use of appropriate statistics and, importantly, an appropriate sample size (which needs to be large enough to enable the detection of a statistically significant difference). Meta-analyses get around some of the need for detailed study of individual investigations and enable information to be integrated by pooling several studies that individually have too few participants, as is commonly the case with psychotherapy research. Meta-analyses yield meaningful conclusions only if the studies that are pooled are homogeneous in terms of their target population, the method of treatment, and the outcome measures used. Fortunately, this is the case for studies of psychological therapies for depression.

A meta-analysis of eight major types of psychological treatments reported on the integrated findings of 308 RCTs with more than 31,000 patients in total (Cuijpers et al., 2021). The review included nineteen studies of psychodynamic psychotherapy and six other modes of treatment. All therapies had significant effects compared with care as usual and waiting list control conditions. This most recent finding confirms a number of previous meta-analyses (Abbass et al., 2014; Barber et al., 2021; Cuijpers et al., 2020; Driessen et al., 2015). This meta-analysis provided an exhaustive comparison of six other contrasting modalities of therapy and showed that the effects of the therapies did not differ significantly from each other. When considered pairwise (head-to-head), all therapies were more effective than care as usual or waiting list control groups, but there were no significant differences between the major therapeutic orientations considered (cognitive-behavioural therapy (CBT), behavioural activation, problem-solving therapy, 'third-wave' CBT, psychodynamic therapy, interpersonal psychotherapy, and non-directive supportive counselling). Only counselling was significantly less effective than CBT, problem-solving therapy, and psychodynamic therapy. This means that a prominent role can be given to patient preference when choosing a therapy (Cuijpers et al., 2021). The conclusions of this meta-analysis reflect the current UK guidelines for the treatment of depression issued by the National Institute for Health and Care Excellence (2022) and other recently published meta-analyses and systematic reviews (Leichsenring et al., 2023; Wienicke et al., 2023).

A systematic umbrella review of meta-analyses and systematic reviews (Barber et al., 2021; Driessen et al., 2015) reported that brief psychodynamic therapy for depression was effective in reducing the severity of depression, and in improving patients' quality of life and interpersonal functioning (Leichsenring et al., 2023). Moreover, this review found that the quality of studies investigating the effectiveness of brief psychodynamic treatment for depression was good and that the risk of publication bias was low. Overall, the available evidence was rated as moderate for comparisons with other active treatments, such as CBT, and good for comparisons with control treatments.

Typically, about 40–50% of patients show a response (defined as a 50% reduction in symptoms of depression) to brief psychotherapies, including brief psychodynamic therapy, and about one-third of patients show remission. These improvements are generally maintained at longer-term follow-up. These findings concerning response and remission are similar to those found for other evidence-based treatments for depression, and indicate the need for longer-term treatment for a subgroup of patients. Importantly, there is preliminary evidence that these findings also generalize to minority groups, although effect sizes may be smaller in these groups, and more research in this context is needed (Driessen et al., 2013). Similarly, more research concerning the cost-effectiveness of brief psychodynamic treatment for depression is needed, although there is preliminary evidence for similar cost-effectiveness to other evidence-based treatments (Town et al., 2020). There is also a need for more research concerning the combination of brief psychodynamic treatment and pharmacotherapy. In a recent meta-analysis of individual participant data, brief psychodynamic treatment combined with antidepressants was more efficacious than a single therapy (i.e. either brief psychodynamic treatment or pharmacotherapy), but the effect size at treatment termination was relatively small ($d = 0.26$, $p = 0.01$) (Driessen et al., 2020).

Traditional meta-analyses are dependent on the quality of study-level information that is reported in a publication. This can lead to an exaggeration of the size of the effect of the treatment under consideration (Tudur Smith et al., 2016). More importantly, meta-analyses are rarely able to provide information about the kind of person who is most likely to benefit from a particular therapy. For that type of information, meta-analyses draw on many studies with relatively distinct populations where effect sizes can be looked at in relation to the average of the study samples. However, these so-called moderation analyses may be misleading because a characteristic at study level may not reflect data at an individual level: no one is an 'average' patient.

In recent years, more and more studies have been undertaken in which individual participant data are used in a meta-analysis based on a substantial number of investigators submitting their raw data for a single combined analysis. Meta-analyses based on pooled individual participant data can standardize data analysis, verify the results from the contributing studies, analyse data that were not originally reported, and, most helpfully, look at potential moderator effects and answer the question of which treatment(s) work best for which patients.

Recently, Wienicke et al. (2023) have collated data from thirteen studies of psychodynamic therapy with over 800 participants. On the basis of this analysis, people with relatively high levels of depression at baseline appear to benefit more from brief psychodynamic therapy than individuals with lower levels of baseline depression. More research is needed to replicate this post-hoc finding.

There is also growing evidence for the efficacy of internet-delivered brief psychodynamic treatment. A recent meta-analysis found that internet-delivered psychodynamic therapy was more effective than control treatments, with a medium effect size ($g = -0.46$, 95%

CI: [−0.73, −0.19], I^2 = 23%, k = 5, n = 359) (Lindegaard et al., 2020). (Internet-delivered DIT is discussed in Chapter 15.)

Finally, there is good evidence to suggest that these findings may generalize to routine clinical practice (Department of Health, 2012; Gaskell et al., 2023). Taken together, these findings confirm that psychodynamic psychotherapy is efficacious for depression, and improvements at individual level on measures of anxiety, general psychopathology, and quality of life suggest that its effect is broader than just an impact on depression. So psychodynamic therapy is 'evidence-based'; but what about DIT specifically?

THE EVIDENCE BASE FOR DIT

DIT is a relatively new therapy compared with other short-term psychotherapies, even within the psychodynamic family of treatments. However, there is evidence supporting its value. At the time of the manualization of DIT over a decade ago, we were keen to establish that practice-based evidence supported its use. In a pilot study in the UK of sixteen participants consecutively recruited from National Health Service (NHS) primary care mental health provision (a programme at that time termed Improving Access to Psychological Therapies (IAPT)), we saw substantial clinical benefits for patients presenting with a mixture of anxiety and depression (Lemma et al., 2011b). The trajectories of individual patients in this small sample were followed so that we could learn more about the way DIT worked. We collected session-by-session outcomes for anxiety and depression over sixteen sessions. When we fitted statistical models to the data, we found that patients with the most severe depression did less well, although all patients improved earlier in the course of therapy. Towards the end of the therapy, patients with the highest scores for depression were more likely to lose the improvements they had made. Interestingly, self-reported anxiety improved even more than self-reported depression during the course of DIT.

A further small experimental study two years later explored whether an implementation provided online could be equally efficacious (Lemma & Fonagy, 2013). In this exploration of the DIT model, online self-help was contrasted with either therapist-facilitated or unfacilitated group meetings. The platform for the intervention was a website dedicated to offering support to individuals with mental health problems, primarily via the provision of educational materials and advice. We introduced random assignment into this trial and, to our surprise, found that with therapist facilitation the intervention achieved 75% remission. Even without therapist facilitation, the online implementation achieved remission in half the participants. Only 25% of participants assigned to self-help alone (without the theoretical and clinical framework of DIT) reached remission. This small pilot study, with only twenty-four participants, has little scientific value other than as a demonstration of principle. However, it does suggest that the psychological model that DIT provides can be helpful to individuals who are actively struggling to find a way through depression.

These preliminary studies were undertaken to establish the feasibility of an RCT (Randomized Evaluation of DIT (REDIT)) to test the superiority of DIT to low-intensity care, which was care as usual within IAPT (Fonagy et al., 2020). The trial also attempted to establish whether it was feasible to randomize participants to either DIT or CBT for a subsequent test of equivalence. This RCT of DIT was a so-called pragmatic trial, which means that the treatment took place more or less under the conditions in which services would be delivered to the same group of patients, and that the sample with whom the treatment was tested was very similar to the population to whom the treatment would be ultimately offered (not specially selected for the study).

In this study, 140 patients were randomized: 68 to the DIT arm, 53 to a control intervention, and 19 to CBT. Of the patients, 39% presented with mild depression, 47% with moderate depression, and 14% with severe depression as scored on the Hamilton Depression Rating Scale. On the Beck Depression Inventory, which categorizes patients in a different way, 6% of the sample scored in the mild range, 23% in the moderate range, and 71% in the severe range. The trial lasted 6 months, with the same time allowed for following up the DIT group.

At 6 months, the treatment effect size was approximately 0.7 of a standard deviation (representing a moderate effect size). Reliable improvement was defined as a pre–post difference on the Hamilton Depression Rating Scale greater than 4.8 and a change on the self-rated Beck Depression Inventory greater than 7.6. About half of the DIT patients showed clinically significant changes, compared with only 9% in the control group. Although all groups improved rapidly over the treatment period, on average the control group reached a plateau between the middle and the end of treatment. Thus, by the end of the treatment there was a substantial difference between the DIT group and the control group. The benefits from DIT were maintained at 12-month follow-up. There was no significant difference between DIT and CBT.

Relative to the control group, DIT patients also showed reductions in both the severity and the distress of general psychopathology and a reduction in social problems, with specific improvements in relation to problems at work and with friends. Finally, DIT patients reported higher health-related quality-of-life scores than control group patients.

This was the first RCT of the effects of DIT on moderate to severe depression performed in the context where this treatment is mostly administered in the UK (at that time within the programme of IAPT services; now within NHS primary care). Although symptomatic improvements were substantial, benefits on measures of attachment and interpersonal problems were less obvious.

A strength of this initial trial is that the control group received a low-intensity treatment that was actually provided as standard within the IAPT system and resembles good-quality routine NHS primary care support, and thus can be considered a bona fide intervention. It is also encouraging that, unlike the initial feasibility study, in this investigation the participants with relatively severe depression also showed significant improvements.

The feasibility study embedded in this investigation was also reassuring. It indicated that participants readily accepted randomization to either DIT or CBT, and per-protocol treatments and assessments were delivered to most participants. When offered randomization to DIT or CBT, no patient refused the therapy, and all took up the treatment to which they were assigned. However, 25% in each group terminated their interventions early, and only 85% of the CBT group and 80% of the DIT group were available for assessment at 6 months. These are indications that a trial to demonstrate the equivalence of these two forms of treatment is feasible.

What should the shape of such a trial be? We already know that CBT and DIT have comparable outcomes in terms of symptoms of depression. The question that perhaps needs answering most urgently is whether training in these two modalities achieves similar outcomes, with similar costs, delivering comparably efficient treatments in terms of the time taken to reach a target improvement (e.g. a 50% reduction in depression). We envisage a study that randomizes clinicians trained in humanistic supportive counselling—the only treatment that appears to be slightly less effective for depression than other treatments—to continue to practise counselling or to be trained to deliver either CBT or DIT during a 1-year training. A careful health economics study could then map the relative cost of training therapists to accredited status along with measuring their therapeutic success over the course of their training and the year that follows.

We have started establishing the feasibility of such an approach with a cohort of twenty-six counsellors undertaking extended DIT training over the course of a year (Khalastchy et al., 2021). The training is comparable in length to what CBT therapists currently undertake. Our preliminary data show that the recovery and remission rates achieved by therapists in training, even when they had no previous background in psychodynamic therapy, are quickly comparable to those achieved in NHS primary care services. We do not know whether trainees would agree to randomization in the way the ideal study design might require.

In another RCT, conducted in China (Wang et al., 2023)[1], patients with depression were randomized to either 16 weeks of DIT plus antidepressant medication (ADM) (DIT + ADM; n = 66), general supportive therapy (GST) plus ADM (GST + ADM; n = 75), or ADM alone (n = 70). Results showed that both DIT + ADM and GST + ADM were superior to ADM alone at treatment termination; no differences were observed between the DIT and GST groups. At 12-month follow-up, DIT was superior to GST + ADM in reducing symptoms of depression, although these follow-up findings must be interpreted with caution given the high attrition during the follow-up phase. This independent replication of the effectiveness of DIT is important not only in itself, but also because it demonstrates that the DIT model can be effectively adapted and implemented in another cultural context.

---

1. In this study, DIT was implemented by clinicians to whom we had taught the model; however, the cases were not supervised by qualified DIT supervisors or trainers.

Other ongoing randomized trials, if successful, have the potential to strengthen the evidence base for DIT. A large multi-site trial designed and led by one of the authors of this book (PL) will contrast CBT and DIT as both normally delivered and blended (i.e. a combination of online work and face-to-face sessions) treatments. Our aim remains improving access to treatment. By reducing therapeutic input, as is typical of blended DIT (see Chapter 15), the number of patients who could benefit from the DIT model could be increased.

We also have some pilot data on DIT for complex care (DITCC) (Rao et al., 2019). In this study, fifteen patients underwent an extended course of DIT (described in Chapter 13). The average inter-session change over twenty-six sessions was about one-third of a point on the Patient Health Questionnaire-9. Perhaps a more meaningful result is that two-thirds of the participants showed improvement on the measure of depression, and in half of these the improvement was clinically highly significant. Interestingly, reminiscent of the pilot study of DIT (Lemma et al., 2011b), the study found that anxiety demonstrated even more marked improvement, with 60% of participants showing clinically significant change and almost three-quarters showing improvement over the period.

There is also evidence from naturalistic studies for the effectiveness of DIT in patients with post-traumatic stress disorder (Chen et al., 2019; Chen et al., 2020; Feldman et al., 2023) and somatoform disorder (Selders et al., 2015), again demonstrating the potential of adaptations of the DIT approach for other disorders and populations. DIT has also recently been piloted in group format, with promising results (Folkes-Skinner & Collins, 2022).

Indications of practice-based evidence outcomes are perhaps most relevant to showing the effectiveness of DIT. Fortunately, the IAPT programme collected outcome data on 98% of patients who were in treatment in the service (Clark, 2018; Department of Health, 2012). Although this evidence is difficult to interpret because patients were referred to different treatment arms according to local beliefs about suitability, and thus 'league tables' of different treatment approaches are most likely misleading, by and large DIT did as well as the other therapies offered in these services.

So, there is practice-based evidence for DIT. Earlier, we mentioned the importance of the breadth of an approach to treatment so it can be seen to be addressing many problems commonly presented by patients attending a service. We are fortunate in relation to DIT in this regard, as its scope has increased considerably since it was introduced, and it is now able to address physical as well as psychological problems that are often seen in community mental health services (Luyten & Fonagy, 2020). Preliminary clinical evidence of the value of this approach is briefly considered in Chapter 14. Patient preference is another important consideration in service implementation. At the time of writing we do not have data on patient preference in relation to DIT, but we believe that the interpersonal focus of DIT would make it a popular choice with patients, along with IPT and third-wave therapies (Cuijpers et al., 2021).

The major current obstacle facing DIT is neither lack of evidence nor lack of popularity. It is that there are currently too few DIT therapists to make a substantial contribution across existing services, although the numbers are increasing. We hope that trials that test the effectiveness of training programmes alongside testing the effectiveness of the therapy will strengthen interest in brief psychodynamic psychotherapy in NHS primary care services. To deliver treatments that adhere to its principles and processes we need adequate measures of adherence and competence. It is to this issue that we will now turn.

RESEARCH ON FIDELITY TO PSYCHODYNAMIC PRINCIPLES IN DIT

When judging the quality of delivery of a manualized psychological treatment such as DIT (Perepletchikova & Kazdin, 2005), treatment fidelity, adherence, and competence need to be considered[2]. Treatment *fidelity* refers to the extent to which the intended treatments are delivered. *Adherence* refers to the part of fidelity that captures the extent to which the pre-specified techniques are used in a specific therapy.

---

2. This section of the chapter is essentially based on the work of Dr Tamara Ventura Wurman, MD, PhD. The research cited is her work on the REDIT study audiotapes. The measure developed by Dr Ventura Wurman (2019) is, to our knowledge, the first to convincingly link therapeutic competence to treatment outcome, and we are privileged to be able to give this important contribution a brief preliminary exposure here.

Competence is a separate aspect of fidelity and refers to the therapist's level of skill in implementing the treatment manual.

Fidelity as a predictor of outcome

It is generally assumed that treatment fidelity will be positively related to outcome. If not, then what is the purpose of writing treatment manuals—such as this book? Surprisingly, the most comprehensive quantitative review of thirty-six studies in this field suggests that fidelity plays only a very small role, if any, in explaining the outcome of treatment (Webb et al., 2010). This meta-analysis found that the effects of adherence and competence on outcome were not significantly different from zero. In defence of the fidelity hypothesis, the meta-analysis also found considerable heterogeneity in studies of the relationship between fidelity and therapeutic outcome. The few studies that examined the correlation between therapist competence and outcome in psychodynamic psychotherapy also reported mixed results (e.g. Barber et al., 1996; Barber et al., 2008; Sandell, 1985; Shaw & Dobson, 1988; Svartberg et al., 1996; Svartberg & Stiles, 1992; Svartberg & Stiles, 1994). Unsurprisingly, there are no generally accepted assessment tools to measure therapeutic competence in psychodynamic therapy. Given how complex such a measure would need to be, it is not difficult to appreciate why, until recently (Ventura Wurman, 2019), no such instrument was available for DIT.

The REDIT trial also planned to assess the influence of adherence and competence, rated from audio-recorded sessions, on depression-related outcomes. A total of 172 audio-recorded DIT sessions were coded to study treatment fidelity (Ventura Wurman, 2019). Two measures were developed specifically to assess treatment fidelity in DIT and were published in the first edition of this book (Lemma et al., 2011a). The mean adherence total score was 19.26 (SD = 3.02), suggesting that most participants received treatments with high levels of adherence (the maximum total adherence score was 21). Likewise, the mean competence total score was high (mean = 161.52, SD = 28.94; maximum total competence score 216), which also suggested that most patients had therapists who displayed, on the basis of these ratings, relatively good competence. Despite the careful rating of a large number of sessions, there was no statistically significant association between the outcome of a treatment and therapists' adherence to key DIT therapist actions, or therapists' competence in delivering these actions with any patient.

Developing a measure of competence

We do not have space in this chapter to comprehensively describe the development of the competence rating scale now used for DIT. An attempt was made to create a simple but theory-based measure of psychodynamic therapeutic competence (Ventura Wurman, 2019) based around the framework of competences for psychodynamic therapies devised by Lemma et al. (2008). This new instrument, the Therapist Competence Scale (TCS), was also informed by a comprehensive thematic analysis of consultations with clinicians considered to be experts in the delivery of DIT. The TCS aimed to capture both general competences, such as engaging the patient, and specific competences required for delivering specific psychodynamic interventions (e.g. interpretations), competences within specific domains (e.g. being attuned and making the patient feel understood), and global competence, which is an intuitive judgement of the overall level of competence shown by the therapist in a session.

The final scale was composed of two subscales and two global ratings. The first subscale included forty-two core competences grouped according to seventeen fundamental aims that psychodynamic psychotherapists are likely to bring to any one session: (1) to create psychic space where it is possible to think together with the patient; (2) containment; (3) to help the patient think for themselves; (4) to foster the patient's epistemic trust (Fonagy & Allison, 2014; Fonagy et al., 2019; see also Chapter 13); (5) to centre the psychotherapeutic work around unconscious processes; (6) to be able to think about themselves in the room with the patient; (7) to promote the patient's psychic and behavioural change; (8) to help the patient grieve; (9) to create an environment of safety; (10) to foster and maintain the therapeutic alliance; (11) to engage the patient in therapy; (12) to promote mentalizing; (13) to have in mind the patient's traits and states of mind; (14) to promote and expand the patient's self-knowledge and self-awareness; (15) to promote and expand the patient's knowledge and awareness of their relational patterns; (16) to help the patient self-regulate emotions; and (17) to manage the patient's defences. A revised version of the competence scale, which we use in DIT at present to evaluate recorded sessions and which is underpinned by Ventura Wurman's (2019) work, is provided in Appendix 3.

The second subscale was made up of thirty-eight 'regrettable' actions and attitudes that therapists can sometimes display in sessions, organized into seven groups: (1) enactments and/or concrete interventions; (2) inability to foster the therapeutic alliance; (3) not adapting the interventions to the patient or context and not considering the consequences of the interventions; (4) lacking the basic skills to intervene; (5) therapists' mental health issues; (6) not accurately understanding the patient; and (7) incompetence in DIT.

Finally, the TCS includes a rating of the complexity presented by the patient. This subscale is based on the model of epistemic trust and epistemic vigilance (Fonagy et al., 2019) and intends to reflect the patient's openness to socially transmitted information, in this case the knowledge and understanding conveyed by the therapist. This subscale aimed to capture the level of challenge presented by a patient as judged by an expert rater, and is influenced by the individual's capacity to work productively in a psychodynamic treatment. The patient complexity subscale can be found in Appendix 4.

In terms of basic psychometrics, the competence subscale of the TCS presented excellent internal consistency (intraclass correlation coefficient (ICC) = 0.994) and a good level of inter-rater reliability (ICC = 0.790). The global competence rating presented a good level of inter-rater reliability (ICC = 0.756), but the inter-rater reliability of the patient complexity rating was only moderate (ICC = 0.524). Obviously of greatest interest to us is the ability of this new measure of clinical skill to identify therapeutic outcome as associated with competence within a session, competence associated with a particular individual therapist or, most ambitiously, competence associated with the rate of change that a therapist can achieve with a patient given the level of severity of their depression or the complexity of the challenge they present to the therapist. The investigation undertaken involved 284 audio-recorded sessions—65 from the initial phase, 169 from the middle phase, and 50 from the ending phase (Ventura Wurman, 2019)—involving 17 therapists and 68 patients.

The findings that emerged were robust. Higher levels of competence in DIT sessions were associated with a faster rate of patient improvement, especially with patients with greater severity of depression at the start of therapy. Across sessions, therapists who were rated as more competent in terms of their recorded interactions produced better outcomes. Importantly, in addition to and concurrently with this linear effect, sessions in which therapists were neither particularly low nor particularly high in competence were the most likely to achieve good outcomes. Furthermore, there was evidence that the most competent therapists worked most effectively with the most complex patients. Less competent therapists had poorer outcomes when treating individuals with high complexity.

Clinical implications

What do these research findings tell us about DIT, how therapists are trained in DIT, and how DIT is implemented? First, we should note that as far as we know, this study is the first published in the psychodynamic literature to establish statistically sound relationships between clinical competence and robust measures of outcome.

When DIT sessions are competently delivered, patients recover more quickly. Greater psychodynamic therapist competence brings about better clinical outcomes. All this is strong evidence for the theoretical approach described in this book. All the competency items were drawn from psychotherapists who are DIT developers or supervisors and who might be expected to highlight aspects of technique embraced within the DIT model. The more these recommendations are implemented, the faster and greater the patients' improvement is.

It is slightly puzzling that high levels of competence in sessions were, on average, linked to slightly worse outcomes than medium levels of competence. Does this suggest that we should encourage therapists not to try too hard? The answer is maybe. The literature on rupture and repair in psychotherapy may be relevant here (Eubanks, Goldfried, et al., 2019; Eubanks, Muran, et al., 2019; Safran & Muran, 2000; Safran et al., 2011). Sessions in which therapists display high levels of competence are also ones where ruptures in the alliance are unlikely to be noted. However, ruptures may trigger a process of repair where explorations between the therapist and patient become deeper. In Chapter 13 of this book we discuss the benefits of the 'we-mode' in terms of opening the therapeutic space for a freer exchange of ideas between a patient and therapist working collaboratively with greater epistemic trust. Thus, it could be that trying too hard to be competent actually deprives our patients of repair and the experience of meeting us where we really are. Seeing our fallibility and our missteps, which can create a rupture, may actually be of greater benefit to our patients than seeing an image of us as always at the top of our game.

This study perhaps underemphasizes the importance of therapist effects because the variability between the therapists in terms of competence was small. There were only seventeen therapists and they came from very similar backgrounds. However, in the research literature, therapist effects only rarely amount to more than 5% of variance in treatment outcome. Given that therapists differ in very many ways besides their competence, it is encouraging that, notwithstanding the small number and homogeneity of the therapists in the study, the competence measures developed identified at least 3% of variance. In other words, competence captures more than two-thirds of the variability directly attributable to therapists in terms of outcome.

WORKING MECHANISMS OF DIT

Although there is growing evidence for the effectiveness of DIT, much remains to be learned in relation to its working mechanisms. In fact, this is currently the case for every type of psychotherapy (Cuijpers et al., 2019). Studies so far suggest that both common factors (working mechanisms shared by all types of psychotherapy) and specific factors (working mechanisms that are specific to psychodynamic therapy) account for the effects of brief psychodynamic therapy for depression (Leichsenring et al., 2023). For example, there is evidence that a positive therapeutic alliance (a common factor) is associated with outcome in brief psychodynamic treatment for depression. At the same time, there is evidence that increases in insight, changes in the use of defence mechanisms, improvements in mentalizing, and increased capacity for emotional experiencing—factors that are more specifically associated with psychodynamic therapy—are related to positive outcomes in the treatment of depression. Hilsenroth et al. (2003) found a strong association between an emphasis on interpersonal relationships and the outcome ($r = 0.57$, $p < 0.01$) in brief psychodynamic treatment of depression, consistent with the strong interpersonal focus in DIT.

However, more research on the working mechanisms of DIT specifically is needed, and the results of several ongoing studies in this context are expected soon. In the meantime, two qualitative studies (Leonidaki et al., 2016, 2018) investigating the effective ingredients of DIT, as reported by patients, suggest that DIT provided patients with more insight into previously hidden aspects of the self; the relational exchange with the therapist challenged intimate fears; patients moved towards a better interpersonal understanding of their difficulties; and the treatment helped them to develop a more coherent narrative of their life and problems. Hence, overall, patients tended to describe an interplay between relational/mentalizing and insight-oriented mechanisms, consistent with the DIT model's proposed theory of change. Importantly, although patients appreciated the activity and direction provided by the DIT therapists, the time-limited nature of DIT was seen as presenting a challenge—but also as presenting opportunity for change. A recent qualitative study in the Netherlands of an adaptation of DIT for patients with Cluster C personality disorders largely replicated these findings (Cuyt et al., 2022).

More research is also needed concerning the effectiveness of DIT for different subgroups of patients. One interesting approach in this regard is to investigate whether DIT is more effective in patients with particular types of interpersonal-affective focus (IPAF), the recurring interpersonal pattern that is connected to the patient's presenting symptoms and is taken as the central focus in DIT (see Chapter 5). To this end, McFarquhar et al. (2023) developed a typology for classifying IPAFs based on contemporary interpersonal approaches. Based on qualitative analysis of transcriptions of audio recordings of DIT sessions from the REDIT trial discussed earlier in this chapter, four types of IPAFs were identified, which were described as: hostile–dominant, hostile–submissive, friendly–dominant, or friendly–submissive. This typology may assist DIT therapists in formulating an IPAF with their patients. Further research is also needed to uncover whether there is an association between these IPAF types and outcome, particularly because previous work (McFarquhar et al., 2018) suggested that pretreatment affiliation is associated with better outcomes than low affiliation, while more hostile–dominant patients might struggle to develop an interpersonal focus and a positive therapeutic alliance, and as a result may show poorer treatment outcome. Whether this is the case in DIT awaits further research.

CONCLUSIONS

The existing research literature broadly supports the validity of DIT, its effectiveness, and its theoretical assumptions. We recognize that much more work is needed but anticipate that ongoing major investigations will deliver more findings soon. Trials of DITCC and DIT training would both be valuable, as would more research on the TCS, which is being used in training and routine practice. Findings inconsistent with our expectations would be particularly welcome, as they could enable us to improve DIT for patients.

REFERENCES

Abbass, A. A., Kisely, S. R., Town, J. M., Leichsenring, F., Driessen, E., De Maat, S., Gerber, A., Dekker, J., Rabung, S., Rusalovska, S., & Crowe, E. (2014). Short-term psychodynamic psychotherapies for common mental disorders. *Cochrane Database of Systematic Reviews, 2014*(7), CD004687. https://doi.org/10.1002/14651858.CD004687.pub4

Barber, J. P., Crits-Christoph, P., & Luborsky, L. (1996). Effects of therapist adherence and competence on patient outcome in brief dynamic therapy. *Journal of Consulting and Clinical Psychology, 64*(3), 619–622. https://doi.org/10.1037//0022-006x.64.3.619

Barber, J. P., Gallop, R., Crits-Christoph, P., Barrett, M. S., Klostermann, S., McCarthy, K. S., & Sharpless, B. A. (2008). The role of the alliance and techniques in predicting outcome of supportive-expressive dynamic therapy for cocaine dependence. *Psychoanalytic Psychology, 25*(3), 461–482. https://doi.org/10.1037/0736-9735.25.3.461

Barber, J. P., Muran, J. C., McCarthy, K. S., Keefe, J. R., & Zilcha-Mano, S. (2021). Research on dynamic therapies. In M. Barkham, W. Lutz & L. G. Castonguay (Eds.), *Bergin and Garfield's handbook of psychotherapy and behavior change* (7th edn., pp. 387–419). John Wiley & Sons.

Cartwright, N., & Munro, E. (2010). The limitations of randomized controlled trials in predicting effectiveness. *Journal of Evaluation in Clinical Practice, 16*(2), 260–266. https://doi.org/10.1111/j.1365-2753.2010.01382.x

Chen, C. K., Ingenito, C. P., Kehn, M. M., Nehrig, N., & Abraham, K. S. (2019). Implementing brief dynamic interpersonal therapy (DIT) in a VA Medical Center. *Journal of Mental Health, 28*(6), 613–620. https://doi.org/10.1080/09638237.2017.1340602

Chen, C. K., Nehrig, N., Wash, L., & Wang, B. (2020). The impact of brief dynamic interpersonal therapy (DIT) on veteran depression and anxiety. *Psychotherapy, 57*(3), 464–468. https://doi.org/10.1037/pst0000282

Clark, D. M. (2018). Realizing the mass public benefit of evidence-based psychological therapies: The IAPT program. *Annual Review of Clinical Psychology, 14*, 159–183. https://doi.org/10.1146/annurev-clinpsy-050817-084833

Cuijpers, P., Ciharova, M., Miguel, C., Harrer, M., Ebert, D. D., Brakemeier, E. L., & Karyotaki, E. (2021). Psychological treatment of depression in institutional settings: A meta-analytic review. *Journal of Affective Disorders, 286*, 340–350. https://doi.org/10.1016/j.jad.2021.03.017

Cuijpers, P., Karyotaki, E., de Wit, L., & Ebert, D. D. (2020). The effects of fifteen evidence-supported therapies for adult depression: A meta-analytic review. *Psychotherapy Research, 30*(3), 279–293. https://doi.org/10.1080/10503307.2019.1649732

Cuijpers, P., Reijnders, M., & Huibers, M. J. H. (2019). The role of common factors in psychotherapy outcomes. *Annual Review of Clinical Psychology, 15*, 207–231. https://doi.org/10.1146/annurev-clinpsy-050718-095424

Cuyt, Y., Kooiman, K., Campens, S., & Luyten, P. (2022). Een kwalitatief onderzoek naar de ervaren werkzaamheid van DIT als multidisciplinaire, dagklinische groepstherapie [A qualitative study of the effectiveness of DIT as a multidisciplinary, day-hospital group therapy]. *Tijdschrift voor Psychotherapie, 48*(4), 296–314.

Department of Health. (2012). *IAPT three-year report. The first million patients.* Department of Health. http://webarchive.nationalarchives.gov.uk/20160302155226/http://www.iapt.nhs.uk/silo/files/iapt-3-year-report.pdf

Driessen, E., Dekker, J. J. M., Peen, J., Van, H. L., Maina, G., Rosso, G., Rigardetto, S., Cuniberti, F., Vitriol, V. G., Florenzano, R. U., Andreoli, A., Burnand, Y., López-Rodríguez, J., Villamil-Salcedo, V., Twisk, J. W. R., & Cuijpers, P. (2020). The efficacy of adding short-term psychodynamic psychotherapy to antidepressants in the treatment of depression: A systematic review and meta-analysis of individual participant data. *Clinical Psychology Review, 80*, 101886. https://doi.org/10.1016/j.cpr.2020.101886

Driessen, E., Hegelmaier, L. M., Abbass, A. A., Barber, J. P., Dekker, J. J., Van, H. L., Jansma, E. P., & Cuijpers, P. (2015). The efficacy of short-term psychodynamic psychotherapy for depression: A meta-analysis update. *Clinical Psychology Review, 42*, 1–15. https://doi.org/10.1016/j.cpr.2015.07.004

Driessen, E., Van, H. L., Don, F. J., Peen, J., Kool, S., Westra, D., Hendriksen, M., Schoevers, R. A., Cuijpers, P., Twisk, J. W., & Dekker, J. J. (2013). The efficacy of cognitive-behavioral therapy and psychodynamic therapy in the outpatient treatment of major depression: a randomized clinical trial. *American Journal of Psychiatry*, *170*(9), 1041–1050. https://doi.org/10.1176/appi.ajp.2013.12070899

Eubanks, C. F., Goldfried, M. R., & Norcross, J. C. (2019). Future directions in psychotherapy integration. In J. C. Norcross & M. R. Goldfried (Eds.), *Handbook of psychotherapy integration* (3rd ed., pp. 474–485). Oxford University Press.

Eubanks, C. F., Muran, J. C., & Safran, J. D. (2019). Repairing alliance ruptures. In J. C. Norcross & M. J. Lambert (Eds.), *Psychotherapy relationships that work. Volume 1: Evidence-based therapist contributions* (3rd ed., pp. 549–579). Oxford University Press.

Feldman, C. L., Schadt, C. D., Wang, B., Polkes, A. J., Ratner, B., & Chen, C. K. (2023). Dynamic interpersonal therapy for U.S. veterans in a primary care setting. *American Journal of Psychotherapy*, *76*(3), 124–127. https://doi.org/10.1176/appi.psychotherapy.20220007

Folkes-Skinner, J., & Collins, L. (2022). Group dynamic interpersonal therapy (GDIT): Adapting an individual interpersonal therapy to a group setting in an NHS IAPT service: a pilot study. *Psychoanalytic Psychotherapy*, *36*(2), 141–156. https://doi.org/10.1080/02668734.2021.2001685

Fonagy, P., & Allison, E. (2014). The role of mentalizing and epistemic trust in the therapeutic relationship. *Psychotherapy*, *51*(3), 372–380. https://doi.org/10.1037/a0036505

Fonagy, P., Lemma, A., Target, M., O'Keeffe, S., Constantinou, M. P., Ventura Wurman, T., Luyten, P., Allison, E., Roth, A., Cape, J., & Pilling, S. (2020). Dynamic interpersonal therapy for moderate to severe depression: A pilot randomized controlled and feasibility trial. *Psychological Medicine*, *50*(6), 1010–1019. https://doi.org/10.1017/S0033291719000928

Fonagy, P., Luyten, P., Allison, E., & Campbell, C. (2019). Mentalizing, epistemic trust and the phenomenology of psychotherapy. *Psychopathology*, *52*(2), 94–103. https://doi.org/10.1159/000501526

Gaskell, C., Simmonds-Buckley, M., Kellett, S., Stockton, C., Somerville, E., Rogerson, E., & Delgadillo, J. (2023). The effectiveness of psychological interventions delivered in routine practice: systematic review and meta-analysis. *Administration and Policy in Mental Health*, *50*(1), 43–57. https://doi.org/10.1007/s10488-022-01225-y

Hilsenroth, M. J., Ackerman, S. J., Blagys, M. D., Baity, M. R., & Mooney, M. A. (2003). Short-term psychodynamic psychotherapy for depression: An examination of statistical, clinically significant, and technique-specific change. *Journal of Nervous and Mental Disease, 191*(6), 349–357. https://doi.org/10.1097/01.NMD.0000071582.11781.67

Kazdin, A. E. (2009). Understanding how and why psychotherapy leads to change. *Psychotherapy Research, 19*(4–5), 418–428. https://doi.org/10.1080/10503300802448899

Khalastchy, J., Abrahamsen, D., Saunders, R., & Fonagy, P. (2021). *Evaluating extended dynamic interpersonal therapy (e-DIT): A mixed methods investigation to identify characteristics associated with successful outcomes of DIT* [MSc Dissertation, University College London].

Leichsenring, F., Abbass, A., Heim, N., Keefe, J. R., Kisely, S., Luyten, P., Rabung, S., & Steinert, C. (2023). The status of psychodynamic psychotherapy as an empirically supported treatment for common mental disorders – an umbrella review based on updated criteria. *World Psychiatry, 22*(2), 286–304. https://doi.org/10.1002/wps.21104

Lemma, A., & Fonagy, P. (2013). Feasibility study of a psychodynamic online group intervention for depression. *Psychoanalytic Psychology, 30*(3), 367–380. https://doi.org/10.1037/a0033239

Lemma, A., Roth, A. D., & Pilling, S. (2008). *Analytic/dynamic competences: Knowledge of the basic principles and rationale for analytic/dynamic therapy*. Research Department of Clinical, Educational and Health Psychology, University College London. https://www.ucl.ac.uk/pals/sites/pals/files/migrated-files/PPC_basic_analytic_competences.pdf

Lemma, A., Target, M., & Fonagy, P. (2011a). *Brief dynamic interpersonal therapy: A clinician's guide* (1st ed.). Oxford University Press.

Lemma, A., Target, M., & Fonagy, P. (2011b). The development of a brief psychodynamic intervention (dynamic interpersonal therapy) and its application to depression: A pilot study. *Psychiatry: Interpersonal and Biological Processes, 74*(1), 41–48. https://doi.org/10.1521/psyc.2011.74.1.41

Leonidaki, V., Lemma, A., & Hobbis, I. (2016). Clients' experiences of dynamic interpersonal therapy (DIT): Opportunities and challenges for brief, manualised psychodynamic therapy in the NHS. *Psychoanalytic Psychotherapy, 30*(1), 42–61. https://doi.org/10.1080/02668734.2015.1081266

Leonidaki, V., Lemma, A., & Hobbis, I. (2018). The active ingredients of dynamic interpersonal therapy (DIT): An exploration of clients' experiences. *Psychoanalytic Psychotherapy, 32*(2), 140–156. https://doi.org/10.1080/02668734.2017.1418761

Lindegaard, T., Berg, M., & Andersson, G. (2020). Efficacy of internet-delivered psychodynamic therapy: Systematic review and meta-analysis. *Psychodynamic Psychiatry*, *48*(4), 437–454. https://doi.org/10.1521/pdps.2020.48.4.437

Luyten, P., & Fonagy, P. (2020). Psychodynamic psychotherapy for patients with functional somatic disorders and the road to recovery. *American Journal of Psychotherapy*, *73*(4), 125–130. https://doi.org/10.1176/appi.psychotherapy.20200010

McFarquhar, T., Luyten, P., & Fonagy, P. (2018). Changes in interpersonal problems in the psychotherapeutic treatment of depression as measured by the Inventory of Interpersonal Problems: A systematic review and meta-analysis. *Journal of Affective Disorders*, *226*, 108–123. https://doi.org/10.1016/j.jad.2017.09.036

McFarquhar, T., Luyten, P., & Fonagy, P. (2023). A typology for the interpersonal affective focus in dynamic interpersonal therapy based on a contemporary interpersonal approach. *Psychotherapy*, *60*(2), 171–181. https://doi.org/10.1037/pst0000462

National Institute for Health and Care Excellence. (2019). *Depression in children and young people: Identification and management. NICE guideline [NG134]*. National Institute for Health and Care Excellence. https://www.nice.org.uk/guidance/ng134

National Institute for Health and Care Excellence. (2022). *Depression in adults: Treatment and management. NICE guideline [NG222]*. National Institute for Health and Care Excellence. https://www.nice.org.uk/guidance/ng222

Perepletchikova, F., & Kazdin, A. E. (2005). Treatment integrity and therapeutic change: Issues and research recommendations. *Clinical Psychology: Science and Practice*, *12*(4), 365–383. https://doi.org/10.1093/clipsy.bpi045

Rao, A. S., Lemma, A., Fonagy, P., Sosnowska, M., Constantinou, M. P., Fijak-Koch, M., & Gelberg, G. (2019). Development of dynamic interpersonal therapy in complex care (DITCC): A pilot study. *Psychoanalytic Psychotherapy*, *33*(2), 77–98. https://doi.org/10.1080/02668734.2019.1622147

Safran, J. D., & Muran, J. C. (2000). The therapeutic alliance. Introduction. *Journal of Clinical Psychology*, *56*(2), 159–161. https://doi.org/10.1002/(sici)1097-4679(200002)56:2<159::aid-jclp2>3.0.co;2-d

Safran, J. D., Muran, J. C., & Eubanks-Carter, C. (2011). Repairing alliance ruptures. *Psychotherapy*, *48*(1), 80–87. https://doi.org/10.1037/a0022140

Sandell, R. (1985). Influence of supervision, therapist's competence, and patient's ego level on the effects of time-limited psychotherapy. *Psychotherapy and Psychosomatics*, 44(2), 103–109. https://doi.org/10.1159/000287900

Selders, M., Visser, R., van Rooij, W., Delfstra, G., & Koelen, J. A. (2015). The development of a brief group intervention (dynamic interpersonal therapy) for patients with medically unexplained somatic symptoms: a pilot study. *Psychoanalytic Psychotherapy*, 29(2), 182–198. https://doi.org/10.1080/02668734.2015.1036106

Shaw, B. F., & Dobson, K. S. (1988). Competency judgments in the training and evaluation of psychotherapists. *Journal of Consulting and Clinical Psychology*, 56(5), 666–672.

Svartberg, M., Seltzer, M., & Stiles, T. C. (1996). Self-concept improvement during and after short-term anxiety-provoking psychotherapy: A preliminary growth curve study. *Psychotherapy Research*, 6(1). https://doi.org/10.1080/10503309612331331568

Svartberg, M., & Stiles, T. C. (1992). Predicting patient change from therapist competence and patient-therapist complementarity in short-term anxiety-provoking psychotherapy: A pilot study. *Journal of Consulting and Clinical Psychology*, 60(2), 304–307. https://doi.org/10.1037//0022-006x.60.2.304

Svartberg, M., & Stiles, T. C. (1994). Therapeutic alliance, therapist competence, and client change in short-term anxiety-provoking psychotherapy. *Psychotherapy Research*, 4(1), 20–33. https://doi.org/10.1080/10503309412331333872

Town, J. M., Abbass, A., Stride, C., Nunes, A., Bernier, D., & Berrigan, P. (2020). Efficacy and cost-effectiveness of intensive short-term dynamic psychotherapy for treatment resistant depression: 18-month follow-up of the Halifax depression trial. *Journal of Affective Disorders*, 273, 194–202. https://doi.org/10.1016/j.jad.2020.04.035

Tudur Smith, C., Marcucci, M., Nolan, S. J., Iorio, A., Sudell, M., Riley, R., Rovers, M. M., & Williamson, P. R. (2016). Individual participant data meta-analyses compared with meta-analyses based on aggregate data. *Cochrane Database of Systematic Reviews*, 9(9), MR000007. https://doi.org/10.1002/14651858.MR000007.pub3

Ventura Wurman, T. (2019). *Therapist competence in dynamic interpersonal therapy and its association with treatment outcome* [PhD Thesis, University College London].

Wang, Y., Yao, J., Koszycki, D., Jiang, W., Fang, F., Wang, M., Tao, J., Zhao, W., Liu, Y., Su, S., Peng, Y., Wang, H., Wang, L., Gao, R., Gu, J., Zhang, J., Bai, Y., Wu, Y., Su, Y., Zhao, Y., Zheng, Z., Chen, S., & Qiu, J. (2023).

Efficacy of dynamic interpersonal therapy for major depressive disorder in China: results of a multicentered, three-arm, randomized, controlled trial. *Psychological Medicine, 53*(15), 7242–7254. https://doi.org/10.1017/S0033291723000788

Webb, C. A., Derubeis, R. J., & Barber, J. P. (2010). Therapist adherence/competence and treatment outcome: A meta-analytic review. *Journal of Consulting and Clinical Psychology, 78*(2), 200–211. https://doi.org/10.1037/a0018912

Wienicke, F. J., Beutel, M. E., Zwerenz, R., Brahler, E., Fonagy, P., Luyten, P., Constantinou, M., Barber, J. P., McCarthy, K. S., Solomonov, N., Cooper, P. J., De Pascalis, L., Johansson, R., Andersson, G., Lemma, A., Town, J. M., Abbass, A. A., Ajilchi, B., Connolly Gibbons, M. B., Lopez-Rodriguez, J., Villamil-Salcedo, V., Maina, G., Rosso, G., Twisk, J. W. R., Burk, W. J., Spijker, J., Cuijpers, P., & Driessen, E. (2023). Efficacy and moderators of short-term psychodynamic psychotherapy for depression: A systematic review and meta-analysis of individual participant data. *Clinical Psychology Review, 101*, 102269. https://doi.org/10.1016/j.cpr.2023.102269

13

Dynamic Interpersonal Therapy for Complex Care (DITCC)

WHO IS DITCC FOR?

Chronic and complex depression is common in both primary and secondary care services. The persistence of this condition often has a devastating impact on patients' relationships and ability to work. They are also more likely to struggle to engage with psychological therapy, all too often feeling hopeless about the possibility of change.

Although evidence is emerging of the effectiveness of dynamic interpersonal therapy (DIT) (see Chapter 12), the clinical experience of DIT therapists has indicated a need to adapt the model for patients with chronic, complex, and severe depression owing to issues related to engagement, risk, and sustainable change with these patients. We found that, before any of the DIT techniques we described in Chapters 3–9 could be employed, focused work to develop a strong enough therapeutic alliance was needed with this patient group. Although these patients typically experienced the identification of an interpersonal-affective focus (IPAF) as helpful, more time was required for the working-through phase because their interpersonal anxieties were more entrenched. Given the prevalence of attachment difficulties and histories of separation trauma in this group, the original sixteen-session model felt too rushed. These experiences led to the development of DIT for complex care (DITCC) and to the first pilot study using this approach (Rao et al., 2019).

Like the original DIT model for mood disorders (see Chapters 3–9), DITCC rests on the assumption that the patient's interpersonal context is central to understanding their behaviour and experience. The DIT therapist focuses on understanding the patient in the context of their current relationships, which might constrain their capacity to function adequately. Patients with chronic depression both impact on and are impacted by their current relationships: their experiences are shaped by the relationships that they encounter and to which they contribute in everyday life. They tend to feel that their capacity to manage relationships is limited and that they cannot alter the personal situations they also need; hence, they feel trapped and helpless.

In many complex cases, the patient shows profound distrust of people with whom they are connected. This includes their relationship with the therapist, which leads to a negative or very unstable transference, acting out, enactments, and impasses in the work. These patients cannot respond flexibly to their (changing) social environment. Instead, they impose a set of expectations, which are tried and tested in previous relationship contexts but not adaptive or responsive to new social information that could potentially change their expectations. Their pre-existing social 'templates' fit their current interpersonal situation poorly, whether it is benign or destructive; this generates relationship difficulties that compound their previous problems, persistently spoiling current and new relationships. Others might react to this by being critical, expressing disappointment, or rebuffing them. This in turn reduces their confidence and trust, and limits their chances of experiencing social connection and enjoyment that could help them correct their expectations. Social isolation is a common consequence. In DITCC, such patterns of behaviour are described as *relationship-interfering behaviours* (RIBs).

The choice between DIT and DITCC is not based on the severity of depression, although depression is likely to be relatively severe in those patients who respond better to DITCC. DITCC is appropriate for people with long-standing relationship difficulties, who are resistant to attempting interpersonal change even though they are aware of their negative relational patterns. We assume that this is because their misinterpretations and relative inflexibility generate RIBs that reinforce their problematic relational templates, and because their past relationship experiences have been particularly painful, leading to avoidance (even when contemplating change).

This state of affairs is common in complex cases of depression. These patients appear relatively inaccessible to brief therapy and often find themselves in secondary community mental health settings. Naturally, their presentations are heterogeneous, with varied diagnostic profiles, but across the diagnoses we see maladaptive expectations of, and emotional reactions to, other people that we understand as having originated in early relationship experiences.

THE COMPLEX CASE: THE FAILURE OF MENTALIZING IN DEPRESSION

The most serious obstacle to improvement in complex cases comes from distrust, a by-product of poor mentalizing, often coupled with truly damaging external experiences (Fonagy & Allison, 2014). As we have learned more about the relationship between distrust and mentalizing, it has become clear that interpersonal relationships— including the psychotherapeutic relationship—are compromised by a combination of failures, perhaps most clearly described by Allen (2021). A person who cannot respond appropriately to social cues is less likely to benefit from benign new environments, including the environment of therapy, and this undermines the potential for them to learn from and to adapt to different contexts. Equally, withdrawing from the community, as is characteristic of complex depression rooted in adversity, deprives the person of opportunities to improve their mentalizing capacity. This is particularly harmful if shame and intense social anxiety lead them to withdraw from close interpersonal interactions that could rekindle their interest and curiosity in seeing themself and others differently. In DITCC, the therapist has to engage the patient's curiosity about their own and others' thoughts and feelings, and help them to take a renewed interest in mentalizing.

In determining who might benefit most from DITCC, we need to assess the likelihood of significant resistance to making changes in relationships, even when the person gains insight about their recurrent unhelpful relational patterns. These patients' limited openness to learning appears as relative inflexibility, and ultimately creates the RIBs that maintain the problematic interpersonal pattern. Take, for instance, a person who feels certain that everyone will dislike them. Anticipating hostility, they react defensively and resentfully to neutral behaviour from others. They might even feel that the apparent neutrality of other people is a deliberate deception, and will repeatedly confuse and antagonize people they meet by being aggressive and distrustful towards them. This tendency will naturally also be deployed in any therapeutic relationship; this is a risk, but also an opportunity to see and address the pattern. The persistence of RIBs can be seen as specifically defensive or as a by-product of a more generalized defensive stance reflecting a catastrophic loss of confidence in what the person can learn from social experience or how they can benefit from social situations. In most cases both of these considerations will apply. Either way, insight alone cannot lead to change.

DITCC considers that the treatment-resistant features of complex depression are rooted in mentalizing difficulties. There are well-known features of depression that suggest substantial difficulties with mentalizing, which in turn can generate the clinical picture just described. Depressed patients with mentalizing difficulties will show greater affective instability, which blurs the relationship between specific stressful experiences and the onset of depression. More striking is the complexity of the emotional pain that depressed patients with mentalizing problems typically experience; this is likely to contain components of rage, sorrow, shame, and panic. These patients often report emptiness, deep self-criticism, diffuse negative emotionality, an underlying fear of being abandoned, and a heavy sense of their static, depressive inner world. They also commonly experience physical symptoms, such as unexplained chronic pain. (Chapter 14 considers in detail the DIT approach to functional somatic symptoms, where these may be a leading feature of a patient's complex presentation.)

From the perspective of mentalizing theory, these features of depression are relatively easy to understand because ineffective mentalizing manifests as developmentally early ways of representing thoughts and feelings of the self and others (see also Chapter 7, which introduces the techniques used in improving mentalizing). Target (2016) provides a detailed clinical example, using the framework of mentalizing and attachment theory (including the developmental failures of mentalizing), of psychodynamic work with a patient with severe depression in the context of personality disorder. This patient was not treated with DITCC, which had not been developed at the time, but the presentation illustrates many of the mentalizing problems we describe here, and correspondingly DITCC contains many elements of the approach that helped the patient over a longer therapy.

The typical emotional manifestations of depression (e.g. a profound sense of failure, expectation of rejection, hopelessness) are experienced in the *psychic equivalence mode*, in which inner reality and physical reality are felt to be the same. The direct experience of an internal state unmediated by the buffer of mentalizing gives it an unshakeable force and intensity. Having difficulty in narrating self-experience leads to a sense of emptiness and greater dependence on others to provide validation and mirroring. Patients' accounts of inner pain and devastation, chronic fatigue, and physical pain are also linked to psychic equivalence, where mental states become embodied and can be experienced as physical realities (see also Chapter 14). This is why, for example, a sense of being rejected can generate real physical pain or the need to create pain through self-harm. Psychic equivalence also explains the surprising lack of curiosity that often characterizes people with severe depression. Why would you try to work out what someone might think or feel when you already believe that you know? Even if they tell you, you will tend not to believe them unless they simply confirm your expectations.

The restricted mentalizing of the *teleological mode* demands concrete observable changes in place of words and ideas (e.g. that people apologize for a past hurt or misunderstanding before resuming contact). For patients with complex problems including depression, being in teleological mode might make them seek physical reassurance, fight to avoid abandonment, and express deep dissatisfaction with psychological therapies. They might feel that their own pain can be relieved only by action—for example, by self-harming, trying to make someone control them, or trying to take charge of others.

Some patients might give repetitive, over-analytical, self-critical, but ultimately empty accounts that indicate the use of hypermentalizing or dominant *pretend mode* function, in which thoughts and feelings are split off from external reality, bringing about dissociative states in extreme cases. The subjective experience might be of meaninglessness. In this mode, patients' tenuous and unconvincing explanations of their feelings might include unrealistic and unwarranted speculations about other people's mental states. In therapy, there might be lengthy, but inconsequential, talk about thoughts and feelings. A vivid fictional example of the dominance of pretend mode, and its slide towards delusion, is provided by the character Blanche DuBois in Tennessee Williams's play *A Streetcar Named Desire*. Early in the play, Blanche presents herself as a refined, respectable, and blameless victim of cruel circumstances; this self-image almost hangs together, except for its quality of exaggeration and self-aggrandizement. Gradually, as facts emerge, her presentation of herself is revealed as a tissue of fantasies. The glamorous dream world that she presented collapses into indignity and desperation, and she finally accepts being revealed as very ill, with nothing real to rely on, inside or out.

The pretend mode can manifest in narratives as intrusive mentalizing when the patient makes unwarranted assumptions about other people's mental states, failing to respect the fact that the mental states of others are hidden. Sometimes the thoughts and feelings the patient attributes to others can seem plausible and even roughly accurate, but the therapist notices that they are assumed without appropriate qualification (rather than 'I can't be certain, but she seems to assume she is right', the patient might say 'She always thinks she knows best').

Poor mentalizing is more obvious when the patient makes great efforts to understand actions in mental-state terms, and might even appear preoccupied with mental-state explanations, but these are off the mark. The patient does not try to check the accuracy of their assumptions about the states of mind of people they are talking about. We have described this tendency as *hypermentalizing*. In some people, pretend mode manifests as destructively inaccurate mentalizing; the patient attempts to deny aspects of observable reality, perhaps in a self-serving manner. For example, the patient might 'explain' other people's negative reactions to their behaviour by attributing convenient but unevidenced mental states (e.g. 'My boss is so envious of my talents'). Most importantly, because people need to feel understood in order to develop enough trust to enable them to learn from others, the mentalizing problems described here will prevent trusting social relationships from evolving—and this includes the therapeutic relationship.

The clinical consequence of distrust and ineffective mentalizing is not simply a lack of therapeutic response. There is also a marked increase in risk of suicide because of hopelessness experienced in both the psychic equivalence and teleological modes (which often go together in patients with severe and complex depression) (Fonagy & Luyten, 2009, 2018). The abnormally intense experience of internal states can bring with it an experience of helplessness because emotions and thoughts make less sense to the patient than their usual states of mind do, which can make them feel out of control and even 'mad'. The psychic equivalence and teleological modes, together with the dissociation linked to the pretend mode, lead to an increase in suicidal ideation and the risk of suicide attempts. For example, shame is a common emotional experience that is strengthened in depression, but when experienced in psychic equivalence it feels literally destructive of the self (*ego-destructive* shame). When feelings are experienced in teleological mode, it can appear that only action can change or relieve them—talking is no good, only death or self-injury can make the feelings go away. Suicidality is, of course, not restricted to this group of patients. Whereas suicidality is directly connected to specific interpersonal circumstances in patients with more treatment-responsive depression, in the group of patients with complex depression whose mentalizing is poor, it is more often directly connected to the subjective experience of complex depression itself. It is not an expression of wanting to die so much as a wish not to live—a need to silence intense feelings of inner pain.

DITCC AND DIT: COMMONALITIES AND DIFFERENCES

Like 'traditional' DIT and other psychodynamic models, DITCC proposes that entrenched relational patterns get in the way of new input from the external world that could challenge or update the internalized developmental models that have been maintaining the status quo in the patient's internal world. However, while DIT assumes that helping the patient to see the maladaptiveness of these models can be enough to lead them to modify their expectations, in DITCC it is assumed that the patient's general attitude to learning from experience also needs to change (Fonagy et al., 2015; Fonagy et al., 2019).

DITCC has two components. The first component overlaps with the DIT principles of identifying an IPAF and highlighting its maladaptive features. The second component directly addresses the situations that generate the individual's distrust of social communications and relationships. How can this distrust be approached in the context of individual psychotherapy? The patients treated in DITCC are often less amenable to the therapeutic approach described in DIT because the therapist themself, just like others in the patient's social world, is regarded with suspicion. Sometimes the therapist finds themself acting in ways that confirms these suspicions. For example, the therapist might unwittingly act in ways that are experienced by the patient as unhelpful or even hostile. They might be working within a dysfunctional mental health system, which can make them untrustworthy—and so not a safe person to learn from—in the patient's eyes. DITCC addresses this challenge directly by specifically focusing on enhancing the patient's trust in the therapist as someone offering a new perspective and possible hope. To do this, the therapist needs to build a coherent understanding of the patient's experience of their social world and of their specific thoughts, feelings, beliefs, and wishes in relation to it. In other words, the therapist must earn the patient's trust by actually learning about and coming to understand the patient's perspective. This process involves clarification and a general enhancing of the patient's sense of agency and control, rather than challenging them or demanding that they change. It also involves the therapist modelling the capacity not to presume that they already know about the patient and what is going on between patient and therapist (the 'not-knowing' stance), and the ability to be open to different points of view (Fonagy et al., 2019).

To help bring about change, the DITCC therapist takes into account and works on the continuing interaction between the patient's internal world of object relations and their current relationships, as the interference with building trusting relationships is believed to occur at this interface. Change occurs because the patient gradually becomes able to abandon their constraining set of expectations, sees their social situation in a more accurate or realistic way, and becomes more able to absorb new information that they feel is *relevant* to them, *reliable*, and *generalizable* to new situations—and so worth remembering. This new learning in turn serves to reduce interpersonal tensions and helps the patient to recover and improve their ability to cope, adjust, and adapt (which we term *resilience*).

DITCC IN PRACTICE

As discussed in the previous section, when working with patients with complex depression in DITCC, the therapist, like others in the patient's social world, is inevitably regarded with suspicion. This distrust will take on various forms, with some patients lacing it with anxiety and an urgent need for the therapist to assuage this, whereas others might be more openly hostile, perhaps contemptuous and rejecting of the therapist's efforts to help them. This can trigger powerful countertransference reactions (e.g. fear of being intrusively overwhelmed or complained about) that make enactments more likely to occur (see Chapter 10). Often enough, the therapist finds themself part of the patient's dysfunctional social system (the treatment context might constitute a large part of the patient's current social world) and they might unwittingly act in ways that the patient experiences as invalidating, rejecting, or discouraging, in so doing repeating the failures of previous treatment efforts. One example of this is the therapist communicating with other professionals who are caring for the patient. In turn, these actions only confirm the patient's belief that the therapist is untrustworthy and is not someone from whom they can learn.

From a psychoanalytic viewpoint, we could characterize these challenges as reflecting the function of underlying personality structures such as a narcissistic structure. Nevertheless, self-absorption and the vulnerability of self-esteem should be treated only as characterizations rather than explanations. Beneath the surface appearance of narcissism lies a lack of confidence in how the individual perceives themself, which propels them towards others for validation. However, the absence of trust in the knowledge that they are seeking from others initiates a vicious cycle: as soon as validation is provided by another, it is instantly devalued by distrust, and the individual has to rely on their self-perceptions, in which they have little confidence. The emergent and familiar pattern of oscillation between demands for reassurance and devaluation of the reassurance that is provided undermines the individual's interpersonal relationships. This fosters tensions that escalate the search for social validation of a fragile and increasingly distorted self-perception from others who are progressively negatively disposed towards the individual.

This means that some modifications are required to the DIT therapist's approach, with more emphasis on the use of mentalizing techniques, including mentalizing the transference and working to improve affect regulation. As in the original DIT model, transference interpretation (see Chapter 8) is used in DITCC, but with a specific focus on the patient's capacity to mentalize. DITCC directly addresses this challenge by concentrating on enhancing the patient's trust in the therapist as a source of social information (which is termed *epistemic trust*). We understand from developmental research that a child's trust in information received from another person is moderated by the extent to which the child already feels recognized as an individual by that person (Csibra & Gergely, 2009). Feeling recognized as an individual (or as a self) enables the ability to listen differently, feel more engaged, and be more open to modifying prior expectations. DITCC systematically focuses the therapist's attention, particularly in the initial stages of treatment, on enhancing their perceived reliability as a source of social understanding for the patient. This is done by ensuring, through contingent responsiveness, that the patient's experiences of themselves are accurately mirrored by the therapist—that is, so that the patient comes to believe that the therapist recognizes, understands, and accepts them as an individual. This involves far more than the therapist being 'nice' or 'agreeable', although this is undoubtedly helpful. Sometimes, the therapist might need to disagree with or distance themselves from the patient's attitude or belief, but they must do so in a manner that clearly communicates their understanding that the patient's belief is what it is—it is something they have learned from their own life, but the therapist can think or believe something different. When such a difference in attitude or belief occurs, it is critical that the therapist recognizes how the patient has understood their experience and expresses empathy with the distress that the patient feels, whether their understanding is correct or not.

The therapist needs to cultivate the patient's sense of agency by enabling them to clearly perceive the correlation between their internal states and their behaviour and broader experience, which has felt like a continuous process of being invalidated as an individual. The therapist can achieve this only if they have a coherent understanding of this aspect of the patient's social world and the specific thoughts, feelings, beliefs, wishes, and desires that underlie it. The therapist must get close to and alongside the patient's experience while also offering their own perspective. The transference, as a new and immediately observable example of the potential for distrust, gives the patient an opportunity to see the therapist as someone providing feedback about the therapeutic relationship while directly experiencing it, rather than hearing about it from a safe distance. The therapist tries to make the patient aware of how the thoughts and feelings they experience create problems for the relationship between them. Trust is also fostered by the patient hearing the therapist describing the situation between them (e.g. that the patient feels let down, and is angry about that). This pattern—in this case of feeling let down and wanting to break off the relationship, in anger—will have been very destructive in the patient's life, in other relationships. It is very powerful for the patient to find that in the therapy, their anger and accusation can be clearly heard and yet the therapist does not reject the patient—even when the patient might reject the therapist. The therapist becomes seen by the patient as a trustworthy source of knowledge and as someone who is dedicated to the patient and to the therapeutic relationship.

The significance of enhanced social understanding stems from the assumption in both DIT and DITCC that self-understanding and social understanding are interconnected: self-understanding is derived from comprehending others' reactions to the self, and the ability to understand others depends on the extension of self-understanding to the other. This could be expressed more simply as: 'I perceive myself as others perceive me, and I understand others by empathizing with their position'. In DITCC, we propose that this learning might occur for the first time within the therapeutic context, where improved social cognition enables the patient to feel understood by another (the therapist). Experiencing this sense of agency—of being an individual understood by someone else—then enhances the patient's capacity to take in new information from the therapist.

Structure of DITCC

The DITCC approach to treating depression is divided into three active phases of treatment, each with particular aims and strategies, and a follow-up phase. As with 'standard' DIT, in DITCC the clinician's interventions aim to link interpersonal processes with the dynamic interplay between different aspects of patients' mental states.

DITCC consists of twenty-six sessions spread over approximately 1 year: twenty weekly sessions followed by six fortnightly sessions, plus an additional two follow-up sessions at monthly intervals, which are optional and dependent on the service context.

- **Phase 1**, the 'set-up and engagement phase', consists of six weekly sessions that are primarily concerned with establishing a working alliance and enhancing the patient's 'readiness' for therapy.
- **Phase 2**, the 'insight phase', comprises fourteen weekly sessions. The early sessions (a maximum of three sessions) in this phase are devoted to the development of the IPAF and setting goals, and the remaining sessions are focused on working through the IPAF and paying close attention to the RIBs.
- **Phase 3**, the 'work-through and ending phase', consists of six fortnightly sessions that focus on actively helping the patient to implement changes in their life. In this phase, attention is paid to the affective experience of the greater challenges of translating the insights generated in therapy into interpersonal change and managing the eventual ending.
- The two **follow-up sessions** are held at monthly intervals and are aimed at supporting well-being and transition.

The model in detail

PHASE 1: SET-UP AND ENGAGEMENT PHASE (SESSIONS 1–6)

The first phase of the treatment is active, supportive, validating, and interpersonally focused. It focuses on establishing a mentalizing therapeutic relationship and identifying maladaptive interpersonal cycles and interpersonal narratives. This phase of the treatment differs most from the 'standard' DIT model to take into account these patients' differing needs. It has three aims:

1. *Engaging the patient in treatment* by providing hope and structure, and working actively with them to support interpersonal change. The patient and the therapist try to collaborate to help the patient identify anxieties and defences that are likely to be triggered when change is encouraged or attempted, which might then obstruct change. This is

essential if the patient is to be helped to risk trying out less maladaptive strategies of interpersonal relating.
2. Addressing interpersonal issues and conflicts relies on *employing strategies for enhancing mentalizing.* The therapist might focus on a range of relationships where the IPAF is enlightening, but the evolving relationship between the therapist and patient is particularly valuable for this group of patients. The degree to which the application of IPAF-based insight is truly illuminating for the patient will directly influence the trust the patient has in the therapy. An aim of focusing on a significant attachment relationship such as the therapeutic relationship is to broaden and build the patient's awareness of how their behaviour is driven by mental states. Generally, we expect that the mentalizing stance adopted for key attachment relationships will generalize beyond the specific interpersonal dynamics of the relationship being addressed in therapy.
3. *Identifying and exploring maladaptive interpersonal cycles* or interpersonal narratives that could undermine change and the change process in therapy. Examples might include regularly dismissing solutions suggested by others; responding to suggestions with suspicion (e.g. seeing everything as disguised self-interest); using emotional exaggeration as a way to reject previously accepted ideas; or forgetting suggestions that have been made. In this phase of the treatment, these strategies need only be non-critically pointed to and named as potential RIBs that could defeat the therapeutic efforts to help the patient.

Phase 2: The insight phase (sessions 7–20)

The second phase is structured to work through interpersonal issues, including issues arising within the patient–therapist relationship. Its primary focus is the recognition and exploration of the IPAF and spelling out its impact on the patient's life, the organization of their social relationships, and the recent onset of symptoms, as well as setting goals relevant to the IPAF. This is along the same lines as in the sixteen-session model (see Chapter 5). Once the IPAF has been agreed between the patient and therapist, the therapist writes to the patient's family doctor/general practitioner to share the IPAF and goals for the therapy, to engage the other professional(s) involved in the patient's care in supporting the treatment.

The insight phase aims to begin to foster resilience by assisting in the development of new ways of managing adversity. In general, it corresponds to the initial and middle phases of the original DIT model, with some initial sessions devoted to the development of the IPAF and the remainder of the sessions committed to working through the IPAF as outlined in the original model.

Work with patients in DITCC calls for a greater-than-usual focus on enhancing adaptations or strengthening resilience. Mentalizing is a key component of resilient adaptation. Having an understanding of the reasons behind someone's actions, if it is reasonably accurate, can help the patient anticipate future behaviours and mitigate their impact, and can help them to develop alternative strategies. Interpersonal problem-solving for someone without robust mentalizing skills is extremely challenging.

Working on mentalizing and problem-solving has a function beyond the immediate at this stage. Implicitly, throughout this process the therapist validates the patient's concerns and acknowledges their point of view. This helps the patient to feel recognized as a person with the capacity to reflect, feel, wish, make decisions, and act accordingly. We regard this as a critical part of the change process. Mentalizing the patient, enabling them to feel that their intentions are understood and respected, is probably the most important tool of any therapeutic relationship, regardless of the type of therapy. It enables the patient, in turn, to treat the therapist as a trustworthy and helpful source of information.

As should be clear, the second phase of DITCC overlaps significantly with the DIT model but places a far greater emphasis on mentalizing and focuses attention on the patient's RIBs. The most significant deviation in structure from the sixteen-session DIT model occurs in session 13, when the 'goodbye' letter would normally be given to the patient. Instead, in DITCC, the patient is given a letter (ideally in session 16) that we refer to as the 'taking stock' letter. The aims of this letter are to outline: (a) the IPAF and RIBs being worked on, (b) the patient's 'defence signature' (i.e. how the patient characteristically defends against the distress associated with the IPAF), (c) the costs of maintaining the status quo, and (d) the ongoing challenges the patient faces.

Phase 3: The work-through and ending phase (sessions 20–26)

This phase comprises six fortnightly sessions. The IPAF that was developed and worked on in Phase 2 describes the nature of the problem. In Phase 3, the therapist actively helps the patient to focus on giving up the maladaptive patterns summarized in the IPAF. Phase 3 provides an opportunity to do further work on defences and resistance to change by focusing on challenging RIBs. This emphasis will have been present to a degree in Phase 2 as well because it is a core feature of the DIT model. However, in DITCC the therapist has an extended period of time to work very actively on supporting interpersonal change through focusing on how the patient's RIBs interfere with interpersonal change. RIBs are a primary focus of intervention in DITCC via two simultaneously active processes. First, we create an increased sense of agency and, through this, increased trust in talking with others (especially, at this stage, through discussion with the therapist). Second, this provides insight into interpersonal processes that interfere with the possibility of change.

Case example

Sam had been working on a very particular pattern of response to any perceived criticism that created collateral damage in his close relationships. The RIB the therapy focused on was how whenever Sam felt he was being judged, he would immediately raise his voice, posture aggressively (which made his partner feel quite fearful), and start to essentially fight back, thereby quickly escalating the situation. When his partner then cried and pulled away from him, he had no way of understanding her reaction other than that she was rejecting him, and he would then withdraw, refuse to speak to her, and become quite despairing as he feared that he had destroyed the relationship. This chimed with Sam's early experience of the loss of his mother: he had argued with her shortly before she died.

Sam had come to understand that this RIB was very costly to him. He reacted in anger out of fear of losing his partner's love: any criticism was felt bound to undermine the fragile trust he had that he could be lovable. Action made him feel he was not helpless but instead in charge. In Phase 2 of his therapy, Sam was helped to become more mindful of how his fear activated this pattern and how it then made his partner pull away because she became afraid of him. Instances in the therapy when Sam reacted angrily to the therapist, for example, when she invited him to reflect on his characteristic lateness, provided important live experiences of how threatening it was for Sam to imagine that the therapist might not be pleased with his behaviour and how he pre-empted her abandonment by withdrawing and not attending the next session.

Over time, Sam became more capable of voicing how he felt in the moment when he perceived a criticism rather that going into what the therapy termed his 'attack mode', which by then he could appreciate was very emotionally costly to him and exposed him to feeling distanced from the people he wanted to be close to.

Endings in DITCC

The last two sessions of DITCC are spaced a month apart. Throughout Phase 3, the therapist keeps the ending of the therapy in mind and makes reference, when appropriate, to the anxieties it generates and the defences that are mobilized. However, it is only in the last two sessions that the therapist *prioritizes* the patient's affective experience of ending.[1] Many of the patients for whom DITCC is intended will have histories punctuated by loss and separation, some of which are very traumatic. This requires careful attention to how the separation from the therapist will affect the patient, and ensuring that this can be reflected on with the therapist.

As in the standard DIT model, the therapist will present the patient with a 'goodbye' letter. This letter will include many components of the 'taking stock' letter provided in Phase 2, but it is expanded to include an additional acknowledgement of what has been achieved in Phase 3, a new emphasis on ending, and the anticipation of challenges ahead and reminders to the patient of the strategies that have helped them during the therapy.

---

1. In some services, two further follow-up sessions, spaced a month apart, have been offered.

The aim is to actively engage the patient in composing the letter with the therapist in the penultimate session (session 25), allowing this to be the focus of the session, so that a final version can be handed to the patient in session 26. The therapist brings a draft letter to the session and then works together with the patient to review its contents and make amendments as necessary. As is always the case with the DIT model, this more task-oriented work still requires sensitive attunement to the patient's feelings as they work on the letter, because it symbolizes the ending of the therapy and the therapeutic relationship.

Techniques in DITCC

DITCC draws on the same techniques as the DIT model but places a greater emphasis, particularly during Phase 2, on working with defences and enhancing mentalizing.

Working with RIBs and defences

The therapist and patient actively work together to support interpersonal change as agreed in the early part of Phase 2 when goals are negotiated. In DITCC, the extended middle phase of the therapy makes this work more possible at a pace that is appropriate for the entrenched nature of RIBs. This work does not involve setting homework as such, but it requires a concerted effort by the therapist to help the patient to identify the anxieties and defences (i.e. the obstacles to change) that are mobilized when change is encouraged, contemplated, or attempted. The path can then be cleared for the patient to experiment with more adaptive ways of relating to others. The therapist actively supports this experimentation.

Working with the patient's defences is particularly important in DITCC because of the intensity of the pain generated in psychic equivalence (e.g. that the fear of a relationship ending is the same as it having ended, and feeling rejected is the same as having been rejected). This pain explains the use of sometimes dramatic defences. In this context, the emphasis should be first on the validation of defences, the recognition of their necessity, and an appraisal of their cost. Validation, as opposed to interpretation, helps the patient feel more compassionate towards themself and will in time contribute to improved regulation of anxiety and shame.

The work on defences involves:

- Recognizing defences and their cost
- Validating the defences to counteract inevitable shame—this helps the patient to feel more compassionate towards themself and to appreciate the need to regulate anxiety and shame, but with an effort to find ways to do this more effectively
- Recognizing strengths
- In-session challenging of defensive behaviours
- With patients whose capacity for self-representation is very limited, it will be important to recognize this and focus primarily on more remedial work on self-representation.

Mentalizing techniques

In Chapter 7, we outlined the core mentalizing techniques. The same techniques are used in DITCC. In DIT, mentalizing techniques are mainly used where the treatment is temporarily not progressing at the desirable rate. The aim of mentalizing techniques in DITCC is much broader and twofold. First, and most obviously, DITCC cannot be implemented effectively unless the patient is potentially able to understand the therapist's communications, which are usually couched in the language of thoughts, feelings, wishes, beliefs, and desires: mentalizing requires focusing on these states and thinking about them as internal mental experiences. The patient's loss of mentalizing, which can be marked by an increase in concrete thinking (psychic equivalence), a demand for action (teleological mode), and/or portraying a fantasy or resorting to inconsequential talk (pretend mode, which includes 'pseudomentalizing'), is an indication that the therapist should set aside their interpretive work and instead focus on helping the patient to recover their capacity to mentalize. Usually this is best achieved by stopping the discourse when mentalizing has gone 'off-line' and 'rewinding' to the last point where the patient was able to use genuine mentalizing.

Second, specific work on the RIB is required to re-establish trust in the therapist's communications. Creating a mentalized version of the dysfunctional communication patterns that disrupt the patient's full recognition of the IPAF (which usually involves beliefs and feelings about the therapist as well as about other significant figures in the patient's life) is essential if the patient is to be enabled to *hear*, and not just listen to, what the therapist is saying. The following techniques are helpful in relation to both these objectives.

Establishing the intervention trajectory in relation to poor mentalizing

The process starts with identifying that mentalizing has lost its effectiveness in therapy. This might be most obvious because it generates discomfort, boredom, anxiety, or confusion in the therapist. At this point, the most important thing to do is to avoid responding naturally by compensating for the lack of mentalizing in the patient by overmentalizing (i.e. trying to mentalize for both parties). Instead, the therapist should take the following steps aimed solely at helping the patient recover mentalizing.

The therapist starts with validation and empathy, ensuring that the patient recognizes that the therapist is doing their best to understand their perspective and emotional experiences. It is essential that empathic validation is genuine. For example, in listening to a patient's story it is critical that there is something in what the patient says that the therapist is able to resonate with and understand. It is often easier to 'get' a basic emotion than a subsequent social or secondary emotion. For example, if a patient tells a story in which they describe feeling angry at being left out of a group, and then got into a complicated rivalry with a member of the group in which they are trying to get revenge, the therapist might feel a bit lost; they might start by saying 'I understand that you felt angry at being left out . . . ?' and then encourage the patient to unpack the rest of the feelings and events, starting from that basic emotional situation.

The critical component of this phase of empathic validation is *contingency of response* in terms of timing, content, intensity, and value. The therapist's response needs to be accurate and proportionate; exaggerated sadness in relation to the patient's account of a disappointing event would be as bad as the absence of empathy.

Having accepted at face value the patient's claimed experience and assured them of this understanding, the therapist can engage in further focused enquiry to help them clarify the nature of the experience fully and, when necessary, challenge what is being described, to make it something both therapist and patient can understand. Events need to be clarified quickly and not in excessive detail. It is essential that the therapist has a clear overall image of what has happened, as they might need to take the patient back to that sequence and 'relive' specific moments. The focus of clarification is the sequence of mental states rather than the chronological sequence of events. The therapist aims to establish a 'recording' of what the patient *experienced*, rather than a 'video' of what *happened*. Clarification ascertains the patient's reflection on events, including their state of mind before the event, how their feelings changed, and how their current state of mind might again differ.

Once the patient has had a chance to elaborate on their assumptions and model of the situation, the therapist might gently present an alternative perspective and encourage the patient to explore thoughts and feelings that they might not have been aware of previously. These thoughts and feelings are *not* presented with an assumption that the patient had been avoiding or denying them (i.e. defending against awareness of the reality), but as alternatives to be put alongside the patient's own model.

The centre of clarification is an emotion, which is usually embedded in the context of a relationship. We label this 'the elephant in the room' to indicate its size (importance) and the lack of awareness of it. Going back to the earlier case example, Sam's potential to be threatening when he himself felt threatened was an 'elephant'. Poor mentalizing is associated with unreliable labelling of emotions. Emotions need to be explored, validated, and normalized, particularly if they are experienced as either excessive or absent. The therapist needs to be aware of the risk of triggering withdrawal by eliciting shame in psychic equivalence, which leads the patient to retreat from the shame of being seen, or perhaps from being misunderstood.

The emotional or affective focus of the session is assumed to be the feeling that disrupted mentalizing in the particular episode being explored. This is mostly not the affect state that is being described in relation to the incident (e.g. the sadness or anger that emerges in relation to an interpersonal rejection by a loved one) but rather the emotion that the patient anticipates experiencing when someone knows about the story (e.g. a sense of humiliation, perhaps specifically in relation to the therapist's attitude about the event).

There is an implicit move through more neutral discourse towards considering how people the patient cares about, including the therapist, might think or feel about the scenario that upset them. Ultimately, addressing distortions in perceptions is critical, particularly in working to remove the RIB, but premature challenge of persistent assumptions about others' reactions will strengthen rather than weaken these assumptions.

Moving towards understanding a relationship in terms of thoughts and feelings is a gradual process. There is a need to lay the groundwork by the use of hints and normalization. Hints such as 'You feel distrustful of everyone, so I would be surprised if you felt you could trust me' are not thrashed out, but are left as pointers.

As the process develops, alternative perspectives in relation to important aspects of attachment relationships can be presented. This might involve:

1. Challenging assumptions about other people's feelings and/or beliefs
2. Enhancing the complexity of mental models of others (e.g. postulating mixed feelings and conflicts)
3. Creating more complex models of the patient's feelings and thoughts about themself in relation to the other person
4. Elaborating second-order mentalizing between self and other (beliefs and attitudes about putative beliefs and attitudes in the relationship: 'What would she think if she realized that this is what I feel?').

When mentalizing and trust are weak or absent, the move towards understanding any critical attachment relationship has to be gentle. We recommend a number of steps for the therapist to consider. Perhaps the best illustration might be the process of mentalizing the relationship with the therapist.

Mentalizing the relationship with the therapist

As ever, the first step in the process is to start with empathic validation.

As a second step, the patient's current experience needs to be specified in the context of the therapist's recent actions: genuine curiosity in relation to what the therapist might have done to provoke an attitude is essential. At this point, correcting or disputing the patient's experience is contraindicated: a well-timed apology expressing sympathy for how the patient was made to feel is more likely to restore and then strengthen their mentalizing. The acceptance of the patient's experience creates a platform for more extensive exploration in the broader context of the patient–therapist relationship in the direction of increased complexity, nuance, and subtlety.

As a picture of what has happened between the patient and therapist evolves and is jointly held by both parties, different perspectives from those initially presented by the patient can be incorporated into the conversation. This moment, which we call the 'we-mode', refers to a feeling of 'we-ness' usually associated with social collaboration, in which both parties feel they are part of a set of thoughts and feelings that are beyond each of their own minds and are shared (Fonagy et al., 2022). The we-mode is an experience that forms the basis for cooperation and commitment to shared goals, and it catalyses the development of epistemic trust (that the therapist can be trusted as a source of perspective and judgement) and trustworthiness (that the patient themself can be trusted). It generates an experience of feeling, thinking, and acting together. At this moment in the therapy, the patient's and therapist's self-identifications are subsumed into the feeling of a social unit or a team, enabling new ways of functioning *together*. The interpersonal landscape is now 'we-structured'. There is no mysterious leap into a mystical interpersonal space of 'we-ness': it is simply the transition from feeling like two individuals talking about a problem to being a team working on it in an integrated way. The we-mode is the key to re-establishing trust and is a mutual creation. It naturally comes and goes, being lost in non-cooperative interactions and then restored in the cultivation of trust, because it remains possible even when it is temporarily lost.

A critical part of establishing the we-mode between the patient and therapist is cautious openness on the part of the therapist about the way the patient's thoughts and feelings have impacted on the therapist's subjective experience. Illustrating how minds can affect minds in this way is central to the process of enhancing mentalizing. Again, we recommend a number of steps for doing this.

- The therapist takes care to review their subjective experience and how it relates to recent aspects of the patient–therapist interaction.
- The therapist anticipates the patient's likely response, imagines how the patient might respond to a statement of the kind they might be about to make, and incorporates this expectation into their explanation.

- In creating a narrative, the therapist clearly marks the experience as their own, at the same time as marking the expected reaction of the patient as based on the therapist's own experience in similar situations (e.g. 'I am finding myself feeling quite hopeless and almost frustrated, but I know that if someone said that to me I might just feel criticized as if this was somehow my fault').
- Monitoring the patient's reactions is key, and ensuring that the reaction is part of the affect focus powerfully supports the underlying aim of enhancing mentalizing.
- The general attitude of the therapist, particularly at times when mentalizing is weak, should be carefully titrated to the patient's capacity to process social attitudes.
- Priority needs to be given to a sharing attitude characterized by a determination by the therapist to be collaborative. The therapist aims to find out what the patient is experiencing, in as much detail and as coherently as is possible. The patient and therapist metaphorically 'sit side by side' to better understand the patient's experience. The therapist's task is to engender curiosity in the patient: this is possible only if the therapist feels curious too. The achievement of joint awareness, and real interest, is the key to establishing the patient's sense of the therapist as someone who is trustworthy.
- The goals of the patient and therapist in the specific here-and-now interaction are shared, and they have an agreed understanding of what is required. If the patient does not see the point of the therapist's questions because they 'know' the reasons already, the conversation will inevitably be characterized by poor mentalizing. Instead, the conversation has to start where the therapist and patient share interests. For instance, if the patient 'knows' about the self, are they interested in why the other might react in the way they appear to be?
- The therapist must monitor the patient's stress level carefully because high arousal often makes good mentalizing impossible. It is the *therapist's* responsibility, not the patient's, to ensure that arousal is kept within a working range. Equally, the therapist must ensure that their own mentalizing

is adequate for the task and is not compromised by their own arousal or their own persistent RIBs.
- Linked to this, cautious openness on the part of the therapist, in particular sharing some of the impact of the patient's actions on their state of mind, can be an important way of strengthening the patient's mentalizing. Making the therapist's mind accessible (albeit restricted to the context of the therapeutic relationship) is essential to enhancing mentalizing—but, of course, this should not extend to sharing personal information.
- Most important is the demand on the therapist to align the complexity of their mentalizing with that of the patient. It is vital to resist the temptation to overcompensate for the patient's 'off-line' mentalizing with overenthusiastic insistence on providing explanations, clarifications, elaborations, and so on. None of these can be processed by a mind that is not open to mentalizing.
- The discourse is always in the present or in working memory. Wherever possible it tries not to take the patient away from current concerns, whether in their past or in the past of the therapy itself.

SUMMARY

The therapist's aim in DITCC is twofold. The first aim is to understand how the patient's general experience of the social world interferes with their capacity to engage in meaningful dialogue with the therapist, which could lead to behavioural and experiential change in relation to the IPAF. The second aim is to actively support the patient in attempting new ways of addressing the interpersonal problems linked to the onset and/or maintenance of their complex depression by an emphasis on RIBs and increasing the patient's capacity to implement the IPAF through increased mentalizing. When the patient is better able to understand their own and others' reactions in mental-state terms, their capacity to trust others and adapt to social situations will increase as their RIBs are identified and addressed, and subsequently reduce in importance. Achieving trust in the context of therapy then often begins to enable trust in the patient's other social relationships.

Achieving moments of joint or shared understanding of events or issues of relevance to the patient is critical to counteract their distrust, hypervigilance, and social withdrawal.

Although it is longer than standard DIT, DITCC is still a brief intervention. We are not attempting to change the patient's personality structure; instead, we use a psychoanalytically informed approach to initiate a level of trust that allows the therapist to implement an insight-oriented approach despite the limitations imposed by a given personality structure and the defensive constellation that underpins it. Instead of tackling the patient's general difficulties, the intervention is restricted to the specific interpersonal situations that disrupt their confidence in social communication and in the possible helpfulness of other people.

REFERENCES

Allen, J. G. (2021). *Trusting in psychotherapy*. American Psychiatric Press.

Csibra, G., & Gergely, G. (2009). Natural pedagogy. *Trends in Cognitive Sciences*, *13*(4), 148–153. https://doi.org/10.1016/j.tics.2009.01.005

Fonagy, P., & Allison, E. (2014). The role of mentalizing and epistemic trust in the therapeutic relationship. *Psychotherapy*, *51*(3), 372–380. https://doi.org/10.1037/a0036505

Fonagy, P., Campbell, C., Constantinou, M., Higgitt, A., Allison, E., & Luyten, P. (2022). Culture and psychopathology: An attempt at reconsidering the role of social learning. *Development and Psychopathology*, *34*(4), 1205–1220. https://doi.org/10.1017/S0954579421000092

Fonagy, P., & Luyten, P. (2009). A developmental, mentalization-based approach to the understanding and treatment of borderline personality disorder. *Development and Psychopathology*, *21*(4), 1355–1381. https://doi.org/10.1017/S0954579409990198

Fonagy, P., & Luyten, P. (2018). Attachment, mentalizing, and the self. In W. J. Livesley & R. Larstone (Eds.), *Handbook of personality disorders: Theory, research, and treatment* (2nd edn., pp. 123–140). Guilford Press.

Fonagy, P., Luyten, P., & Allison, E. (2015). Epistemic petrification and the restoration of epistemic trust: A new conceptualization of borderline personality disorder and its psychosocial treatment. *Journal of Personality Disorders*, *29*(5), 575–609. https://doi.org/10.1521/pedi.2015.29.5.575

Fonagy, P., Luyten, P., Allison, E., & Campbell, C. (2019). Mentalizing, epistemic trust and the phenomenology of psychotherapy. *Psychopathology*, *52*(2), 94–103. https://doi.org/10.1159/000501526

Rao, A. S., Lemma, A., Fonagy, P., Sosnowska, M., Constantinou, M. P., Fijak-Koch, M., & Gelberg, G. (2019). Development of dynamic interpersonal therapy in complex care (DITCC): A pilot study. *Psychoanalytic Psychotherapy*, *33*(2), 77–98. https://doi.org/10.1080/02668734.2019.1622147

Target, M. (2016). Mentalization within intensive analysis with a borderline patient. *British Journal of Psychotherapy*, *32*(2), 202–214. https://doi.org/10.1111/bjp.12211

14

Dynamic Interpersonal Therapy for Patients with Functional Somatic Disorders

Patients with persistent somatic symptoms or functional somatic disorders (FSDs) can be encountered by practitioners working across the different medical specialities (Burton et al., 2020). They comprise a large subset of patients across the different tiers of health care. The largest meta-analysis to date, covering thirty-two studies in twenty-four countries (total $N = 70,085$ patients), estimated that up to 50% of patients in primary care present with at least one somatic complaint that cannot be readily explained by medical causes, and approximately 30% of patients fulfil criteria for somatic symptom disorder (Haller et al., 2015).

This chapter describes specific adaptations that are made to the dynamic interpersonal therapy (DIT) model for patients with FSDs depending on their position on the spectrum of severity. Patients situated towards the less severe end of the spectrum are likely to benefit most from a combined focus on mental representation and mental process (Fonagy et al., 1993; Luyten, Blatt, et al., 2013) that is typical of the standard sixteen-session DIT model described in this book. The sixteen-session model combines a focus on identifying and working through distortions in the content of mental representations (i.e. the interpersonal-affective focus (IPAF)) with a focus on improving the process of mentalizing. Patients at the less severely affected end of the spectrum typically have the capacity for insight and mentalizing, as well as epistemic trust (the capacity to trust knowledge conveyed by others, including mental health professionals, which we have discussed in Chapter 13) needed for such a combined approach. Patients who have more severe impairments in mentalizing and higher levels of epistemic mistrust struggle to establish a therapeutic alliance, and do not have the necessary mentalizing capacities to benefit from DIT in 16 sessions. Although systematic research is currently lacking, our clinical experience suggests that treatment of these patients requires a greater emphasis on fostering mentalizing (and thus a process focus), particularly in the initial phase. This necessitates a longer treatment of up to twenty-six sessions, as in DIT for complex care (DITCC), which is described in Chapter 13 (see also Rao et al., 2019), or up to forty sessions or more in patients at the more severe end of the spectrum.

THE DIT APPROACH TO UNDERSTANDING PATIENTS WITH FUNCTIONAL SOMATIC DISORDERS

Introduction

Several psychodynamic treatment approaches for patients with FSDs have been developed and empirically evaluated (Abbass et al., 2020; Abbass et al., 2021). Brief psychodynamic therapy is at least as effective as other *bona fide* psychological therapies for these patients, including cognitive-behavioural therapy. Effects are larger for brief psychodynamic therapies longer than twelve sessions and brief dynamic treatments that include a strong focus on emotional experience, which is a key part of DIT and especially DIT adapted for the treatment of patients with FSDs (DIT-FSD). In patients whose disorder is more severe, research findings support the effectiveness of multidisciplinary, multicomponent treatments (Koelen et al., 2014). In this context, a pilot study has provided preliminary evidence for a multicomponent, group-based DIT programme for patients with FSDs (Selders et al., 2015). Brief psychodynamic treatment has also been shown to influence the neurobiological circuits that are central in the development of FSDs, including the stress, reward, and mentalizing systems (Abbass et al., 2014).

DIT presents an integrative psychodynamic approach to the treatment of FSDs. This chapter will outline the particular emphasis given to the role of attachment, impairments in mentalizing, and problems with epistemic trust when treating patients with FSDs. Over the years, as treatment originators and clinicians, we have learned to adopt the not-knowing, enquiring stance with genuine sincerity in relation to patients in general, and in particular with those patients who present with chronic somatic symptoms. For any given patient, it is virtually impossible to gauge the respective role of biological versus psychological factors and their interactions in the patient's presenting problems, particularly in the early stages of treatment, as the DIT therapist's knowledge of the patient and their problems is extremely limited. The DIT therapist should therefore model humility in relation to the cause of the patient's symptoms and be careful not to apply a schematic, and most likely incorrect, understanding of the patient's somatic problems ('Oh, this is probably another case of stress-related problems'). Of course, as treatment progresses, both the patient and therapist will arrive at a better understanding of the patient's presenting problems, but even then, the question of the respective roles of biological and psychological factors typically remains open for discussion. Moreover, the crucial difference from any *a priori* assumptions about the roles of biological and psychological factors made by the therapist is that the patient and therapist will together—in the 'we-mode'—arrive at a better understanding about the roles of these factors during the course of the treatment. The we-mode represents a particular type of co-mentalizing (or *relational mentalizing*) in which intentional states can be shared and joined together with a common purpose—in this case, a shared understanding of the origins of the patient's problems.

DIT therapists should therefore also routinely refer patients presenting with chronic somatic symptoms for a thorough medical screening (except, of course, when the patient has recently had such a screening) to exclude obvious and important causes of somatic symptoms (e.g. a chronic infection or a brain tumour). The fact that the therapist insists that the patient undergoes a medical screening also communicates to the patient that the therapist takes the possible role of biological factors seriously, countering the patient's possible feelings of epistemic mistrust. We might say something like, 'It is clear that biological factors may play an important role in explaining your symptoms; I therefore think it is important that you undergo a thorough medical screening. This may of course not get to the bottom of it, but then we can at least exclude some known causes of symptoms like the ones you have.' Moreover, if all the tests turn out to be negative, this does not mean that biological factors are *not* playing any role in the patient's condition; as science advances, new discoveries about the origins of FSDs will be made, and thus it will never be possible to exclude a potential role for biological factors.

A contemporary psychodynamic approach to FSDs

The DIT approach to FSDs, schematically depicted in Figure 14.1, focuses on issues concerning attachment, mentalizing, and epistemic mistrust.

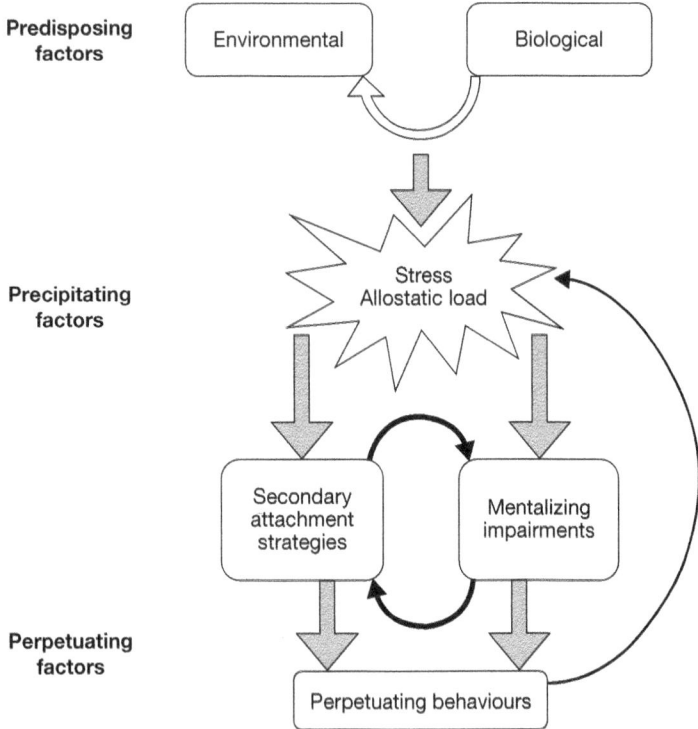

Figure 14.1 Factors that predispose to, precipitate, and perpetuate functional somatic disorders.

ATTACHMENT ISSUES AND THE IPAF

FSDs are part of a spectrum of disorders that result from complex interactions among biological and environmental factors (Tak & Rosmalen, 2010). FSDs typically reflect a chronic overburdening of the stress system as a result of physical and/or psychological stress and conflict, leading to a state of *allostatic load* (McEwen, 2007) (see Figure 14.1), which disrupts the dynamic equilibrium (*allostasis*) that characterizes the stress-regulation system and several key neurobiological systems associated with the stress response, such as the immune and pain-regulating systems and associated biomediators.

It is here that the role of the attachment system, as a key regulator of the stress system, needs to be considered (Maunder & Hunter, 2015). Specifically, the attachment system is activated in response to any type of distress, leading to seeking proximity to attachment figures either in reality (i.e. seeking others for comfort, support, and care in times of need) or at the representational level (i.e. activating representations of attachment figures and memories linked to secure attachment experiences). When attachment figures are available and responsive (either in reality, at the representational level, or both), the individual feels understood, supported, and cared for, which typically leads to effective down-regulation of distress. Developmentally, experiences such as these also give rise, gradually and progressively, to increasing feelings of agency and efficacy in the face of adversity, based on the underlying belief that others will be there in times of need and that the individual will be able to deal with difficulties encountered in life. Hence, co-regulation in relation to attachment figures remains an essential feature of normative stress and emotion regulation across the lifespan (Diamond et al., 2003; Sbarra & Hazan, 2008). At the neurobiological level, this involves the activation of a powerful mesocorticolimbic dopaminergic reward system, which underlies both the rewarding features associated with secure attachment experiences and agency and autonomy, and the down-regulation of the hypothalamic–pituitary–adrenal axis and the sympathetic nervous system involved in the stress response (Luyten & Fonagy, 2018).

Persistent somatic symptoms, either alone or in combination with premorbid psychological distress, fundamentally disrupt the normative down-regulation of distress, as even attachment figures who are available are unable to provide much relief from chronic pain and/or fatigue. As a result, physical stress and psychological stress become closely intertwined. This is demonstrated by studies showing that many patients with FSDs show a pattern of overactivity to 'prove' their self-worth, become involved in counterproductive behaviours (e.g. disregarding their physical limitations), and develop a pattern of excessive rumination, often in combination with sleep problems, leading to a chronic overburdening of the stress system (Luyten, Van Houdenhove, et al., 2013; Van Houdenhove & Luyten, 2008). Moreover, many patients with FSDs encounter invalidating responses from others ('Are your symptoms real? We all feel tired sometimes, you need to pull yourself together'), leading to further difficulties and setting in motion a particularly vicious cycle characterized by increasing levels of emotional distress, conflict, and feelings of being misunderstood and invalidated. As a result, the individual begins to function in a constant state of fight/flight, which may switch to a 'freeze' state, in which they finally give up and feel completely beyond help.

Moreover, as the primary attachment strategy—that is, the normative (co-)regulation of distress—increasingly fails, the individual is forced to shift to the use of *secondary attachment strategies* (Mikulincer & Shaver, 2007) in an attempt to down-regulate distress. These secondary attachment strategies consist of hyperactivation of the attachment system (involving anxious efforts to find understanding, support, and relief, expressed in increasingly demanding behaviour) on the one hand, or deactivation of the attachment system (denying the need for attachment, with the patient resorting to a stance emphasizing independence, strength, and invulnerability) on the other (Cassidy & Kobak, 1988; Mikulincer & Shaver, 2007). The latter strategy is also often expressed in high levels of perfectionism, persistence, overactivity, and the 'all-or-nothing' (or 'boom-and-bust') pattern of behaviour that is typical of many patients with FSDs, to compensate for their underlying feelings of inferiority and vulnerability and their attachment needs (Luyten et al., 2011). In individuals with more severe attachment disruptions, usually from earlier in their lives, a combination of attachment-hyperactivating and attachment-deactivating strategies may occur, leading to cycles of idealization and denigration in their relationships. This extends to their relationships with therapists and other health professionals.

These considerations are highly relevant when formulating the IPAF of patients with FSDs, particularly as these secondary attachment strategies bring some temporarily relief but at the same time are associated with high interpersonal and metabolic costs. The typical IPAFs at the start of treatment of patients who primarily rely on attachment-hyperactivating strategies, attachment-deactivating strategies, or a combination of both are described in Table 14.1.

The role of (embodied) mentalizing

The state of allostatic load and over-reliance on secondary attachment strategies in patients with FSDs also gives rise to impairments in their capacity for mentalizing, and particularly their capacity for *embodied* mentalizing (see Figure 14.1). Embodied mentalizing is the ability to interpret the body as the seat of emotional life and as an intrinsic part of one's own self. It is a common experience for somatic symptoms, such as pain, to be experienced as an 'attack' from within on one's capacity to reflect on the self, and the embodied self in particular; patients often describe their symptoms in terms of an 'internal object' (e.g. referring to their illness as an enemy or a thing they need to negotiate with) that is constantly threatening them from within (Schattner et al., 2008).

Research based on different theoretical traditions, focusing on areas ranging from the role of alexithymia to problems with emotional awareness (Jurist, 2005; Lane et al., 1990; Lumley et al., 2017; Luyten et al., 2019; Taylor & Bagby, 2013), has demonstrated that a significant proportion of patients with FSDs have problems with embodied mentalizing, either because of pre-existing problems or as a result of chronic somatic symptoms, or a combination of the two. These problems pertain to one or, in most cases, several components of embodied mentalizing:

1. **Problems recognizing the relationship between bodily sensations and emotions:** many patients with FSDs seem to be unable to relate bodily experiences to inner mental states ('How do I feel? Tense, bad all the time, that's about it'), and some patients even deny that they feel anything at all ('How do I feel? I feel nothing. I am in pain, that's what counts').

Table 14.1 PROTOTYPICAL IPAFS AS A FUNCTION OF ATTACHMENT STYLE IN PATIENTS WITH FUNCTIONAL SOMATIC DISORDERS

Attachment style	Self	Others	Affect	Defensive function
Attachment-hyperactivating strategies	Weak, vulnerable, neglected, misunderstood	Rejecting, unavailable	Depressed, anxious, helpless, tense	Defence against feelings of frustration/anger
Attachment-deactivating strategies	Strong, invulnerable, self-reliant	Critical, not having the same high standards, disappointing	Empty, tense	Defence against wish to be cared for, supported, and loved
Attachment-hyperactivating/ deactivating strategies	Weak/vulnerable versus strong/attacking	Rejecting versus critical	Depressed, anxious, helpless, tense	Oscillating between defences against anger and wish to be cared for

2. **Problems recognizing emotions as their own:** while some patients with FSDs are easily 'infected' by others' emotions, others deny that they feel depressed, sad, or vulnerable: 'I have never needed anyone's help or support; I have always been strong and independent, and I will overcome this too'.
3. **Problems reflecting on and modulating emotions:** some patients are easily overwhelmed by emotions and/or are quickly triggered to respond in teleological mode, leading to enactments ('Yes, but what are you going to *do* about this?').
4. **Problems sharing emotions appropriately:** many patients with FSDs, particularly in the early stages of treatment, will feel that it is a sign of weakness to share their emotions with others; others, by contrast, will almost immediately share even their most traumatic experiences or most difficult emotions, assuming an inappropriate level of familiarity with their therapist.

These impairments in embodied mentalizing give rise to an increasing pressure to externalize experiences that cannot be successfully mentalized or understood as psychological. In the first instance, an oscillation between hypomentalizing and hypermentalizing ensues. *Hypomentalizing* is often expressed in psychic equivalence functioning ('Why are you asking me how I feel? There is a virus causing my problems, your questions are irrelevant. I feel awful, how would you feel if you were in my shoes?'), which may be associated with a denial of the importance of mental states. Psychic equivalence functioning in patients with FSDs is often combined with teleological mode functioning ('Can we focus on physical, biological factors, please, as they are the real causes of my problems?'). This in turn leads to excessive mentalizing or *hypermentalizing*, which is often expressed in very elaborate narratives about biological factors and/or mental states that lack any grounding in subjective experience.

Yet, these hypomentalizing–hypermentalizing cycles provide little or no relief and leave the patient with unmentalized feelings such as anxiety, depression, rejection, anger, and disgust, which are then externalized in an attempt to restore self-coherence and get rid of these painful feelings ('Why are you not listening to me? I am telling you what's wrong with me, but you keep asking me these irrelevant questions about my life. You clearly do not understand me. As a therapist, you should know better. Are you just like all the others, suggesting that it's all in my mind?').

Epistemic mistrust

The above considerations also shed a different light on the notion that patients with FSDs are 'difficult to treat'. This notion is neither accurate nor helpful. The high levels of epistemic mistrust and even epistemic vigilance (an often hypercritical alertness to the trustworthiness and believability of others) are understandable, given the high prevalence of attachment-related or complex trauma and associated problems with epistemic trust in these patients. For individuals growing up in an abusive and/or neglectful environment, mistrusting others is an understandable adaptation strategy. Moreover, many patients will have had repeated experiences of invalidation from others, including health professionals ('We can't find anything physically wrong with you, perhaps it's all in your mind'; 'Your condition is most probably the result of excessive stress'), which further erodes their epistemic trust in health professionals. Health professionals often still rely on unhelpful diagnostic labels (e.g. 'medically unexplained syndrome') and obsolete models of the origins of FSDs (e.g. assuming that these problems are 'psychosomatic'), and completely underestimate these patients' strong need for empathic validation and understanding (Blom et al., 2012) to counter their epistemic mistrust. Indeed, while the patient remains in a state of epistemic mistrust, any attempt to explain a treatment model to them will be met with suspicion and is likely to be at best ineffective and at worst iatrogenic (Luyten & Abbass, 2013). Hence, as described in more detail in the next section of this chapter, empathic validation and normalization of feelings of despair and epistemic mistrust are particularly important in the first phase of DIT. At the same time, however, the DIT therapist should also be aware that, in a desperate attempt to find help and relief, the patient may temporarily abandon their epistemic mistrust and cling on to the therapist (or to complementary and alternative medicine) as their 'last resort', which may lead to even stronger disappointment, criticism, and increased epistemic mistrust if the therapist does not recognize and address this idealization.

DIT-FSD

Background and basic principles of DIT-FSD

The following sections describe the adaptations to the sixteen-session format of DIT-FSD. This format can be extended to twenty-six sessions, as in DITCC (see Chapter 13), for patients with more severe disorders, or to a more open-ended format in the most severely affected patients. However, even in the case of patients with the most severe presentation, setting a time limit (e.g. forty sessions) is often more productive than open-ended treatment, as most of these patients benefit from a structured approach that activates their underlying dynamics and at the same time provides a clear, time-limited framework that counters regression.

The initial phase (sessions 1–4): engagement and case formulation

As noted above, patients with FSDs function almost continuously in a 'fight/flight' or 'freeze' state because of their inability to effectively regulate (or co-regulate) often high levels of arousal and distress; they therefore typically present with severe problems with (embodied) mentalizing and poor epistemic trust at their first consultation with the therapist, and frequently hold the expectation that the therapist will also be unavailable, or even unwilling, to help co-regulate their distress. This is why in DIT-FSD, particularly in the earliest phase of treatment, there is a very strong *process* focus (i.e. a focus on the recovery of mentalizing and on engaging the patient by developing epistemic trust) rather than a focus on the *content* of the patient's dynamics (i.e. the IPAF). This process focus in DIT-FSD is deliberate: most patients first need to recover their capacity for mentalizing and start to trust their therapist before they can begin to reflect on possible connections between their presenting symptoms and interpersonal issues. Moreover, as discussed earlier, most of these patients have a history of negative encounters with health professionals, characterized by experiences of not being understood and/or not being taken seriously. Although these narratives about rejection and not feeling understood may be related to their IPAF (and in many cases they are, and thus should also be seen as reflecting a strong cautionary tale (see Chapter 4)), any hint on the part of the therapist that there might be a relationship between these experiences and the patient's attachment history is likely to far exceed their mentalizing capacity. Particularly in the initial phase of DIT-FSD, there is therefore a strong focus on avoiding iatrogenic interventions that inadvertently worsen or complicate the problem to be treated. Premature interpretations that rely on a capacity for insight that the patient simply does not (yet) have should be avoided at all costs.

Similarly, equally premature attempts to convey a particular illness theory to the patient may lead to early dropout or stormy transference/countertransference issues (e.g. idealization–denigration cycles, regressive dependency, or sadomasochistic transferences) (Luyten & Abbass, 2013). In the course of DIT-FSD, the understanding of the patient's illness is arrived at through consensus, rather than through conflict or through the therapist conveying (implicitly or explicitly) a particular illness theory. Moreover, this illness theory, which gradually develops during treatment based on experiences in the here-and-now of the therapeutic session, must recognize both the patient's subjective experience and the complexity of the origins of the patient's symptoms.

It is therefore important that the therapist first responds to feelings of invalidation (often in combination with more general feelings of epistemic mistrust and even epistemic vigilance) by strong and empathic validation and normalization of those understandable feelings (which we think of as 'understanding misunderstanding' and empathizing with feeling misunderstood). This typically entails recognizing the reality of the patient's suffering ('You do not have to convince me of the reality of your illness, I can clearly see that you are suffering'), without necessarily agreeing completely with the patient's illness theory. Hence, empathic validation includes distinguishing between the patient's mind and the therapist's mind, thus modelling the not-knowing, inquisitive stance ('I do not know precisely what is wrong with you—how could I know, we have only just met—but I want to find out together with you. For now, I can clearly see you are in pain'). As noted earlier, it is therefore important to refer patients routinely for a thorough medical screening (other than in those cases where the patient has recently undergone such a screening), while also acknowledging that this is not the therapist's field of expertise (in so doing, modelling not knowing everything, and therefore in a sense being with the patient in not yet having an answer).

In some patients, explicitly addressing the cautionary tale of what might 'go wrong' in relation to the therapist is needed and may prevent early dropout or poor outcome. Indeed, the therapeutic relationship tends to activate strong anxieties in these patients, including anxieties rooted in their attachment history; these typically include expectations of being ridiculed, abused, rejected, or abandoned. An open discussion of these anxieties will lead to the patient experiencing greater feelings of being understood and being recognized as an agent, which also fosters curiosity in the therapist's mind and epistemic trust.

Empathic validation and normalizing interventions typically decrease the patient's level of arousal, thus improving their mentalizing capacities and activating interpersonal narratives and material in the here-and-now of the therapeutic session. These narratives lead the way to the joint formulation of the IPAF and a more interpersonal focus, which is based not on what the therapist might suggest is 'wrong' with the patient, but on the actual felt experiences of the patient concerning the connection between bodily states and symptoms and repetitive interpersonal patterns ('Now I come to think about it, this has been the story of my life. I have always been criticized, I was never good enough'). Formulating the IPAF with the patient is therefore the second core focus of the initial phase of DIT-FSD. Empathic validation and normalization come first and lead to the activation of attachment memories, which then enable a greater focus on the content of the patient's dynamics.

In this regard, the DIT therapist should be very alert to the type of secondary attachment strategy that the patient uses to deal with distress, not only because these observations will help in formulating the IPAF with the patient (see Table 14.1), but also because this material provides crucial information about the type of impairments in (embodied) mentalizing that are typical of the patient as well as the interventions that are likely to be effective in improving embodied mentalizing.

Although more insight-oriented interventions are possible in the first phase of DIT-FSD, a process-oriented, validating, and mentalizing focus is still very much in the foreground in this phase. For example, patients with FSDs often depict the self as strong and independent, while they experience others as critical and disappointing, reflecting the use of attachment-deactivating strategies. Yet, these patients often had no other choice in life than to become self-reliant and critical of themselves and others because their parents were emotionally unavailable. Moreover, their strong—but defended against—wishes to be loved and cared for by others often help the therapist to remain empathic with the patient, even when the patient questions and criticizes them.

Finally, with regard to the joint formulation of treatment goals, the DIT therapist again needs to be aware of the importance of acknowledging and validating the patient's wish for changes in physical symptoms and functioning. Because of their training, DIT therapists are often more focused on formulating goals with regard to psychological (and especially interpersonal) issues; patients with FSDs may be very sensitive to this (implicit) bias and are liable to experience it as another rejection, or another experience of being misunderstood or silenced.

The middle phase (sessions 5–12): fostering embodied mentalizing and working through

The middle phase of DIT consists of working through the IPAF and consolidating therapeutic progress. The patient is encouraged to recognize their own IPAF pattern in their daily life between sessions and, based on the work in the therapy, the patient becomes increasingly able to understand its developmental origins, and its advantages and disadvantages (i.e. the emotional 'cost'). Both the patient and therapist increasingly come to understand and accept the patient's pattern as an adaptation strategy that, although understandable, is associated with a high emotional cost and also a substantial physical cost (e.g. pain, fatigue, or restlessness).

A major obstacle to achieving this understanding in patients with FSDs is their often profound impairment in the capacity for embodied mentalizing. It is only when the patient begins to realize the high personal, interpersonal, and metabolic costs of this repetitive pattern of relating to themselves and others *in the here-and-now of the session* that the patient can begin to change.

It is the therapist's task to carefully explore the potential relationships between bodily experiences and unmentalized states of mind

Table 14.2 BASIC PRINCIPLES FOR FOSTERING EMBODIED MENTALIZING

Principle	How?
Not-knowing, inquisitive stance	Be constantly curious about mental states that may underlie bodily experiences, be open to potential meanings, and model misunderstanding
Use of own mind by the therapist	Develop and share hypotheses with the patient about possible feelings linked to particular bodily experiences or expressions (i.e. draw attention to somatic markers of emotions)
Embodied interventions	Use marked mirroring of the patient's bodily expressions
Focus on internal mental states and not behaviour	Stop and explore possible internal mental states linked to somatic markers of emotions
Work at the optimal level of arousal of the patient	Use empathic validation and normalizing interventions when the arousal level is too high; explore internal mental states if the arousal level is too low
Use brief, simple interventions	Focus on the here-and-now of the embodied experience of the patient based on 'micro-slicing' of specific experiences

(Luyten & Fonagy, 2020), using the not-knowing, inquisitive stance and basic mentalizing principles (Table 14.2).

These interventions typically start with the therapist drawing attention to so-called somatic markers of emotions, that is, non-conscious bodily expressions of emotions (Table 14.3). Promoting embodied mentalizing involves the following sequence (named by the mnemonic RADLE), which focuses on **R**ecognizing, **A**mplifying, and **D**ifferentiating between emotions, **L**inking these emotions to the interpersonal dynamics associated with the onset and persistence of symptoms, and marking the **E**motional cost of problems with embodied mentalizing.

Table 14.3 SOMATIC MARKERS OF INNER MENTAL STATES

Facial markers	Frowning, blinking fast, scowling, smiling, blushing, crying
Vocal markers	Speaking very loudly or quietly, stuttering, sudden changes in pitch of voice, quavering voice
Specific bodily markers	Hand clenching, headaches, tension in the shoulders/neck/arms/legs/chest, sighing, sweating, vomiting, fainting, dizziness, restless legs, psychogenic non-epileptic seizures, pseudoparalyses
Body posture markers	Leaning back or forward, making self seem bigger or smaller

Recognizing emotions

Patients with FSDs are often initially almost completely unable to reflect on their bodily and physical sensations ('How do I feel now? I wouldn't know, I just feel tense and tired'). The first task for the DIT therapist is therefore to carefully attend to potential somatic markers of emotions in the patient—that is, undifferentiated, and thus unmentalized, bodily experiences that reflect specific emotions. As the patient is often unable to reflect on these experiences, the DIT therapist must use their own mind to generate hypotheses about these unmentalized bodily experiences and test them against the patient's experience, using marked mirroring. The therapist highlights ('marks' as belonging to the patient) the mental states of the patient contingently in the here-and-now ('mirroring'). Taking the example of an attachment-deactivating patient, the therapist enquires how the patient felt when he had to give a presentation to his team and his co-workers asked him lots of critical questions. The patient replies: 'That's a difficult question, I don't know, I just felt tired, I'd had enough.' While the patient is speaking, the therapist notices him clenching his hands and sighing (potential somatic markers of emotions). The therapist adds: 'I can imagine you must have felt somewhat criticized because of all these questions, which seemed to overwhelm you, as I noticed that while you were talking about your co-workers' response you became tense all over your body, you clenched your hands tightly together, you took a deep breath, and you sighed.' It is important to realize that the therapist is offering this as a hypothesis about the mental states underlying the patient's reactions. As we all have experienced in our own development, attempts at marked mirroring are prone to error. The therapist's not-knowing stance thus implies humility: 'Ah, you didn't feel criticized, but insulted. It's good that you pointed this out; you see how easily I can be mistaken about how you are feeling.'

Many patients with FSDs have experienced serious deficits in marked mirroring in relation to their attachment figures. Therapists may therefore need to point out that patients feel uneasy when someone is genuinely interested in and attempts to mirror their internal mental states, as this activates often ambivalent attachment-related memories in them ('I've noticed that every time I point out that you might be feeling something you might be unaware of, you seem to become slightly uneasy. Is that correct? Does it remind you of experiences you've had before?'). Moreover, it is important that the therapist's attempts at marked mirroring are embodied, just as the marked mirroring provided by attachment figures in early child development is embodied—that is, attachment figures use their bodies to mirror the child's internal mental states, and do so in a modulated way that helps the child to understand and co-regulate their experiences. For instance, the attachment figure widens their eyes when they mirror the child's surprise, or they raise their voice when they mirror indignation. When working with patients who show impairments in embodied mentalizing, it is vital that the therapist is clearly embodied, as otherwise there is a risk that the patient will not feel any connection between bodily states and emotions, and the whole exercise becomes purely cognitive (and is conducted in pretend mode).

AMPLIFYING EMOTIONS

For the same reasons, the therapist then needs to amplify the identified emotions one by one, again using embodied marked mirroring: 'Ah, so you felt *insulted* in the first place; how did that feel?' This strong affect focus is essential in DIT-FSD to foster embodied mentalizing because patients with FSDs are typically largely unaware of their unmentalized bodily experiences (despite the therapist thinking that they must be aware of them, based on patients' often strong non-verbal reactions).

DIFFERENTIATING EMOTIONS

For patients with impairments in embodied mentalizing, it is crucial that they realize that unmentalized bodily experiences almost invariably involve several emotions that are related to one another and typically also to the IPAF. In the example given earlier in this chapter (see 'Recognizing emotions'), the patient felt ridiculed and insulted by his co-workers asking so many questions, and this feeling led to strong feelings of anger (expressed in his sighing and clenching his hands when recounting the incident), followed by guilt about being angry, after which he 'shut down' and felt completely exhausted. Hence, it is the task of the therapist to explore with the patient each of the unmentalized emotions, amplify them, and discover how they are causally linked. Brief recapitulation followed by checking back needs to be used between each of these links ('So, first you felt insulted, which then led to anger and then to guilt because of your anger; is that about right?'). As a result of this process, the patient no longer experiences the self solely in terms of a physical self but also as a psychological self, and develops second-order representations and *mentalized affectivity*, the capacity to reflect on and modulate embodied emotional experiences.

Linking emotions to prototypical ways of relating to the self and others and their connection with presenting symptoms

In the middle phase of treatment, the repeated 'micro-slicing' of embodied experiences invariably leads the patient to realize in the here-and-now of the therapeutic session and between sessions that they have a prototypical pattern of relating to the self and others that is associated with the occurrence, intensity, and, typically, the first onset of their somatic symptoms. It is thus not so much that the DIT therapist attempts to convey to the patient a particular illness theory about the origin of the patient's symptoms, but rather that the patient and therapist 'discover' together in the course of the treatment whether there is a relationship between interpersonal events and somatic symptoms. This leads the patient and therapist to revisit questions concerning the origin of the patient's symptoms and problems. Often, patients express their gratitude for the therapist not forcing a particular illness theory on them at the start of the treatment, and for taking their symptoms seriously ('I remember our first session, you really believed that I was ill; it was then that I had the feeling you might be able to help me').

Highlighting the emotional cost of problems with (embodied) mentalizing

Finally, as the relationship between (interpersonal) experiences and unmentalized emotions becomes clearer, both the advantages and disadvantages of problems with embodied mentalizing can increasingly be discussed. In the above example, for instance, the patient and therapist together might begin to understand that the patient has had a lifelong pattern of feeling ridiculed, which always infuriated him, but he had to 'shut down' feelings of frustration and anger because he feared retaliation—originally by his father, but later by his peers and others, particularly authority figures. This led to a pattern of 'self-silencing' in combination with harsh self-criticism and a tendency to avoid thinking about himself. However understandable this response may have been given his attachment history, all he felt now were feelings of emptiness, fatigue, and vague feelings of frustration and bodily tension and pain, which increasingly incapacitated him.

In most patients with FSDs, there is a distinct shift from a process- or mentalizing-oriented focus to a more content- or insight-oriented focus in the middle phase. The DIT therapist is increasingly able to use the full spectrum of middle phase interventions: (a) supportive interventions (i.e. support, empathic validation), (b) interventions aimed at fostering (embodied) mentalizing; (c) expressive interventions, including interpretation; and, importantly, (d) directive techniques, such as encouraging the patient to experiment with new ways of relating to the (embodied) self and others.

As in the original DIT model, in DIT-FSD there is a limited focus on the transference relationship, particularly in the early stages of treatment. However, in the middle and ending phases, discussion of the link between material that emerges in the therapeutic relationship and the IPAF is often used to further clarify the link between unmentalized emotions and the IPAF. Moreover, when the transference relationship is overly negative (or positive), it is often vital that the patient's underlying anxieties be addressed.

Finally, it is important to realize that such a focus on somatic markers of emotions and the embodied attitude of the therapist in DIT-FSD may not come naturally for some therapists. The active attitude that also makes use of their own body often feels uncomfortable for some therapists initially, especially those who are themselves less in touch with their own embodied self or who defensively avoid such a focus. We have found supervision based on videotaped recordings of sessions particularly useful in this regard.

The ending phase (sessions 13–16): empowerment and improvement

The ending phase in DIT-FSD focuses on empowering the patient to continue the process of therapeutic change after the end of treatment. As is typical of DIT, this process is initiated by the therapist sharing a draft 'goodbye' letter with the patient. The patient is invited to read this letter aloud in the session. Consistent with the focus of DIT-FSD, there is a greater focus than in 'standard' DIT on problems with embodied mentalizing and the patient's illness theory in the goodbye letter for these patients. As described in Chapter 9, the goodbye letter tends to reactivate the patient's IPAF. This provides another opportunity for the patient and therapist to review the extent to which the patient is aware that their typical pattern of responding is indeed reactivated in response to the goodbye letter and the impending end of the treatment.

Empowering the patient to continue the process of therapeutic change during the ending phase and after the end of treatment is particularly important in DIT-FSD, as many patients with FSDs have a lifelong history of either dependency or compulsive self-reliance, both of which will tend to cut them off from the process of *salutogenesis* (the capacity to derive benefit from the social environment; Antonovsky, 1996). In some patients, strong termination reactions may occur (e.g. a worsening of symptoms). It is important to work through such reactions and relate them to the IPAF and the fantasies around ending. In cases where the patient and therapist agree that therapeutic change is still unsatisfactory, it is advisable to add a few booster sessions at a lower frequency (e.g. every two weeks or once a month) rather than switch from time-limited to open-ended treatment. Again, empowering the patient to be able to continue the process of therapeutic change is essential in DIT-FSD; extending treatment sessions with no agreed end date often leads to an unhealthy dependency on the therapist and the treatment. It is always a good idea to discuss these issues with a colleague or in supervision to prevent enactments on the part of the DIT therapist.

CONCLUSIONS

This chapter presents adaptations to the DIT model for treating patients with FSDs based on a contemporary, integrative psychodynamic approach to the conceptualization of patients with persistent somatic complaints. DIT-FSD focuses on these patients' impairments in attachment, embodied mentalizing, and epistemic trust, and particularly the influence of these impairments on the establishment of a therapeutic alliance. Compared with the original DIT model, DIT-FSD involves a greater emphasis on empathic validation to reduce the potential for iatrogenic treatment effects, a stronger focus on the impact of secondary attachment strategies in dealing with unmentalized feelings of conflict and distress, and a greater focus on fostering embodied mentalizing.

REFERENCES

Abbass, A., Lumley, M. A., Town, J., Holmes, H., Luyten, P., Cooper, A., Russell, L., Schubiner, H., De Meulemeester, C., & Kisely, S. (2021). Short-term psychodynamic psychotherapy for functional somatic disorders: A systematic review and meta-analysis of within-treatment effects. *Journal of Psychosomatic Research, 145*, 110473. https://doi.org/10.1016/j.jpsychores.2021.110473

Abbass, A., Town, J., Holmes, H., Luyten, P., Cooper, A., Russell, L., Lumley, M. A., Schubiner, H., Allinson, J., Bernier, D., De Meulemeester, C., Kroenke, K., & Kisely, S. (2020). Short-term psychodynamic psychotherapy for functional somatic disorders: A meta-analysis of randomized controlled trials. *Psychotherapy and Psychosomatics, 89*(6), 363–370. https://doi.org/10.1159/000507738

Abbass, A. A., Nowoweiski, S. J., Bernier, D., Tarzwell, R., & Beutel, M. E. (2014). Review of psychodynamic psychotherapy neuroimaging studies. *Psychotherapy and Psychosomatics, 83*(3), 142–147. https://doi.org/10.1159/000358841

Antonovsky, A. (1996). The salutogenic model as a theory to guide health promotion. *Health Promotion International, 11*(1), 11–18. https://doi.org/10.1093/heapro/11.1.11

Blom, D., Thomaes, S., Kool, M. B., van Middendorp, H., Lumley, M. A., Bijlsma, J. W., & Geenen, R. (2012). A combination of illness invalidation from the work environment and helplessness is associated with embitterment in patients with FM. *Rheumatology (Oxford)*, *51*(2), 347–353. https://doi.org/10.1093/rheumatology/ker342

Burton, C., Fink, P., Henningsen, P., Löwe, B., Rief, W., & Euronet-Soma Group. (2020). Functional somatic disorders: Discussion paper for a new common classification for research and clinical use. *BMC Medicine*, *18*(1), 34–34. https://doi.org/10.1186/s12916-020-1505-4

Cassidy, J., & Kobak, R. R. (1988). Avoidance and its relation to other defensive processes. In J. Belsky & T. Nezworski (Eds.), *Clinical implications of attachment* (pp. 300–323). Routledge.

Diamond, D., Stovall-McClough, C., Clarkin, J. F., & Levy, K. N. (2003). Patient-therapist attachment in the treatment of borderline personality disorder. *Bulletin of the Menninger Clinic*, *67*(3), 227–259. https://doi.org/10.1521/bumc.67.3.227.23433

Fonagy, P., Moran, G. S., Edgcumbe, R., Kennedy, H., & Target, M. (1993). The roles of mental representations and mental processes in therapeutic action. *Psychoanalytic Study of the Child*, *48*(1), 9–48. https://doi.org/10.1080/00797308.1993.11822377

Haller, H., Cramer, H., Lauche, R., & Dobos, G. (2015). Somatoform disorders and medically unexplained symptoms in primary care. *Deutsches Ärzteblatt International*, *112*(16), 279–287. https://doi.org/10.3238/arztebl.2015.0279

Jurist, E. L. (2005). Mentalized affectivity. *Psychoanalytic Psychology*, *22*(3), 426–444. https://doi.org/10.1037/0736-9735.22.3.426

Koelen, J. A., Houtveen, J. H., Abbass, A., Luyten, P., Eurelings-Bontekoe, E. H., Van Broeckhuysen-Kloth, S. A., Buhring, M. E., & Geenen, R. (2014). Effectiveness of psychotherapy for severe somatoform disorder: Meta-analysis. *British Journal of Psychiatry*, *204*(1), 12–19. https://doi.org/10.1192/bjp.bp.112.121830

Lane, R. D., Quinlan, D. M., Schwartz, G. E., Walker, P. A., & Zeitlin, S. B. (1990). The Levels of Emotional Awareness Scale: A cognitive-developmental measure of emotion. *Journal of Personality Assessment*, *55*(1–2), 124–134. https://doi.org/10.1080/00223891.1990.9674052

Lumley, M. A., Schubiner, H., Lockhart, N. A., Kidwell, K. M., Harte, S. E., Clauw, D. J., & Williams, D. A. (2017). Emotional awareness and expression therapy, cognitive behavioral therapy, and education for fibromyalgia: A cluster-randomized controlled trial. *Pain*, *158*(12), 2354–2363. https://doi.org/10.1097/j.pain.0000000000001036

Luyten, P., & Abbass, A. (2013). What is the evidence for specific factors in the psychotherapeutic treatment of fibromyalgia? Comment on 'Is brief psychodynamic psychotherapy in primary fibromyalgia syndrome with concurrent depression an effective treatment? A randomized controlled trial'. *General Hospital Psychiatry*, 35(6), 675–676. https://doi.org/10.1016/j.genhosppsych.2013.07.007

Luyten, P., Blatt, S. J., & Fonagy, P. (2013). Impairments in self structures in depression and suicide in psychodynamic and cognitive behavioral approaches: Implications for clinical practice and research. *International Journal of Cognitive Therapy*, 6(3), 265–279. https://doi.org/10.1521/ijct.2013.6.3.265

Luyten, P., De Meulemeester, C., & Fonagy, P. (2019). Psychodynamic therapy in patients with somatic symptom disorder. In D. Kealy & J. S. Ogrodniczuk (Eds.), *Contemporary psychodynamic psychotherapy: Evolving clinical practice* (pp. 191–206). Academic Press. https://doi.org/10.1016/B978-0-12-813373-6.00013-1

Luyten, P., & Fonagy, P. (2018). The stress-reward-mentalizing model of depression: An integrative developmental cascade approach to child and adolescent depressive disorder based on the Research Domain Criteria (RDoC) approach. *Clinical Psychology Review*, 64, 87–98. https://doi.org/10.1016/j.cpr.2017.09.008

Luyten, P., & Fonagy, P. (2020). Psychodynamic psychotherapy for patients with functional somatic disorders and the road to recovery. *American Journal of Psychotherapy*, 73(4), 125–130. https://doi.org/10.1176/appi.psychotherapy.20200010

Luyten, P., Kempke, S., Van Wambeke, P., Claes, S., Blatt, S. J., & Van Houdenhove, B. (2011). Self-critical perfectionism, stress generation, and stress sensitivity in patients with chronic fatigue syndrome: Relationship with severity of depression. *Psychiatry: Interpersonal and Biological Processes*, 74(1), 21–30. https://doi.org/10.1521/psyc.2011.74.1.21

Luyten, P., Van Houdenhove, B., Lemma, A., Target, M., & Fonagy, P. (2013). Vulnerability for functional somatic disorders: A contemporary psychodynamic approach. *Journal of Psychotherapy Integration*, 23(3), 250–262. https://doi.org/10.1037/a0032360

Maunder, R. G., & Hunter, J. (2015). *Love, fear, and health: How our attachments to others shape health and health care*. University of Toronto Press.

McEwen, B. S. (2007). Physiology and neurobiology of stress and adaptation: Central role of the brain. *Physiological Reviews*, 87(3), 873–904. https://doi.org/10.1152/physrev.00041.2006

Mikulincer, M., & Shaver, P. R. (2007). *Attachment in adulthood: Structure, dynamics and change*. Guilford Press.

Rao, A. S., Lemma, A., Fonagy, P., Sosnowska, M., Constantinou, M. P., Fijak-Koch, M., & Gelberg, G. (2019). Development of dynamic interpersonal therapy in complex care (DITCC): A pilot study.

Psychoanalytic Psychotherapy, *33*(2), 77–98. https://doi.org/10.1080/02668734.2019.1622147

Sbarra, D. A., & Hazan, C. (2008). Coregulation, dysregulation, self-regulation: An integrative analysis and empirical agenda for understanding adult attachment, separation, loss, and recovery. *Personality and Social Psychology Review*, *12*(2), 141–167. https://doi.org/10.1177/1088868308315702

Schattner, E., Shahar, G., & Abu-Shakra, M. (2008). 'I used to dream of lupus as some sort of creature': Chronic illness as an internal object. *American Journal of Orthopsychiatry*, *78*(4), 466–472. https://doi.org/10.1037/a0014392

Selders, M., Visser, R., van Rooij, W., Delfstra, G., & Koelen, J. A. (2015). The development of a brief group intervention (dynamic interpersonal therapy) for patients with medically unexplained somatic symptoms: a pilot study. *Psychoanalytic Psychotherapy*, *29*(2), 182–198. https://doi.org/10.1080/02668734.2015.1036106

Tak, L. M., & Rosmalen, J. G. M. (2010). Dysfunction of stress responsive systems as a risk factor for functional somatic syndromes. *Journal of Psychosomatic Research*, *68*(5), 461–468. https://doi.org/10.1016/j.jpsychores.2009.12.004

Taylor, G. J., & Bagby, R. M. (2013). Psychoanalysis and empirical research: The example of alexithymia. *Journal of the American Psychoanalytic Association*, *61*(1), 99–133. https://doi.org/10.1177/0003065112474066

Van Houdenhove, B., & Luyten, P. (2008). Customizing treatment of chronic fatigue syndrome and fibromyalgia: the role of perpetuating factors. *Psychosomatics*, *49*(6), 470–477. https://doi.org/10.1176/appi.psy.49.6.470

15

Internet-Delivered Dynamic Interpersonal Therapy (i-DIT) for Depression and Anxiety

Many patients with depression or anxiety do not seek treatment, delay seeking treatment, drop out of treatment, or do not receive adequate treatment (Cuijpers et al., 2010; Luyten & Fonagy, 2014; Rost et al., 2019). These factors lead to high levels of unmet need among people with depression. Internet-delivered treatments might play an important role in filling this treatment gap (Andersson et al., 2019). The start of the Covid-19 pandemic in 2020 focused many treatment services and researchers, more than previously, on how to make therapies available online or in a blended format. Internet-delivered treatments are offered either (a) as unguided self-help, in which users work through the intervention themselves, unaided; (b) as guided self-help, in which administrative or therapeutic support is provided during the intervention by telephone, text, or chat messages; or (c) in a blended format, in which work on the online programme is integrated into and alternated with in-person face-to-face sessions. Each of these formats may connect with patients who are otherwise difficult to reach with more traditional forms of psychotherapy. Although there is good evidence to suggest that the effectiveness of online treatments increases with increasing support from a therapist (Andersson et al., 2019; Richards & Richardson, 2012), unguided self-help may be particularly effective for patients with considerable reflective capacities and high levels of agency and autonomy, and might also help those who are unwilling to seek any in-person help for their mental health problems (Andersson et al., 2019; Bendelin et al., 2011). Blended therapy may be appropriate for an even larger group of patients, as it includes face-to-face sessions (and thus therapist support) while also enabling patients to work on their problems themselves at a time and location that is convenient for them (van der Vaart et al., 2014), thereby offering 'the best of both worlds'. Findings across therapy modalities suggest that therapist support may be particularly important for facilitating the therapeutic process, including addressing factors that impede progress in treatment, while the internet-based, self-help components help to foster feelings of agency and autonomy, as patients are more in charge of their own therapeutic process than in traditional face-to-face therapy. Indeed, some studies suggest that blended therapy may be as effective as traditional face-to-face therapy, and, as blended therapy is typically associated with a 30–50% reduction in therapist time, it is also more cost-effective (Thase et al., 2018). Compared with unguided internet-delivered therapies, blended treatment may also be better able to reach digitally and socioculturally disadvantaged and minority groups, although these groups remain under-represented in studies of e-mental health and effective uptake of e-health (Stone & Waldron, 2019). Indeed, the digital and language skills required for engagement with e-mental health interventions are beyond the reach of many people, particularly those in some minoritized ethnic groups. This is an important concern in mental health care in general (Lund et al., 2018).

Whereas until recently most internet-delivered treatments were rooted in cognitive-behavioural approaches, there is a growing body of research documenting the effectiveness of psychodynamic internet-based treatments (Andersson et al., 2019; Lindegaard et al., 2020). A recent meta-analysis involving 1080 patients showed that internet-delivered psychodynamic therapy was more effective than control conditions in reducing depression ($g = 0.46$) and anxiety ($g = 0.20$), and in improving quality of life ($g = 0.46$). These effects were maintained or increased at follow-up and were similar to those typically found for brief face-to-face psychotherapy (Cuijpers et al., 2020). These results are in line with findings concerning the effectiveness of internet-delivered psychotherapy more generally. An individual participant meta-analysis of guided internet-based interventions, involving twenty-four randomized controlled trials (and a total of 4889 participants), showed that these interventions were associated with recovery rates similar to those achieved by face-to-face interventions (Karyotaki et al., 2018).

Despite limitations, there is clearly emerging evidence for the effectiveness of internet-delivered treatments and their potential to fill the gap in the treatment of depression and related conditions. As we describe in Chapter 12, an online version of dynamic interpersonal therapy (DIT) with therapist facilitation was shown in a small pilot study to be very promising, with substantial recovery rates.

Based on these findings, unguided i-DIT, guided i-DIT (supported through online chat with a therapist), and blended i-DIT have been developed. At the time of writing, various studies investigating the efficacy and cost-effectiveness of blended i-DIT and unguided i-DIT are in progress. This chapter describes the structure of i-DIT and outlines the specific competences needed to deliver i-DIT and blended i-DIT in particular, including assessment of patients' suitability for i-DIT and managing resistance to online work. This chapter is therefore written with practising DIT therapists in mind, with a focus on helping them, if appropriate, to acquire the necessary skills and competences to deliver i-DIT.

THE STRUCTURE OF BLENDED I-DIT

As shown in Figure 15.1, the structure of blended i-DIT is largely similar to that of face-to-face DIT, except blended i-DIT consists of eight face-to-face sessions and eight online modules for the patient to complete between the face-to-face sessions. Face-to-face sessions are typically scheduled every two weeks to give patients enough time to complete the online modules and work on the issues discussed in treatment. This schedule also means that the treatment length of blended i-DIT is the same as the sixteen-session DIT model. Of course, it is possible to adapt this approach, for example, by increasing the number of face-to-face sessions or online modules. Blended i-DIT can also be offered, with some modifications, in a group format. We have found that it is often more effective if patients enter the DIT group with an interpersonal-affective focus (IPAF) formulation, as it may take a lot of group time to arrive at a formulation for each member, although this approach may work in smaller or slow-open groups.

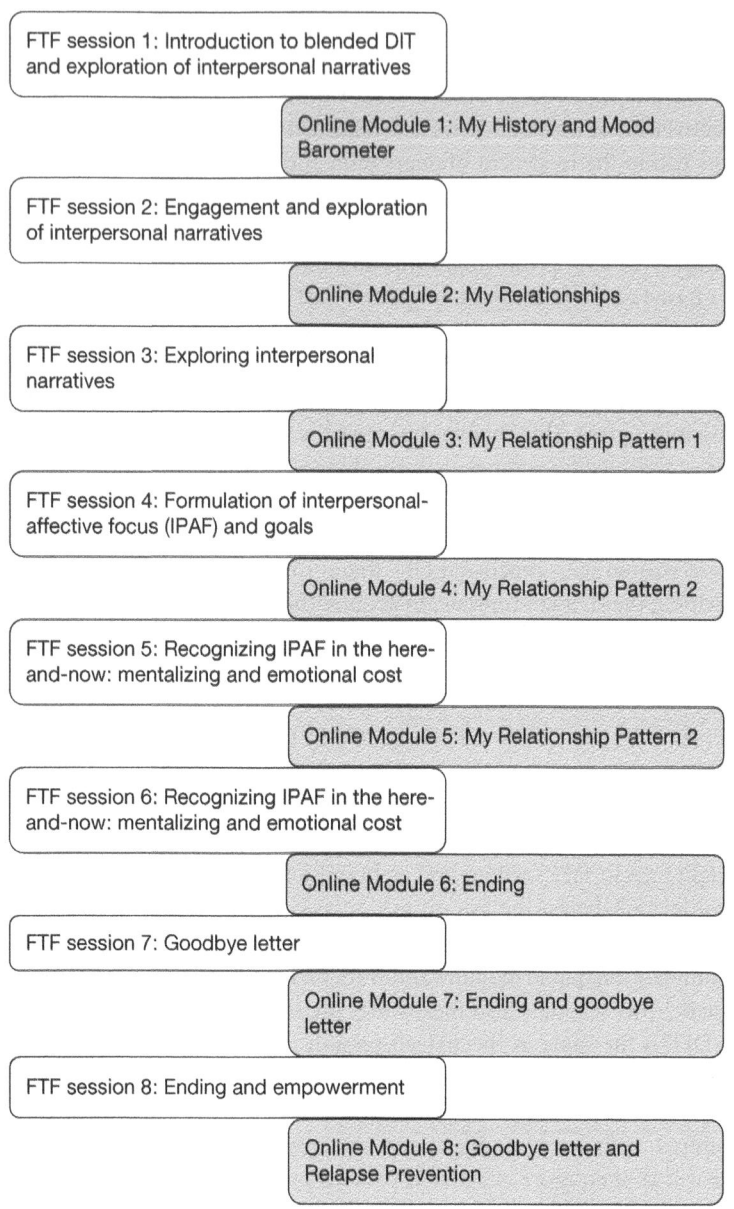

Figure 15.1 Structure of blended i-DIT. Note: FTF = face-to-face.

The initial phase of blended i-DIT also focuses on engagement and case formulation. For many patients, it may be desirable to extend this phase of the treatment, as they may find it too overwhelming to be introduced to both the overall DIT approach and blended i-DIT in particular in the first session. This is often also too cumbersome for DIT therapists, who, in addition to all the tasks of the first DIT session, have to provide the patient with the necessary information on accessing the online modules. This information includes how to log in and set and change their password, and an explanation of what the patient should do if they experience any problems accessing or completing the modules. Hence, for many patients, either the initial phase should be extended by one or two sessions or, even better, the DIT therapist should assess the patient's suitability for i-DIT and introduce the patient to blended i-DIT at the end of an intake phase consisting of two or three intake sessions, during which the patient is provided with all the necessary information about blended i-DIT. This approach includes giving the patient a flyer containing information about i-DIT, which they can read before the start of the first therapy session.

Whatever specific treatment format is used, at the end of the initial face-to-face therapy session, the first online module ('My History and Mood Barometer') is introduced to the patient. This module focuses on the developmental history of the patient (including important events and stressors and their impact on the patient) and the patient's presenting psychological symptoms and problems.

The patient's responses to the different tasks that make up the first online module are then taken as a starting point for the second face-to-face session, as they enable the therapist to focus on interpersonal narratives related to important life events and experiences, as well as the patient's presenting symptoms, consistent with the interpersonal focus of DIT ('I was struck by the fact that you described that your father died when you were 11. Can you tell me a bit more about what happened then, and what effect it has had on you?'). A face-to-face session in blended i-DIT typically begins by reviewing the patient's online responses and thus is slightly more structured than traditional face-to-face DIT. Similarly, at the end of each face-to-face session, a new online module is introduced to the patient. The second online module, 'My Relationships', focuses on important relationships in the patient's life, using an interactive task that involves the patient positioning important people in their life in an interpersonal circumplex. This module also includes the relationship questionnaire (described in more detail in Chapter 4), which assesses the patient's attachment style. Once the patient has completed this questionnaire, the results are presented in a graph. Patients often bring a printout of their interpersonal map and attachment-style graph to the next face-to-face session, which is a starting point for further exploration of their interpersonal narratives. Alternatively, the therapist reviews the patient's responses in the third face-to-face session on a tablet or laptop, and together the therapist and patient reconstruct the patient's thoughts and feelings while they were completing the second module. As in 'traditional' DIT, this process contributes to a more precise formulation of the patient's typical interpersonal patterns and their relationship to presenting symptoms. It is important to note that many of the patient's responses (e.g. to the relationship questionnaire) are automatically copied into subsequent exercises and modules. It is important for the therapist to encourage the patient to update their responses (if needed) based on what is discussed in each face-to-face session. These changes can be made during or after the face-to-face session.

At the end of the third face-to-face session, the DIT therapist introduces the online module 'My Relationship Pattern 1', which focuses on the patient's self- and other-representations, the emotions linking the two, and the potential adaptive or defensive function of this pattern. In this module, patients arrive at their own IPAF formulation, which is then discussed in the fourth face-to-face session, during which the patient and therapist jointly formulate and agree on the IPAF and goals for treatment. At the end of the fourth session, the next module, 'My Relationship Pattern 2', is introduced to the patient. This module contains specific exercises to foster the patient's mentalizing in general, and specifically about the identified IPAF, by asking the patient to recognize the IPAF playing out in their daily life. In addition, the patient is invited to reflect on the possible advantages and disadvantages ('cost') of this pattern as it occurs in relationships with significant others (including the therapist), and on how the patient could change this pattern.

These issues form the focus of face-to-face session 5, after which the patient revisits the 'My Relationship Pattern 2' module in an effort to consolidate their mentalizing skills and reflect on the advantages and the cost of the IPAF. The patient's reflections are discussed in face-to-face session 6, which often also involves a conversation about new ways of relating to the self and others, and the difficulties that may arise when trying to do this. At the end of this session, the next online module ('Ending') is introduced, which invites the patient to reflect on their progress in treatment before the next face-to-face session.

The patient brings their thoughts and feelings with regard to their progress and any areas of disappointment in the treatment to session 7, in which the therapist also introduces the goodbye letter and invites the patient to read it together with them (see Chapter 9). As expected, this session also includes a discussion of changes that might need to be made to the letter. After the session, the letter is uploaded to the online system by the therapist and is thus available to the patient.

The eighth and final face-to-face session discusses any other changes that the patient would like to make to the goodbye letter, and also introduces the final online module, focusing on relapse prevention—that is, planning how the patient will continue the work that has begun, and helping the patient to recognize any signs of relapse. Hence, blended i-DIT has a very strong focus on empowering the patient to continue the therapeutic process after the end of the treatment. To this end, the online system and all the modules remain available for the patient to access for at least a year after the end of treatment.

SPECIFIC COMPETENCES NEEDED TO DELIVER BLENDED I-DIT

Delivering blended i-DIT requires a number of specific competences. In this section, we discuss these competences, illustrate them with concrete examples, and explain how they are linked to each other, in that they all relate to the overall capacity of the DIT therapist to combine and integrate online work and face-to-face sessions into a single, coherent treatment approach. Although some DIT therapists may struggle initially to achieve this integration, most develop the necessary competences quickly through supervision, preferably based on videotaped sessions and delivered in small groups so that participants can learn from one another.

Assessment of suitability

In addition to the general criteria around suitability for DIT set out in Chapter 1, both practical and psychological criteria are weighed up when assessing a prospective patient's suitability for i-DIT. In terms of practical criteria, although this may seem self-evident, patients need not only good access to the internet but also sufficient computer and language literacy to benefit from internet-delivered treatments. Notwithstanding that the vast majority of patients seen in economically developed countries have access to the internet, it is always a good idea to explore these issues in some detail with the patient, as problems with internet access or with computer/language literacy have been associated with dropout from internet-based treatments (Johansson et al., 2015). For instance, many patients are able to access the internet only via a smartphone (which might limit their ability to complete online exercises because of the small screen) or use a device that they have to share with other family members and/or that is located in a busy area of their home, so that they have little opportunity to complete the online modules in private. i-DIT is written in accessible language and contains many examples to support patients in completing the online modules; however, it still requires sufficient computer literacy and language capacity to complete the online work. In this regard, it is important that the DIT therapist is open about their own computer literacy. Patients often find it quite helpful and validating when the therapist acknowledges their own struggles with the online world, and with i-DIT in particular ('Don't worry too much about it; the first time I had to log into the system I felt a bit anxious as well, particularly as I'm not really a computer wizard, so I can relate to your doubts').

Besides these important practical factors in considering patients' suitability for i-DIT, there is emerging practice-based evidence that i-DIT may considerably expand the group of patients who might benefit from the DIT approach. Moreover, in contrast to many therapists' beliefs, suitability for i-DIT is not restricted to patients with 'mild to moderate' problems only, and certain patients with more severe problems can benefit from the approach. In assessing suitability, it is helpful to distinguish between the following five groups of patients.

1. **Patients presenting with mild to moderate psychological problems, relatively good reflective capacities and epistemic trust, who have an interest in interpersonal and affective themes.** These patients may be particularly suited for i-DIT. These are typically patients with high levels of autonomy and agency. Particularly when they also have a preference for self-sufficiency, these patients tend to prefer unguided or guided self-help, as they prefer to address their problems on their own or with minimal therapist support. When their ambivalence towards accepting help from others is less prominent, these patients are good candidates for blended i-DIT. This group of patients has also been described as 'doers', as they prefer an active approach to addressing their psychological difficulties and are able to translate and generalize the skills that they acquire in treatment to their everyday life (Bendelin et al., 2011).
2. **Patients presenting with more severe psychological problems and/or greater impairments in mentalizing and epistemic trust.** This group of patients is not necessarily disqualified from i-DIT. With these patients, more work during the intake and initial phases of i-DIT is needed to address their ambivalence towards psychotherapy (including, but not limited to, i-DIT) and their underlying anxieties. In the case of i-DIT, these anxieties are typically related to their IPAF (e.g. that they 'are being left on their own' in more dependent patients, or 'will not able to live up to expectations' in more self-critical patients). Yet, when these patients are given sufficient empathic validation, and their underlying anxieties are addressed and linked to their IPAF, where appropriate, most are suitable for i-DIT, particularly guided or blended i-DIT. In fact, as illustrated later in the section 'Motivating patients to engage in online work', a discussion of these anxieties often contributes to an initial IPAF formulation and the patient realizing the emotional cost of their typical pattern of relating to the self and others (e.g. by realizing how anxious they are about trying out something new).
3. **Patients with a marked borderline level of functioning.** These patients are characteristically less amenable to i-DIT as they tend to lack the necessary reflective capacities needed for unguided self-help, or are likely to develop

split transferences between work with their therapist and online therapy. Such fragmented transferences are difficult to manage and integrate. For instance, the patient might increasingly idealize the therapist and devalue online work ('It is just childish, I want to talk to you, can we just stop the online work?') or they might begin pointing to perceived inconsistencies ('It is not clear what you expect from me. I completed the online exercises, I thought we were going to discuss them here today, but now you have started talking about something else'). They might also report severe instances of self-harm or interpersonal trauma in the online exercises, but deny that these happened or minimize them in their subsequent in-person session with their therapist. Patients with less profound borderline features experience fewer problems in this regard and thus might be suited to i-DIT. Similarly, when i-DIT is integrated into a more comprehensive treatment approach (e.g. a specialist outpatient programme for patients with borderline personality disorder), the internet-delivered treatment might form an important component of the overall package.
4. **Patients who show a combination of more severe psychological problems, often in combination with a history of substantial trauma, but who often also have remarkable resilience.** Internet-delivered DIT, in particular blended i-DIT, may be of particular benefit in this group. For these patients, the fact that they can work on their difficulties on their own helps them develop feelings of agency and resilience.
5. **Patients with chronic mental health difficulties, and/or patients who have been disappointed by more traditional mental health care approaches.** Perhaps somewhat surprisingly, these patients seem to derive some benefit from internet-delivered treatments. This is also our experience with i-DIT, in particular unguided i-DIT. More research is needed to clarify the reasons for this, but it seems that online work provides these patients with a new way to address their psychological difficulties in combination with a sense of agency and control.

Of course, as we have pointed out in relation to suitability for psychotherapy more generally (Chapter 1), much research remains to be done to investigate factors associated with suitability for i-DIT. These studies also promise to shed more light on the potential harmful effects of internet-delivered treatments (Johansson et al., 2015).

Motivating patients to engage in online work

From experience so far, many patients respond positively when the therapist proposes blended i-DIT as a treatment option. Patients are generally keen to find out more about the online modules, and particularly like the fact that online work implies that they are more in control of their own therapy than they would be in traditional face-to-face therapy. In fact, anxieties and concerns about blended i-DIT are often considerably greater in DIT therapists training in the approach than in patients.

However, even when patients meet the suitability criteria for blended i-DIT discussed earlier, they might raise concerns about blended treatment either at the start or during the course of treatment. The DIT therapist needs to be open to these concerns and empathically validate them based on a realistic and nuanced approach towards the possibilities and challenges of blended therapy, supporting the patient's agency and autonomy ('I'm sure it will not always be easy, I can see that given what you just told me, but I will be here to help you and I trust that you can do it'). This approach is, of course, consistent with the overall approach of DIT, with its emphasis on fostering autonomy and agency. Hence, particularly in the initial phase, acknowledging and discussing potential obstacles and difficulties is a key component of blended i-DIT. The DIT therapist might also consider logging into the online system in face-to-face sessions with the patient, using a tablet or laptop, so that the patient feels supported and the therapist can monitor the patient's responses to the online system in vivo. As discussed in more detail below, although some of the difficulties might be purely practical (e.g. 'When should I complete the online work?'), even practical concerns are often related to the patient's IPAF. In this respect, a discussion of the patient's responses to the online system as a whole, and to its modules and exercises, generates considerable interpersonal narratives in the here-and-now of the session that will help in developing the IPAF (for instance, 'How will my husband react to this? He isn't used to me doing something on my own').

Introducing blended i-DIT and the rationale behind this treatment approach requires the DIT therapist to feel confident and comfortable with the approach themself. Potential concerns or anxieties in this respect need to be addressed in training and supervision. This also leads naturally to a discussion of resistance to online work, both in the patient and in the therapist, and how to manage it when it arises.

Recognizing and dealing with resistance to online work

Many therapists starting to use blended i-DIT feel uncomfortable when patients come to a session and say that they have not completed their online work or struggled to do so ('I am sorry but I didn't complete the module. I was just so busy'). Rather than exploring the reasons behind this behaviour and its potential relationship with the patient's IPAF, we have noted that many DIT therapists who are new to blended i-DIT tend to disregard the incomplete module ('OK, I see, so let's see what we can do then in this session. How has your week been since we met last time? It seems you have been very busy'). Or even worse, the therapist dismisses the potential value of online work and thus colludes with the patient's resistance ('Yes, I can see you have had a tough week and then on top of that you needed to complete these online exercises. Don't worry about it, let's just talk about it here today, I'm sure that's a lot easier').

In blended i-DIT it is important first to acknowledge the patient's difficulties in completing the online work and then to carefully explore what prevented the patient from completing the online exercises, using 'micro-slicing', that is, a detailed reconstruction with the patient in the here-and-now of the session of the patient's thoughts and feelings immediately before and while attempting to complete the online exercises. These thoughts and feelings are almost invariably related to the IPAF, and thus are helpful not only in clarifying the patient's resistance to online work but also in developing the formulation. Some examples include:

- The grandiose patient who becomes annoyed every time they think about the online modules: 'Surely I don't fit into any of these categories' or 'This is beneath me; I'd rather talk to you than answer childish questions online; this is clearly developed for morons.'
- The perfectionistic patient who spends hours completing an exercise, trying to be as comprehensive as possible, and finally gives up feeling guilty and ashamed: 'My therapist will be so disappointed in me, they will think I'm stupid.'
- The dependent patient who feels alone or even abandoned by the therapist while completing the online modules, and increasingly feels like a failure for 'not being able to answer even the most obvious questions about myself. It is just yet more proof that I'm useless.'

Hence, the patient's response to the online work typically contains transference tracers. Take the example of a dependent patient with marked passive-aggressive features, who is very collaborative and eager to please in the face-to-face sessions but fails to do the online work before each session, every time shamefully apologizing, 'I have really done my best, but everything has been so hectic, and I couldn't concentrate. I know you will be disappointed in me, but please don't be, I really gave it my all.' Detailed micro-slicing, however, revealed that every time this patient logged into the online system, she began to feel frustrated and annoyed because it reminded her of her mother, who had always insisted that she had to do her homework. The patient and therapist were then able to arrive at a deeper understanding of the patient's IPAF and how this influenced her response to both the online work and the therapeutic relationship. It also allowed clarification of the cost of her IPAF: by placating while at the same time feeling frustrated and angry (i.e. a pattern of passive aggression), she denied herself opportunities for change and growth.

Addressing resistance to online work involves the following sequence:

1. Empathic validation and normalization of the patient's difficulties in completing online modules
2. Exploring the patient's feelings and thoughts, rewinding to when the patient started to complete the online exercises

and/or when the patient thought about completing them, through micro-slicing
3. Linking these feelings and thoughts to the patient's IPAF
4. Validating and accepting the thoughts and feelings as understandable, but also as exacting an emotional cost
5. Inviting the patient to complete the online exercises together in the session.

As we have noted, DIT therapists who deliver blended i-DIT need to explore their own (often unconscious) attitudes towards online work, including potential idealization ('Blended treatment is so much better than traditional therapy') and reducing anxiety by limiting direct contact with patients, as well as possible resistance to and denigration of digital media ('Blended therapy is not the real thing; it will never be able to replace the talking cure'). These attitudes may also interact with the patient's IPAF, reinforcing the resistance.

It is important in this context to note that most therapists' training has a strong (and often exclusive) focus on traditional face-to-face treatments only. It is therefore once again important to realize that most patients have fewer reservations about online work than many therapists assume. DIT therapists who feel uncomfortable or uneasy about using a laptop or tablet in the session with the patient can also print out the online exercises or use a flipchart to discuss the exercises. Patients will rarely find this odd; on the contrary, they almost always appreciate the therapist taking the time to work together with them in completing the exercises, and will often want to take a picture with their smartphone of the work they have done with the therapist on the printed exercises or the flipchart.

Formulation of the IPAF

One of the main differences between fully face-to-face DIT and blended i-DIT is that most patients will come to the face-to-face session (typically the fourth face-to-face session in the model trajectory depicted in Figure 15.1) with their own IPAF formulation. Hence, rather than formulating the IPAF together with the therapist in the third or fourth session, as would be the case in 'traditional' DIT (as discussed in Chapter 5), many patients will memorize or perhaps print or take a screenshot of the IPAF formulation that they completed online and bring it to the face-to-face session. The patient and therapist then work together in the session to review and refine the IPAF, in a similar fashion to the work typically done in face-to-face DIT.

It is crucial that the DIT therapist validates the patient's efforts in formulating their IPAF online in i-DIT. For many patients, formulating their own recurring pattern of 'self-affectively-interacting-with-other' is an eye-opener or 'Aha!' moment, of which they are often very proud. It is usually the case that a patient can hardly wait to see their therapist after completing the online module on formulating the IPAF: 'I am now finally beginning to understand why I behave the way I do in relationships.' Hence, even though the therapist might consider the initial IPAF arrived at by the patient to be 'wrong' (particularly if the potential defensive function of the IPAF is missing, as is often the case, or it has a defensive self-representation and is protectively formulated), it is important to validate the patient's efforts and feelings. Whatever the initial IPAF formulation the patient has developed, it is a good starting point to begin reconstructing in the session how the patient arrived at it. This process also enables the therapist to carefully and empathically challenge aspects of the formulation, where appropriate, and, together with the patient, arrive at a better understanding. Hence, the patient is never 'wrong', but the patient and therapist may jointly improve the formulation in the treatment session when reviewing it together. This process also demonstrates the 'we-mode' of functioning that we believe is central in all human communication—including psychotherapy. The patient is then invited to reflect on the work done in the session and to make any changes to the IPAF formulation agreed on in the session by adding them to the online system. This is also required because the system will automatically copy this formulation into the exercises in subsequent modules.

Balancing the content focus and the process focus

The considerations and examples outlined in the previous sections also illustrate the greater process focus in blended i-DIT compared with DIT delivered only in person. In 'traditional' face-to-face DIT, the therapist has to attend to issues related to both the content and the process of therapy. In blended i-DIT, much of the content of the therapy (e.g. information about the patient's developmental history and important attachment figures, the initial IPAF formulation, and the patient's own perception of the advantages and the emotional cost of their IPAF) is generated by the patient themself, based on the online exercises they complete after the first few in-person sessions. The therapist can be freed up to facilitate the patient's treatment by fostering the patient's progress and helping them whenever there are blockages in treatment.

Again, many DIT therapists may struggle initially with this altered role, which requires a different balance between a focus on content and on process. For instance, some DIT therapists may tend to 'repeat' all the work the patient has done online in the next face-to-face session, and then find themselves conflicted at the end of the session because they have run out of time to explore some of the issues that emerged during the session. We recommend that the face-to-face sessions in blended i-DIT start with a review of the work the patient has completed online, carefully attending to exercises the patient struggled to (or was unable to) finish. In this regard, blended i-DIT is slightly more structured than fully face-to-face DIT; the material that is discussed in sessions still emerges from the patient, but often as much—or even more—of what is discussed derives from the patient's online work as from what the patient brings to sessions.

Managing the ending phase

Because blended i-DIT typically involves fewer face-to-face sessions than fully in-person DIT, it is often associated with a greater activation of the patient's IPAF than occurs in traditional DIT during the ending phase. This also implies that the DIT therapist's concerns and anxieties, like those of the patient, may be even greater than in traditional DIT. For example, one DIT therapist had the feeling that she had denied her patient an effective treatment: 'I should have offered the patient more sessions, as I usually do in [fully] face-to-face DIT.' Upon further exploration in supervision, she realized that this was a strong countertransferential response to the activation of her patient's IPAF, in which themes of abandonment and separation were central.

It is therefore important for the DIT therapist to discuss and explore the patient's response to the ending of treatment in quite some detail. To support this process, there is a specific online module in blended i-DIT exploring the patient's response to ending, in addition to work around the goodbye letter. This module focuses on the patient's opinions about what they have accomplished in treatment, what factors may have contributed to this progress, and what the patient had hoped for but not experienced or received so far in the treatment. The patient's responses to this module are then discussed with the therapist in the next face-to-face session, which allows for a detailed and nuanced evaluation of the treatment and provides another opportunity to review the work that has been done together. For many patients, this is an important occasion to realize that they will need to continue their work after the face-to-face sessions have ended. As shown in Figure 15.1, in this session (session 7) the therapist also introduces the goodbye letter, which may already incorporate the patient's work around ending, and asks the patient to read the letter together with the therapist in the session. Here, the DIT therapist is on familiar ground, as the central task is to explore the patient's conscious and unconscious responses to the letter. The goodbye letter (with any changes that have been made during the session) is then uploaded on to the online system so that the patient can review the letter and suggest further changes, which are then discussed in the last face-to-face session. Before this closing session, the patient is also invited to complete the final online module, which focuses on relapse prevention (i.e. how the patient is planning to consolidate the changes made in therapy, how to recognize signs of relapse, and what to do if these signs occur).

As is the case with traditional DIT, the number of face-to-face sessions in blended i-DIT is not set in stone. Hence, the patient and therapist might agree to schedule one or more booster sessions after the end of the course of blended i-DIT, or they might agree to extend the treatment. In this regard, i-DIT may serve as an important bridge to more intensive psychotherapy, particularly for patients who have had difficulty seeking help for their mental health problems. However, the DIT therapist should always be aware of the risk of acting out when considering extending the treatment, and thus it is always a good idea to discuss potential extensions with a colleague or supervisor.

CONCLUSIONS

i-DIT may contribute to filling the existing treatment gap for individuals with mental health problems. The different types of i-DIT—unguided i-DIT, guided i-DIT, and blended i-DIT—may reach different types of individuals struggling with mental health difficulties, and may considerably expand the number of people who might benefit from the DIT approach. Most DIT therapists will experience few problems in acquiring the skills and competences needed to deliver i-DIT. In supervision, issues related to assessing patients' suitability for i-DIT, recognizing and dealing with resistance to online work, and concerns and anxieties about ending are often central and typically require the most attention. Despite the steep learning curve, most DIT therapists quickly begin to appreciate the way that i-DIT enables patients to work on their psychological difficulties between therapy sessions at times and in places that are most convenient or comfortable for them, and provides them with a sense of agency and autonomy from the start.

REFERENCES

Andersson, G., Titov, N., Dear, B. F., Rozental, A., & Carlbring, P. (2019). Internet-delivered psychological treatments: from innovation to implementation. *World Psychiatry*, *18*(1), 20–28. https://doi.org/10.1002/wps.20610

Bendelin, N., Hesser, H., Dahl, J., Carlbring, P., Nelson, K. Z., & Andersson, G. (2011). Experiences of guided Internet-based cognitive-behavioural treatment for depression: a qualitative study. *BMC Psychiatry*, *11*, 107. https://doi.org/10.1186/1471-244x-11-107

Cuijpers, P., Karyotaki, E., de Wit, L., & Ebert, D. D. (2020). The effects of fifteen evidence-supported therapies for adult depression: A meta-analytic review. *Psychotherapy Research*, *30*(3), 279–293. https://doi.org/10.1080/10503307.2019.1649732

Cuijpers, P., van Straten, A., Bohlmeijer, E., Hollon, S. D., & Andersson, G. (2010). The effects of psychotherapy for adult depression are overestimated: a meta-analysis of study quality and effect size. *Psychological Medicine*, *40*(2), 211–223. https://doi.org/doi:10.1017/S0033291709006114

Johansson, O., Michel, T., Andersson, G., & Paxling, B. (2015). Experiences of non-adherence to Internet-delivered cognitive behavior therapy: A qualitative study. *Internet Interventions*, 2(2), 137–142. https://doi.org/10.1016/j.invent.2015.02.006

Karyotaki, E., Ebert, D. D., Donkin, L., Riper, H., Twisk, J., Burger, S., Rozental, A., Lange, A., Williams, A. D., Zarski, A. C., Geraedts, A., van Straten, A., Kleiboer, A., Meyer, B., Unlu Ince, B. B., Buntrock, C., Lehr, D., Snoek, F. J., Andrews, G., Andersson, G., Choi, I., Ruwaard, J., Klein, J. P., Newby, J. M., Schroder, J., Laferton, J. A. C., Van Bastelaar, K., Imamura, K., Vernmark, K., Boss, L., Sheeber, L. B., Kivi, M., Berking, M., Titov, N., Carlbring, P., Johansson, R., Kenter, R., Perini, S., Moritz, S., Nobis, S., Berger, T., Kaldo, V., Forsell, Y., Lindefors, N., Kraepelien, M., Bjorkelund, C., Kawakami, N., & Cuijpers, P. (2018). Do guided internet-based interventions result in clinically relevant changes for patients with depression? An individual participant data meta-analysis. *Clinical Psychology Review*, 63, 80–92. https://doi.org/10.1016/j.cpr.2018.06.007

Lindegaard, T., Berg, M., & Andersson, G. (2020). Efficacy of internet-delivered psychodynamic therapy: Systematic review and meta-analysis. *Psychodynamic Psychiatry*, 48(4), 437–454. https://doi.org/10.1521/pdps.2020.48.4.437

Lund, C., Brooke-Sumner, C., Baingana, F., Baron, E. C., Breuer, E., Chandra, P., Haushofer, J., Herrman, H., Jordans, M., Kieling, C., Medina-Mora, M. E., Morgan, E., Omigbodun, O., Tol, W., Patel, V., & Saxena, S. (2018). Social determinants of mental disorders and the Sustainable Development Goals: A systematic review of reviews. *Lancet Psychiatry*, 5(4), 357–369. https://doi.org/10.1016/S2215-0366(18)30060-9

Luyten, P., & Fonagy, P. (2014). Psychodynamic treatment for borderline personality disorder and mood disorders: A mentalizing perspective. In L. Choi-Kain & J. Gunderson (Eds.), *Borderline personality disorder and mood disorders: Controversies and consensus* (pp. 223–251). Springer.

Richards, D., & Richardson, T. (2012). Computer-based psychological treatments for depression: a systematic review and meta-analysis. *Clinical Psychology Review*, 32(4), 329–342. https://doi.org/10.1016/j.cpr.2012.02.004

Rost, F., Luyten, P., Fearon, P., & Fonagy, P. (2019). Personality and outcome in individuals with treatment-resistant depression: Exploring differential treatment effects in the Tavistock Adult Depression Study (TADS). *Journal of Consulting and Clinical Psychology*, 87(5), 433–445. https://doi.org/10.1037/ccp0000391

Stone, L., & Waldron, R. (2019). *Great Expectations* and e-mental health: The role of literacy in mediating access to mental healthcare. *Australian*

Journal of General Practice, 48(7), 474–479. https://doi.org/10.31128/ajgp-11-18-4760

Thase, M. E., Wright, J. H., Eells, T. D., Barrett, M. S., Wisniewski, S. R., Balasubramani, G. K., McCrone, P., & Brown, G. K. (2018). Improving the efficiency of psychotherapy for depression: Computer-assisted versus standard CBT. *American Journal of Psychiatry, 175*(3), 242–250. https://doi.org/10.1176/appi.ajp.2017.17010089

van der Vaart, R., Witting, M., Riper, H., Kooistra, L., Bohlmeijer, E. T., & van Gemert-Pijnen, L. J. (2014). Blending online therapy into regular face-to-face therapy for depression: Content, ratio and preconditions according to patients and therapists using a Delphi study. *BMC Psychiatry, 14*, 355. https://doi.org/10.1186/s12888-014-0355-z

16
Future Directions for Dynamic Interpersonal Therapy

Sixty years ago, Malan (1963) posed the question of why the secret of brief psychotherapy, which early analysts possessed, had been lost. After all, we know that many of Freud's original cases were seen for fewer than sixteen sessions; however, since then the tendency has mostly been for analytic work to increase in length (Malan, 1963). Gustafson (1997) posited that the average lifespan of a school of brief therapy is twenty years at best, as if brief psychotherapy is doomed to be as short-lived as its modality. Dynamic interpersonal therapy (DIT) is now in the second decade of its existence; we hope that this second edition conveys the way the model has evolved over the first ten years or so—which might bode well for its continuing life. As we have demonstrated, in the past decade, the DIT model has been adapted to working in different contexts, and it will continue to do so in the future. It now makes use of techniques including mentalizing, directive, and supportive interventions to reach a wider population of depressed and anxious patients. DIT has also been adapted to working with other patient populations, such as patients with functional somatic disorders (discussed in Chapter 14), and across new formats, such as internet-delivered DIT (i-DIT) and blended DIT (see Chapter 15). DIT for complex care (DITCC) was developed out of the experience of working in the sixteen-session model as a way of accommodating greater complexity in treatment-resistant depression and with patients with trauma and characterological presentations (Chapter 13).

We are also aware of the various ways DIT has been applied in the meantime, including adaptations with art therapists, adolescents and young adults, individuals with brain injury, older adults, perinatal work, post-traumatic stress in veterans, and group DIT, among others (e.g. Chen et al., 2020; Folkes-Skinner & Collins, 2022; Havsteen-Franklin et al., 2021; Landström et al., 2019; Ryan & Yeates, 2022; Wilson & Esposito, 2018).

We have extended the training model (outlined in Appendix 5) to include therapists and counsellors without psychodynamic backgrounds, by teaching them the DIT model alongside a foundation training in brief psychodynamic psychotherapy. The initial results have been very promising in suggesting that the model can be attained and applied effectively by this group of clinicians (Khalastchy et al., 2021). Looking ahead, we want to sketch out some of the areas for the future development of DIT.

THE BROADENING SCOPE OF DIT

We imagine that the format for blended DIT and i-DIT might make it more accessible to other populations. i-DIT has the potential to offer more cost-effective ways of reaching a wider population. We are aware that this may feel controversial for those who do not wish to embrace technological changes, and hope that we can apply these adjustments without losing sight of the overarching psychoanalytic stance that informs DIT. Further training needs to be developed to ensure that DIT therapists have the necessary competence to adjust to this blended and digital form of DIT. The potential of artificial intelligence in DIT is another area that could be explored in the future, for example, the use of large language models to support clinicians to achieve a deeper understanding of language processing and statistical patterns to help identify the interpersonal-affective focus (IPAF) or assist with supervision.

We have seen a few different applications of group DIT, and are currently involved in a pilot study of group DIT. We feel confident that the interpersonal focus of DIT could benefit from the group setting. We hope to develop further training to cover the way the model could be delivered in different group formats, and we anticipate that this will borrow from some of the i-DIT online modules (see Chapter 15) to ensure that face-to-face individual sessions have the most impact.

We can foresee DIT fitting within a wider group of variations of the treatment offer. Perhaps a shorter form of DIT could be developed for more straightforward presentations of depression and/or anxiety, or for particular patient groups who may benefit from a more streamlined approach, such as university students or adolescents. Similarly, we are encouraged by the development of DITCC, which demonstrates that the model can be extended to allow meaningful engagement with patients with more complex needs and might almost seamlessly transition into specialized treatments for these patients, such as mentalization-based treatment.

There is increasing evidence for a general psychopathology factor or p factor, a single dimension underlying various mental disorders that accounts for the co-occurrence of different forms of psychopathology (Caspi & Moffitt, 2018), similar to how 'g' represents a general intelligence factor (Spearman, 1927). This understanding shifts the focus from categorically distinct disorders towards a more dimensional perspective on mental health. DIT might offer a particularly interesting transdiagnostic approach, firmly rooted in psychoanalytic thinking and research, for patients across the spectrum of psychopathology. This perspective might help DIT therapists in the future to formulate a more comprehensive and nuanced understanding of their patients' experiences, and facilitate a more personalized approach to treatment, including identifying the optimal length of treatment for each patient and the specific techniques that might be particularly effective in each phase of treatment. Research is needed to investigate these assumptions, but the move that we are currently witnessing in the field of psychotherapy from a focus on specific diagnoses to a more transdiagnostic understanding of the person is entirely consistent with the DIT approach, as it is based on a common guiding set of principles in case formulation and treatment that cut across specific diagnoses. These trends are consistent with efforts to develop a modular approach in psychodynamic treatments (Leichsenring & Schauenburg, 2014), and more research is needed to investigate the effectiveness of such an approach. Establishing the cost-effectiveness of DIT is another important area for future research, particularly given the increasing pressure on mental health services worldwide.

All of these new developments with DIT open up avenues for further research. Our priority is to develop a systematic programme of research into the cost-effectiveness of the different variants of DIT, which will also include a focus on mechanisms of change in DIT and ways to identify the patients who can be expected to benefit from each variant.

TRAINING IN DIT

The start of the Covid-19 pandemic brought about a seismic shift in the way we delivered DIT training—and, indeed, the therapy itself. Many DIT trainings are currently carried out online, with the training methods used in person substituted (and, as far as possible, replicated) by making the most of remote teaching platforms, breakout rooms, and online quizzes. This change has brought gains and losses. One of the important benefits of online training is the geographical parity it offers in relation to access to training: trainees can attend from all around the world. Online training also widens access as it reduces the financial burden (e.g. travel costs) that in-person training imposes and opens access to people with disabilities (e.g. mobility restrictions) or health considerations (e.g. vulnerability to infection) that make in-person attendance difficult. However, some people experience difficulties in maintaining concentration on the screen for extended periods of time and engaging with other course participants. To address these issues, we use blended and hybrid approaches to teaching days, to allow participants to meet in person where possible. We also encourage breaks and take care to teach in short stints, and include many applied exercises and opportunities to discuss clinical work in small groups.

Training of supervisors has also developed, with additional supervisor training days to cover the key competences of DIT supervision, such as evaluation of observed sessions using the competence framework (see Appendix 3) and other evaluations of clinical skills, working in small-group supervision, issues of confidentiality, and contracting in DIT supervision. The training trajectory is explained in detail in Appendix 5. The future of the DIT model largely depends on our capacity to train the next generation of supervisors and trainers, and we should continue to develop our thinking about the role and nature of training in the DIT model. Further innovation in this regard is to be expected, and should make full use of current and future technological advances.

Accreditation is an important issue in the current era of managed care. In the UK, the existing five-day DIT training was reaccredited by the British Psychoanalytic Council in 2022, and the extended twenty-day DIT training was kite-marked by the same council in late 2021. The Anna Freud Centre currently holds the lists of DIT practitioners and supervisors, and hopes to develop further the network of DIT clinicians in the UK and beyond. In this regard, efforts to cultivate an international community of DIT practitioners, supervisors, trainers, and researchers need to be stepped up.

CONCLUSIONS

We are aware that DIT has reached across some of the globe, with courses having been taught and DIT being practised across most of Europe, the USA, and Australia, and more recently extending into Scandinavia, China, and South America. At the same time, new adaptations of DIT are being developed and empirically evaluated. Notwithstanding Gustafson's (1997) caution that perhaps all brief models of psychotherapy have a limited shelf life, for now we are hopeful that DIT will continue to grow and flourish.

REFERENCES

Caspi, A., & Moffitt, T. E. (2018). All for one and one for all: Mental disorders in one dimension. *American Journal of Psychiatry*, *175*(9), 831–844. https://doi.org/10.1176/appi.ajp.2018.17121383

Chen, C. K., Nehrig, N., Wash, L., & Wang, B. (2020). The impact of brief dynamic interpersonal therapy (DIT) on veteran depression and anxiety. *Psychotherapy*, *57*(3), 464–468. https://doi.org/10.1037/pst0000282

Folkes-Skinner, J., & Collins, L. (2022). Group dynamic interpersonal therapy (GDIT): Adapting an individual interpersonal therapy to a group setting in an NHS IAPT service: a pilot study. *Psychoanalytic Psychotherapy*, *36*(2), 141–156. https://doi.org/10.1080/02668734.2021.2001685

Gustafson, J. P. (1997). *The complex secret of brief psychotherapy: A panorama of approaches*. Jason Aronson.

Havsteen-Franklin, D., Oley, M., Sellors, S. J., & Eagles, D. (2021). Drawing on dialogues in arts-based dynamic interpersonal therapy (ADIT) for complex depression: A complex intervention development study using the Medical Research Council (UK) phased guidance. *Frontiers in Psychology, 12*, 588661. https://doi.org/10.3389/fpsyg.2021.588661

Khalastchy, J., Abrahamsen, D., Saunders, R., & Fonagy, P. (2021). *Evaluating extended dynamic interpersonal therapy (e-DIT): A mixed methods investigation to identify characteristics associated with successful outcomes of DIT* [MSc Dissertation, University College London].

Landström, C., Levander, L., & Philips, B. (2019). Dynamic interpersonal therapy as experienced by young adults. *Psychoanalytic Psychotherapy, 33*(2), 99–116. https://doi.org/10.1080/02668734.2019.1641834

Leichsenring, F., & Schauenburg, H. (2014). Empirically supported methods of short-term psychodynamic therapy in depression – towards an evidence-based unified protocol. *Journal of Affective Disorders, 169*, 128–143. https://doi.org/10.1016/j.jad.2014.08.007

Malan, D. H. (1963). *A study of brief psychotherapy*. Plenum Press.

Ryan, A., & Yeates, G. (2022). Neuropathological inertia and re-mobilisation of cathexes: Brief psychodynamic therapy after basal ganglia lesions. In C. Salas, O. Turnbull, & M. Solms (Eds.), *Clinical studies in neuropsychoanalysis revisited* (pp. 155–178). Routledge.

Spearman, C. (1927). *The abilities of man: Their nature and measurement*. Macmillan.

Wilson, C., & Esposito, M. (2018). Dynamic interpersonal therapy and older people. *FPOP Bulletin: Psychology of Older People, 142*, 49–52. https://doi.org/10.53841/bpsfpop.2018.1.142.49

APPENDIX 1

Patient Information Leaflet: Dynamic Interpersonal Therapy (DIT) for Depression and Anxiety[1]

WHAT IS DIT?

DIT is a time-limited (sixteen sessions) psychodynamic therapy that has been specifically developed for the treatment of depression and anxiety. One of the main ideas in psychodynamic therapy is that when something is very painful we can find ourselves trying to ignore it (it's a bit like the saying 'out of sight, out of mind'). Most of the time we know when we're doing this, but sometimes we can bury something so successfully that we lose sight of it completely. This is why difficult experiences in the past can continue to affect the way we feel and behave in the present. DIT provides people with a safe place to talk openly about how they feel and to understand what might have contributed to them becoming depressed and/or anxious.

An example shows how this might work. Someone who was repeatedly rejected by their parents may stop themself thinking about how painful this is. As an adult they might become depressed, and withdraw from relationships, feeling that it is safer to be alone and not having to depend on anyone. Although not getting close to anyone helps them to feel safer, they might also feel lonely and get depressed as a result.

How would a DIT therapist help such a person? By helping them to talk freely about themself and their relationships it might become clear that whenever someone tries to get to know them, they fear the worst and push them away, just to make sure that no one ever gets close enough to hurt or disappoint them again. In the course of day-to-day life people don't necessarily notice how they are behaving or

---

1. Written by Tony Roth and Alessandra Lemma.

responding to others because this becomes second nature—'the way things are'. By drawing their attention to this pattern in their relationships, therapy would help them to understand themselves better and change the way they respond. This pattern, and how it can help them to understand their depression, then becomes the focus of the therapy.

WHAT DOES THERAPY INVOLVE?

Everyone's therapy will be a bit different, but we have tried to describe some of the important things that a capable therapist will do and what they will help you focus on.

STARTING OFF

All therapists should be able to help you feel respected and comfortable. Many people find it difficult to talk about their problems with someone they do not know, and it is important that your therapist can make you feel that they are to be trusted, and can help you manage if you talk about things that upset you or about which you feel embarrassed. Talking openly about yourself for the first time to a new person can feel difficult and you may be worried about what your therapist thinks about you. Your therapist will be interested in how you experience them and will help you to make sense of any worries you may have about starting therapy. They should give you the feeling that they know that starting therapy can be difficult and that they understand what life is like for you.

GETTING A PICTURE OF WHAT YOU NEED ('ASSESSMENT')

Your therapist will need to get as good a picture as they can of what you are finding difficult in your life and how this is affecting you and people close to you. They will ask some questions, but they should also make it clear that you only need to give as much information as you feel comfortable with. Many people find that as therapy gets going they are able to talk more openly, and in the early stages you shouldn't find yourself under pressure to say more than you want.

Although your therapist will need to gather some basic information about you and your life, and your current and past relationships in particular, some of the time they will wait for you to talk. This is because they are interested in hearing about what is on your mind rather than asking you lots of questions. Sometimes your therapist may remain silent, waiting for you to speak. This may well feel a bit uncomfortable— for example, you may feel unsure what to say. However if this gets too uncomfortable, your therapist will help you talk.

At the start of therapy your therapist will ask you to complete some questionnaires. These will give them a better idea of the sorts of problems you have (by asking about the sorts of difficulties you have), as well as how badly these affect you (by asking how much each problem affects you). Your therapist will discuss the results of these questionnaires with you. They will ask you to complete the questionnaires again every session because this helps you and your therapist see what progress you are making. This is very useful, because not everyone makes progress at the same rate. If the questionnaires show that you are not benefiting from therapy it gives you and your therapist a chance to think about why this might be.

EXPLAINING HOW DIT MIGHT WORK FOR YOU

Early on your therapist should explain how DIT works, and help you to think through how the approach makes sense of what you are finding difficult in your life. The experience of the assessment should also give you an idea of how the therapy works, what is expected of you and what you can expect of the therapist. The main thing is that the therapist needs to help you see the ways in which ideas from DIT could be relevant to you and what you want help with. That does not mean you need to be 100% convinced at this stage—it's more that the idea of DIT needs to make some sense to you if you are going to get the best out of it.

SHARING IDEAS ABOUT WHAT YOU WANT TO ACHIEVE

When your therapist has enough information they will begin thinking with you about what would be most helpful for you to focus on over the sixteen sessions. This is also an opportunity to agree with your therapist about what you want out of the therapy. In DIT the therapist will typically aim to help you to work on a recurrent pattern in your relationships.

LENGTH AND FREQUENCY OF TREATMENT

Your therapist will talk with you about the fixed number of sessions you can expect to have. This will typically be sixteen sessions. The therapy usually takes place once a week. Your therapist will discuss with you any planned breaks and what happens if you cancel sessions.

WHAT CAN YOU EXPECT OF YOUR THERAPIST

Your therapist is responsible for ensuring that your meetings take place at a regular time, in a setting where you can be sure of confidentiality. Wherever possible they should let you know if they expect to be away or need to change the time of your therapy. Sometimes people find breaks from the therapy hard to manage. When this happens your therapist should discuss this with you and help you to understand why this may feel particularly difficult.

ENDING THE THERAPY

Many patients find that ending the therapy is difficult. This is because the relationship that develops between you and your therapist can become quite important. Ending therapy can feel like a big loss and you are likely to experience a range of feelings about it. Your therapist will realize and understand this, and you should expect them to help you to explore your feelings, including any worries you might have about how you will cope in the future. They should help you think about how you would manage if things became difficult again. After all, the aim of DIT isn't to remove your problems—everyone has problems that they need to deal with. The hope is that you will have learned how to manage better, and so avoid problems becoming major difficulties again.

SOME IMPORTANT FEATURES OF PSYCHODYNAMIC THERAPY

1) One important feature of DIT is that it uses what happens in the relationship between therapist and patient to help think about the problems in your life. An example would help. Remember the person we described at the start of this leaflet, who worries about getting rejected by people. As they settle into therapy they might start to worry that the therapist will reject them too—for example, they could become convinced that the therapist wasn't really interested in them. Because this would provide a clear illustration of where things go wrong in the patient's relationships, the therapist might comment on their concern. By discussing the similarity between the worries they have about the therapist and the worries they have in general, the patient would start to get a better picture of what happens to them in relationships. In practice this means that the therapist will often draw your attention to what you are currently feeling in the session. The idea is that by exploring the relationship between you and your therapist, you can get a better understanding of what is troubling you.
2) As discussed earlier, you may find that your therapist is a bit more 'silent' than you might be used to. For example, at the beginning of each session your therapist will greet you, but beyond this they may not ask questions. Instead they will wait to hear from you about what is on your mind. This is not because they are being 'unfriendly', but because they want you to have some space to work out what is on your mind. This can take a while to get used to, but your therapist will understand how hard it can be and should help if you find this particularly difficult.
3) Another feature of DIT is that the therapist won't always answer your questions directly. Sometimes they may be

interested in what lies behind your questions. For example, someone who is very worried about starting therapy may not feel able to say this straightforwardly. Instead they may ask lots and lots of questions about what therapy involves. Rather than answering all of these directly, the therapist may notice that behind the questions is a worry about beginning therapy. Helping the patient talk about this, rather than answering all the questions, is probably a more helpful way forward.

APPENDIX 2

DIT Checklist

Therapist's Name: _____ DIT Case No. _____

Session Number	To Do	✓
Before starting	Give your supervisor copy of CV and your line manager's details (where applicable)	
	Sort out recording equipment and how to get recordings to your supervisor in compliance with your workplace's Information Governance requirements	
Every session	Outcome measures: PHQ-9 and GAD-7 Record each session Listen back to your session and make process notes for supervision Reading to support your DIT work Regular reviewing of the training booklet and DIT manual	
1	Audio consent form (beginning of session)	
By session 2	Agree remaining session times and breaks	
By session 3	Relationship questionnaire	
3	Bring provisional IPAF to supervision	
4 (usually)	Negotiate IPAF with patient	
4 (usually)	Give IPAF recording to supervisor to rate	
4 (usually)	Agree goals related to IPAF	
Middle phase	Give recording to supervisor to rate (1st DIT patient)	
12	Bring draft of goodbye letter to supervision	

Session Number	To Do	✓
13 (usually)	Share goodbye letter with patient	
14 or 15	Redo relationship questionnaire and compare	
Ending phase	Give recording to supervisor to listen (1st DIT patient)	
14 and 15	Revise goodbye letter	
16	Give patient final version of goodbye letter	
End of treatment	Delete all recordings	

PHQ-9, Patient Health Questionnaire nine-item depression scale; GAD-7, seven-item Generalized Anxiety Disorder scale.

APPENDIX 3

DIT Competence Rating Scale[1]

■ **Absent:** The feature described is either not present in the session and/or it is not possible to assess (Score = 0)

□ **Limited:** Therapist demonstrates significant absence of skill or inappropriate performance, which is likely to have negative therapeutic consequences (Score = 1–2)

■ **Competent:** Therapist's performance is appropriate with evident degree of skill. However, therapist either demonstrates competency in a limited way, restricted to a specific aspect of the competency or particular moment in the session, or there are problems/inconsistencies in therapist's performance of the specific competency (Score = 3–4)

□ **Good–Advanced:** Therapist consistently demonstrates high level of skill with only few/minor problems. Therapist demonstrates ability to carry out the competency in a range of ways and varying complexity during session. Therapist demonstrates breadth and depth in performance of the competency (Score = 5–7)

1. With thanks to Tamara Ventura Wurman for her work on a DIT therapist competence framework (Ventura Wurman, 2019) on which this scale is based.

SCORING	Absent Score: 0	Limited: Score: 1–2	Competent: Score: 3–4	Good–Advanced: Score: 5–7
1. BUILDING AND MAINTAINING THERAPEUTIC ALLIANCE • Engages the patient with therapy (particularly in the INITIAL PHASE) • Fosters and maintains the therapeutic alliance • Containment: helping the patient feel understood • Fosters the patient's epistemic trust, including explaining rationale behind DIT COMMENTS:				
2. HOLDING THE DIT STANCE AND PSYCHODYNAMIC FRAME • Creates a psychic space where it is possible to think together with the patient • Creates an environment of safety • Holds in mind the patient's traits and state of mind when intervening • Promotes and expands the patient's self-knowledge and self-awareness • Promotes psychic and behavioural change • Holds the psychodynamic frame (consistency, reliability, neutrality, anonymity, abstinence) COMMENTS:				

SCORING	Absent Score: 0	Limited: Score: 1–2	Competent: Score: 3–4	Good–Advanced: Score: 5–7
3. INITIAL PHASE: ELICITING INTERPERSONAL MAP AND NEGOTIATING IPAF • Elicits interpersonal narratives to explore experiences of self, other, and linking affect • Works with the relationship questionnaire to recognize attachment patterns • Maps repeated patterns across different relationships, past and present • Works collaboratively to negotiate IPAF with patient to arrive at shared focus for DIT • Shares the defensive function of the IPAF with the patient • Establishes goals with the patient after agreeing the IPAF COMMENTS:				
4. WORKING WITH UNCONSCIOUS PROCESSES, INCLUDING TRANSFERENCE AND COUNTERTRANSFERENCE • Maintains awareness of unconscious processes • Therapist is able to think about themself in the room with the patient • Focuses discussion on relationship between patient and therapist in order to further exploration of IPAF • Recognizing and managing the patient's defences and resistance, including avoidance of important topics and shifts in mood; taking up cost of defences COMMENTS:				

SCORING	Absent: Score: 0	Limited: Score: 1-2	Competent: Score: 3-4	Good–Advanced: Score: 5-7
5. FACILITATING MENTALIZING • Helps the patient to think for themself (patient understands themself) • Promotes flexible mentalizing • Helps the patient explore, express, and self-regulate emotions COMMENTS:				
6. KEEPING FOCUS ON THE AGREED PATTERN (IPAF) • Continues to refine the IPAF over the course of DIT • Promotes and expands the patient's knowledge and awareness of their relational patterns • Helps patient make connection between symptoms and interpersonal events • Takes up the reverse of the IPAF, where possible COMMENTS:				
7. ENDING PHASE OF DIT • Writes and shares the goodbye letter in a collaborative manner, which is refined over the ending phase • Repeats the relationship questionnaire and reviews changes since the start of therapy • Helps the patient grieve (i.e. facilitates expression of anxieties and fantasies about ending; helps patient review the work that has been accomplished and engages patient in anticipating future difficulties/areas of vulnerability) COMMENTS:				
GENERAL COMMENTS:				

APPENDIX 4

DIT Patient Complexity Subscale[1]

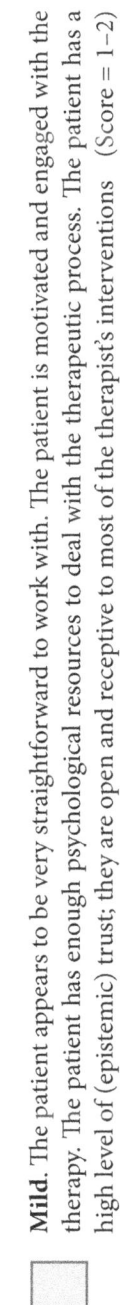

Mild. The patient appears to be very straightforward to work with. The patient is motivated and engaged with the therapy. The patient has enough psychological resources to deal with the therapeutic process. The patient has a high level of (epistemic) trust; they are open and receptive to most of the therapist's interventions   (Score = 1–2)

Moderate. The patient is at times challenging to work with. The patient may be ambivalent towards therapy. The patient has some psychological resources to deal with the therapeutic process. The patient has a moderate level of (epistemic) trust; they receive some of the therapist's interventions but remain closed to others   (Score = 3–4)

Severe. The patient appears to be challenging to work with. The patient may be unmotivated or disengaged from therapy. The patient appears not to have the necessary psychological resources to deal with the therapeutic process. The patient has a high level of (epistemic) vigilance, and has difficulty hearing and listening to the therapist's interventions
(Score = 5–6)

1. With thanks to Tamara Ventura Wurman for her work on a DIT therapist competence framework (Ventura Wurman, 2019) on which this scale is based.

APPENDIX 5

Training and Supervision Model for DIT

Here we set out the way the DIT model has been taught, assessed, and supervised since its inception. The original DIT training is designed to take place over five days, with teaching carried out over the first four days and the final day used for pass-out role plays and an optional lecture in the application of DIT in the primary care setting. We will also look at recent developments in the extended twenty-day DIT training model that teaches DIT to therapists without established psychodynamic competences. Most psychoanalytic and psychodynamic trainings have in common a three-pronged approach to qualification: theory, supervised practice, and personal psychotherapy or analysis. We have replicated this approach for the five-day DIT training, and modified it in the extended twenty-day DIT training to be more inclusive and outward-reaching in trying to attract NHS staff to acquire this modality.

ELIGIBILITY TO TRAIN AS A DIT THERAPIST

The training requires applicants to demonstrate that they meet a set of entry-level criteria to be able to participate in the five-day DIT training. This establishes that the therapist meets the set of psychodynamic competences established by Lemma et al. (2008).

1. Completion of a minimum of a year's course in psychodynamic/analytic theory

This should last a minimum of one year and lead to professional membership of a recognized body such as the UK Council for

Psychotherapy (UKCP), British Psychoanalytic Council (BPC), British Association for Counselling and Psychotherapy (BACP), or Health and Care Professions Council (HCPC) in the UK. The course of psychoanalytic theory should consist of at least forty-five hours of teaching. In addition to that, there would be accompanying reading of prescribed texts for the course. This could be in the context of a psychodynamic counselling course, counselling or clinical psychology training with an evidenced psychodynamic syllabus that meets these requirements, psychodynamic psychotherapy training, child and adolescent psychotherapy training, group analytic training, psychoanalytic psychotherapy training, and/or psychoanalytic training.

2. Evidence of a minimum of 100 hours of supervised psychodynamic psychotherapy or psychodynamic counselling with adult patients

We require a letter from the psychodynamic supervisor to attest to these hours and verify the therapist's level of experience in this area. The supervisor needs to be psychodynamically or psychoanalytically trained to the minimum entrance level required for this training. We ask supervisors, in providing this reference, to comment on the therapist's ability to meet the basic and specific competences of psychodynamic psychotherapy (Lemma et al., 2008), as follows:

BASIC PSYCHODYNAMIC COMPETENCES

- Knowledge of basic principles and rationale of psychodynamic approaches
- Ability to assess the likely suitability of a psychodynamic approach
- Ability to engage the client in psychodynamic psychotherapy
- Ability to derive a psychodynamic formulation
- Ability to establish and manage the therapeutic frame and boundaries
- Ability to work with unconscious communication
- Ability to maintain a psychodynamic focus

- Ability to identify and respond to difficulties in the therapeutic relationship
- Ability to work with both the client's internal and external reality.

SPECIFIC PSYCHODYNAMIC COMPETENCES

- Ability to make dynamic interpretations
- Ability to work in the transference
- Ability to work with the countertransference
- Ability to recognize and work with defences.

3. Evidence of at least one year of personal therapy with a psychoanalyst, psychodynamic psychotherapist, or psychodynamic counsellor

We require a letter from the psychodynamic psychotherapist, psychodynamic counsellor, or psychoanalyst attesting that the therapist has completed at least one year of a minimum of once-weekly psychodynamic psychotherapy/counselling. Alternative forms of psychodynamic psychotherapy will be considered on their individual merits, for example, group analytic therapy.

4. At least two years of relevant clinical work experience

This is required to demonstrate the generic therapeutic competences set out in the framework, namely: knowledge and understanding of mental health problems; knowledge of and ability to operate within professional and ethical guidelines; knowledge of a model of therapy and the ability to understand and employ the model in practice (in this case, psychodynamic therapy); ability to engage the client; ability to foster and maintain a good therapeutic alliance and to grasp the client's perspective; ability to deal with the emotional content of sessions; ability to manage endings; ability to undertake generic assessment, including identifying suitability for the intervention; and ability to make use of supervision.

The five-day DIT course does not focus on teaching the basic psychodynamic competences; therefore, we require therapists to provide this evidence to demonstrate that they have established these capacities before undertaking the training.

PRE-COURSE PREPARATION

Before attending the course, therapists are invited to undertake pre-course reading, and a recommended DIT reading list is provided in advance of the training. This includes research papers into the effectiveness of DIT and related theoretical papers that inform the model. Therapists are also asked to bring a clinical case, which they will use during the early stages of the training for applied work and role plays. The therapists are given guidance about the type of patient to select for the purposes of the training. The patient is ideally someone they have met a few times and about whom they know some of the history and key interpersonal narratives, past and present. It is advisable not to bring a case that is very well known as they may become bogged down in too much detail. Similarly, we suggest that the case is not overly complex, to make learning as easy as possible during the training. Inevitably, some participants bring unsuitable cases to think about during the training, and this can be a useful exercise in reflecting on who is best suited to brief psychodynamic psychotherapy.

Participants are asked to anonymize details of their patients as far as possible. In addition, everyone is asked to sign a confidentiality agreement, in keeping with General Data Protection Regulation requirements. We also ask everyone to keep notes on other people's patients in a separate area from their course notes so that these can be handed in and destroyed at the end of the training.

We have found it useful to let participants know who will be teaching on the course in advance so that they can alert us to any boundary issues should they know one of the trainers. If there are existing work relationships with course participants, we recommend that they work in different small groups throughout the training.

ETHOS OF THE TRAINING

As we have demonstrated, the DIT model is a semi-structured approach that has at its heart a commitment to unconscious processes and the unfolding of the transference. The teaching of the course walks a similar tightrope, with a need to cover the key areas of knowledge and skills development while also being receptive to the emergent qualities of the model and the needs of the particular group of participants. The trainers are asked to keep both goals in mind throughout the training and to build in sufficient time for discussion of role plays, group exercises, demonstration videos, general questions, and reflections. Trainers are also encouraged to bring clinical examples of their own to illustrate the model. We encourage them to provide examples that reflect a range of cultural diversity.

We also want trainers to emphasize that DIT is not a mentalizing treatment per se. Rather, it is a brief psychodynamic model of therapy that uses mentalizing techniques when the patient's mentalizing capacity is compromised to ensure that the interventions are as effective as possible. Notwithstanding this, we understand that one of the main outcomes of DIT should be an improvement in the patient's capacity to mentalize self and other more flexibly, as captured by the patient's ability to step out of the restrictions of their interpersonal-affective focus (IPAF).

Where possible, trainers will go around small groups of participants to provide support and input to their discussions. The training can also be a useful way to train supervisors in the model by providing them with experience in small-group supervision, where they are asked to think with the group about the clinical material they are presenting and apply the DIT model to it. Supervisors are invited to shadow the training in support of their continuing professional development (CPD) requirements as well as towards qualifying as DIT trainers.

STRUCTURE OF THE TRAINING

We will now give a breakdown of how the training is delivered.

Theoretical background in DIT

The training begins by explaining the impetus for the development of DIT in the context of the public health service in the UK and the

Improving Access to Psychological Therapies (IAPT) initiative in operation at the time, as well as in the context of mood disorders. This is discussed in Chapter 1. In our experience, participants have varied exposure to the theories upon which the DIT model is based. While many are familiar with object-relations theory, fewer psychodynamic and psychoanalytic therapists are taught Sullivan's interpersonal psychoanalysis, Bowlby's attachment theory, or Fonagy and Hepworth's mentalizing theories and techniques. The model is oriented around these four theoretical pillars, and the start of the training establishes this foundation for DIT.

We include in the teaching on attachment theory the way we use Bartholomew and Horowitz's (1991) relationship questionnaire as a self-reported attachment style questionnaire. The questionnaire can seem confusing to patients and therapists alike, and while we do not return to teach this topic during the rest of the training, it is important that these concepts are continually linked to the rest of the model. The trainer should aim to link the patient's attachment style to the emerging IPAF, for example, when participants present their case examples to the group, by asking them to consider the patient's likely attachment style. In this way, concepts are repeated and connected across the training so that they become meaningfully related, rather than being seen as a form-filling exercise. We expect participants to undertake further reading to familiarize themselves with new measures such as the relationship questionnaire, so that they feel able to explain the differences between the various categories of attachment to their patients.

Case example of DIT treatment trajectory

We have found it useful to provide an example of a course of DIT treatment at the start of the training to orient therapists to the model and what is possible to achieve by the end of sixteen weeks of therapy. With time, we have found other, more engaging ways of getting the group to start thinking about the approach by providing some patient material and then asking the group to get into smaller groups of three or four people to discuss what they see as an emerging pattern. This allows the group to be introduced to the concepts in a live and applied way from the start. We can then share with the group the course of treatment by reading the 'goodbye' letter from the ending phase of DIT. The use of a carefully selected clinical example provides a standardized and accessible way of engaging the group in discussion. It gives participants a chance to work together in smaller groups and get to know one another, thereby facilitating a learning environment.

Individual introductions that include a sense of each therapist's interest in the model, their background training, and their hopes and fears in relation to the course are another useful start to the training. However, this can be time-consuming with a larger training group, so trainers may find ways of sharing this information more succinctly, for example, by a show of hands or through a small-group exercise where participants from each group feed back to the larger group.

Initial phase

We then move on to teaching about the first four sessions of DIT, which form the foundation of the rest of the work. It is important to give sufficient time to the initial phase during the training course, as without a good grasp of these concepts, the rest of the course can easily flounder. We do this through a series of role-play exercises that build on the concepts in a stepwise manner while also teaching key concepts linked to this phase of DIT. These include the DIT stance, establishing a therapeutic alliance with the way the cautionary tale is taken up, the therapeutic contract, the interpersonal map and eliciting interpersonal narratives, the relationship questionnaire and the use of sessional measures, culminating in formulating and sharing the IPAF. Demonstration videos are shared with the group to show these skills in action.

The course involves applied work in the model through role plays and skills demonstrations in the larger group. The role plays take place in small groups, with two members playing a DIT therapist and a patient while the remaining participants observe and provide feedback after the role play. In this way, we encourage the group to develop an IPAF for each patient, culminating in an exercise where they practise negotiating that IPAF with the patient. Participants are also asked to practise answering the question 'How will DIT help me?' as a way of conveying to the patient a succinct understanding of the model. There is also an exercise in setting goals for treatment that are achievable and realistic for this brief therapy.

We invite the small groups to share the emerging IPAFs with the rest of the group. This allows the trainer to demystify the central concept of the IPAF, and for the group to notice emerging commonalities in the patients' interpersonal patterns.

There can be some resistance to role plays, with certain participants rising to the challenge and discovering hidden acting talents while others feel exposed and nervous. Applying knowledge and practising skills through role plays is an important part of learning the DIT model. In our experience, the participants quickly get used to the role play format and find it a useful adjunct to their learning.

Middle phase

This part of the training focuses on the various techniques that are employed in the working-through stage of DIT, including judicious use of mentalizing techniques, working with defences and resistance, working with affect, and the use of interpretations and taking up the transference as these both link to the IPAF. We spend some time thinking about how to use the outcome measures as a way into thinking about the events of the past week, which can then illuminate the activation of the IPAF. While recognizing that the IPAF is important, we also want to encourage change in relation to the goals that have been agreed with the patient. Where change is resisted, this is also explored in the middle phase. The training examines difficulties that can arise in the course of work as well as introducing the way we think about diversity within the DIT model.

Ending phase

This section of the teaching occurs as the training itself is coming to an end. We think about the change in focus during the last four sessions of DIT, the use of the goodbye letter, which introduces a summary and review of the work the therapist and patient have undertaken together, and the importance of taking up the unconscious phantasies around ending during this stage.

Suitability for DIT

The training concludes by looking at questions of suitability for brief work, with a view to identifying who might make an appropriate training patient. Reference can be made to the therapists' case examples brought to the course to illustrate the adaptations to the model as well as the challenges posed when working with patients with more complex difficulties. The model has been adjusted for working with greater complexity in DIT for complex care (see Chapter 13), and it is also used with patients with functional somatic disorders (see Chapter 14), older adults, adolescents, and individuals with organic brain damage, body dysmorphic disorder, postpartum depression, or anxiety disorders (in particular social anxiety and generalized anxiety), among others.

Accreditation

The next steps towards accreditation are discussed so that participants understand how to take the training further to become a DIT therapist, supervisor, or trainer, as well as the ongoing CPD requirements. Participants are given access to a practitioner-restricted website with various online resources, including case study examples and the detailed case study marking scheme.

Pass-out role play

On the fifth day of training, participants take part in a brief role play with an actor taking the part of a DIT patient. Participants are required to demonstrate key skills to move on to supervision in the model, namely: whether they can demonstrate the DIT stance; whether they can investigate the patient's interpersonal map and draw links between different interpersonal domains so as to explore possible interpersonal and affective patterns; and whether they can give a good enough explanation of the way the DIT model works.

Supervised practice and case study

To qualify as a DIT therapist in the UK, participants are required to see two training patients with individual supervision for each of the sixteen sessions. A minimum of thirty minutes of supervision is required for each of the sixteen sessions of DIT. This can be delivered one-to-one or in small groups, where participants have the advantage of listening to other people's clinical material and gaining breadth of experience. Supervision can be given remotely or in person. The supervisor rates three sessions from the initial, middle, and ending phases of DIT with the first training case, and the IPAF session of the second training case. These sessions are rated against the revised competence framework (see Appendix 3) and supervisees are given detailed feedback around the areas of the model that they need to focus on developing. The supervisor in DIT has both a facilitative/educative and an evaluative function. Chapter 10 refers to some of the difficulties that can arise for therapists learning the DIT model. In some instances, the therapist might be asked to see another case towards accreditation, or they may have to put supervision on hold while they spend time developing competence in an identified area, such as working in the transference or holding the analytic frame.

Once both training cases have been completed to a satisfactory standard, the therapist writes up one of the cases and submits it for marking. The case study should demonstrate an understanding of the model and an ability to formulate an IPAF using the patient's history and to apply psychodynamic/analytic theory to illuminate that formulation. The therapist is also asked to reflect on the learning points in the model as part of the case study. This can include observations about the experience of supervision in the DIT model; adjustments that had to be made to acquire the model; aspects of the model that felt challenging and/or rewarding; the challenges posed by particular patients; and any changes the therapist would make with the benefit of hindsight.

CONTINUING PROFESSIONAL DEVELOPMENT AND POST-QUALIFYING SUPERVISION IN DIT

When someone is advised that they have attained DIT accreditation, we provide information about what is required for them to maintain that accreditation in the UK. There is an expectation that they will see a minimum of one DIT patient each year. They are also asked to undertake at least half a day of CPD each year. This can be made up of courses in DIT, self-study including reading related to DIT, and supervision. In relation to supervision, newly qualified DIT therapists are required to continue with a qualified DIT supervisor for the first year post-qualification to consolidate their grasp of the model. There is an expectation that they will have one hour of supervision for every twelve hours of DIT therapy they offer. With a caseload of three DIT patients, that usually works out to one hour of supervision each month. On completion of the first year, they can move on to peer supervision with other qualified DIT therapists. There are regular CPD courses in aspects of DIT, including refresher courses, top-up training on mentalizing techniques in DIT, and working with affect, as well as working with particular patient groups. We are building a DIT network to support DIT therapists in developing their research and clinical interests in the model.

EXTENDED, TWENTY-DAY DIT TRAINING MODEL

The twenty-day DIT training course is an extended version of the five-day training. It was developed to reach a wider audience of therapists who do not meet the criteria of pre-existing psychodynamic competences. As a result, the training model has been modified to ensure that these competences can be taught and acquired over the course of twenty teaching days, together with close supervision of three clinical cases. In essence, it is a foundation course in DIT. Participants write up each case as a clinical log and also produce a reflective essay at the end of the course. There is no requirement for experience of personal psychodynamic psychotherapy, although this is preferred, and we encourage participants to access this therapy during the training.

The training consists of:

- **Pre-course reading and podcasts**—this provides the theoretical basis of DIT. Assessment of this component via a multiple-choice questionnaire is a prior condition for attendance on the course.
- **Twenty teaching days**—the teaching includes an introduction to key psychoanalytic concepts, teaching the DIT model, and opportunities to apply the model through small-group work and discussion. There are typically eight teaching days in the first term, with the remaining twelve days spread out across the second and third terms and scheduled every fortnight or more during term time. Participants are asked to set learning objectives each term, and to keep a journal of their experience across the training so they can draw on this for the reflective essay.
- **Close supervision of three training cases, with a clinical log written up for each completed case**—supervisors watch two video recordings from each training case and provide detailed feedback to supervisees. One of the assessed recordings will always be the session in the initial phase of DIT in which the IPAF is negotiated. It is expected that supervisees will show steady progress from each clinical case and demonstrate an ability to take on board, integrate, and apply the feedback they receive in supervision as part of their learning.

Training methods in the twenty-day DIT training

The training days are divided into four sessions, with at least half of the time taken up with active learning using role plays and clinical presentations. Experiential exercises in the form of role plays and responsive interaction with video content form a core component of training to link teaching material to clinical context and interpersonal experience.

Some points are best illustrated through watching a demonstration and/or video clip, from which therapeutic techniques can be individually rated by each participant, with the ratings and observations then discussed in a larger group.

One of the advantages of the twenty-day DIT training is that it allows participants to revisit aspects of the model as they acquire experience in using it. Concepts can be refined over time, and learning is further supported by recommended reading, including key theoretical papers in psychodynamic and psychoanalytic concepts.

REMOTE TEACHING DURING THE COVID-19 PANDEMIC, AND BEYOND

The start of the Covid-19 pandemic in 2020 disrupted the five-day DIT training and necessitated moving it online. We found we were able to approximate the delivery of in-person training with an online format, using virtual breakout rooms for small-group work together with screen-sharing PowerPoint presentations and demonstration DVDs as well as tailor-made online quizzes. While the online training is not quite the same as in-person training, feedback demonstrated that participants valued the chance to continue with their learning and were able to engage well with the process. Supervision has typically been delivered remotely via telephone or online platforms, and this has continued through the pandemic in support of the training. Adjustments have had to be made to avoid too many consecutive teaching days, as we have found that being online for more than two days in a row is rather demanding on our capacity to focus and attend. As with similar arguments about remote psychotherapy, there is a case for applying Lombard and Ditton's (2006) prerequisites for creating the illusion of non-mediation, namely where there is sufficient imagination to sustain disbelief, the desire to connect in this way, and the ability to focus attention in the face of competing demands and distractions (Essig & Russell, 2021; Russell, 2015).

The twenty-day DIT training is designed to reach therapists working in NHS primary care health settings across England. The move to remote learning has eliminated the need to travel to training sessions, thereby making the course more accessible and egalitarian. At the same time, not everyone finds remote learning easy. Technical challenges—for example, a poor internet connection, inadequate equipment, or lack of privacy—have interfered with some people's ability to attend reliably. We have also been mindful of the way in which personal circumstances have been far more present when training people in DIT during the pandemic. This can result in therapists' sensitivity to particular aspects of the model, notably the ending phase, when grappling with their own experiences of loss. When training a group that has not had personal psychotherapy as an entry requirement, care needs to be taken to ensure there is adequate support should problems arise during training. This is even more incumbent on the trainer working remotely, when the online disinhibition effect (Suler, 2005) can lead to greater levels of self-disclosure than might take place during in-person training. We now provide teaching on the adjustments to working remotely in the DIT model and the importance of paying attention to our embodied countertransference even when working online.

REFERENCES

Bartholomew, K., & Horowitz, L. M. (1991). Attachment styles among young adults: A test of a four-category model. *Journal of Personality and Social Psychology*, *61*(2), 226–244. https://doi.org/10.1037/0022-3514.61.2.226

Essig, T., & Russell, G. I. (2021). A report from the field: Providing psychoanalytic care during the pandemic. *Psychoanalytic Perspectives*, *18*(2), 157–177. https://doi.org/10.1080/1551806x.2021.1896300

Lemma, A., Roth, A. D., & Pilling, S. (2008). *The competences required to deliver effective psychoanalytic/psychodynamic therapy*. Research Department of Clinical, Educational and Health Psychology, University College London. https://www.ucl.ac.uk/pals/sites/pals/files/ppc_clinicians_background_paper.pdf

Lombard, M., & Ditton, T. (2006). At the heart of it all: The concept of presence. *Journal of Computer-Mediated Communication*, *3*(2), JCMC321. https://doi.org/10.1111/j.1083-6101.1997.tb00072.x

Russell, G. I. (2015). *Screen relations: The limits of computer-mediated psychoanalysis and psychotherapy*. Karnac Books.

Suler, J. (2005). The online disinhibition effect. *International Journal of Applied Psychoanalytic Studies*, *2*(2), 184–188. https://doi.org/10.1002/aps.42

INDEX

For the benefit of digital users, indexed terms that span two pages (e.g., 52–53) may, on occasion, appear on only one of those pages.

The user is also referred to the Abbreviations List in the preliminary pages

Tables, figures, and boxes are indicated by *t*, *f*, and *b* following the page number

Abbass, A 254–55, 304
accreditation for DIT 237–38
'acting out' 45, 216
addictive behaviours 45
Adult Attachment Interview 159
affect
 hyperactivation 46
 regulation 285–86
  early 36–37
 suppression 46
affect focus 66–67, 170–71
 see also interpersonal-affective focus (IPAF)
aggression 27–28, 49, 116, 133–34, 216–17, 279–80, 291
 passive 339
 unconscious 50, 116
Akhtar, S 29, 96
allostasis 306*f*, 307, 309
analytic frame, holding in brief work 237
analytic listening 157–60
Andersson, G 327–29
Anna Freud Centre 351

Antonovsky, A 322
Appendices
 competence rating scale 361
 patient checklist 359
 patient complexity subscale 365
 patient information leaflet 353
 supervision and training protocol 367
attachment 6, 307
 as a key regulator of stress system 307
 perspective on defences 45–46
 related concerns 10–11
 secondary attachment strategies 308
attachment behavioural system 8, 31, 32, 33, 34, 43, 90*f*, 97, 158–59, 216
attachment models, distorting mentalizing re external relationships 34–35
attachment strategies
 deactivating 46

attachment strategies (*cont.*)
  hyperactivating 45–46
  interpersonal contexts yielding information 90*f*
attachment styles 8, 31, 32, 33, 34, 43, 90*f*, 94–95
  personality disorders and 94–95
  prototypical IPAFs 310*t*
attachment theory
  Bowlby's development of 33
  failure of mentalizing 280–81
  IWMs 31
attachment-history-based cognitive-affective schemata 10–11
autobiographical memories 31

Bakermans-Kranenburg, M J 11
Balint, M 28–29
Barber, J P 254–55, 263
Bartholomew, K 91–92, 372
Bateman, A 29
Beck Depression Inventory 258
Bendelin, N 327–28, 335
Bifulco, A 10–11
Binder, J L 3
Blatt, S 9, 10–11, 45–46, 303–4
blended and i-DIT 329–33
  see also i-DIT
Blom, D 312
body modification 45
borderline personality disorder (BPD) 68–69, 247, 335–36
Bowlby, J 31–33, 45–46, 371–72
Bretherton, K 31, 32
brief psychodynamic therapy
  continuum of models 246
  cost-effectiveness 255–56
  internet-delivered 256–57
  see also DIT; meta-analytic evidence base of psychological treatment

Brown, G W 11
Burton, C 303

caregivers 31
Cartwright, N 253–54
Caspi, A 349
Cassidy, J 308
Centre for Outcomes Research and Effectiveness 37–38
character armour 42–43
character development 33
character disorders 27
Chen, C K 261, 347–48
China, randomized controlled trials of DIT 260
clarification 163, 164–66, 296
  'elephant in the room' 296
Clark, D M 21, 261
classic and romantic visions of humanity 29
classic triad, neutrality, with abstinence and anonymity 219–20
classification systems, concession to pragmatism 4
Cluster C personality disorders 268
cognitive analytic therapy (CAT), goodbye letter 207–15
cognitive-behavioural therapy (CBT) 259–61
  compared with DIT 12–13, 161, 179, 254–55, 258–59, 260, 261, 304, 311
communication, unconscious 40–42
communication analysis 178
competence
  core and specific competences 37–38
  framework for effective delivery of psychodynamic therapy 245–46
  see also DIT, competence

Therapist Competence Scale
    (TCS) 264, 265, 269
complex care *see* DIT for complex
    care (DITCC)
compliant patient 230–31
computers
  internet-delivered DIT
    formats 327–28
  see also i-DIT
confrontation 162–64
Conradi, H J 10–11
consent for DIT, information
    on 98–100
conversion 45
counselling
  training DIT model 348
  vs major therapies 254–55
countertransference 41, 48–49
  ability to work with 48–49
  basis for intervention 249
  complementary response to 49
  defined 19
  detecting unconscious
    processes 41
  dimensions 220–21
  emotional impact of patient's
    presentation 19
  'hate in the' 39–40
  hypotheses about problematic
    interpersonal
    patterns 126
  id, ego, and superego 48–49
  interpersonal-affective
    patterns 144*f*
  neutral position 48–49
  role-responsive position 49
  source of information 46–47,
    220, 249
  therapist's own 81, 95–96, 124
  two-way unconscious
    communication 48
  see also transference

Covid-19 pandemic 327–28, 350
Crittenden, P M 31, 32
Csibra, G 286–87
Cuijpers, P 254–55, 267,
    327–29
cultural context of DIT 95–96
curiosity, lacking in psychic
    equivalence mode 281
Cuyt, C 268

deactivating attachment
    strategies 46
defence mechanisms 42–45
  ability to recognize and work
    with 42–45
  attachment perspective 45–46
  primitive 38–39
defences
  conceptualization 45–46
  costs 153
  neurotic defences 44
  object-related defences 150–51
  strategies for exploring 152*f*
  working with 150–53
defensive responses 45
denial 43
depersonalization 44
depressed phantasies 204–5
depression and/or anxiety
  intrapersonal/interpersonal
    dimensions 9, 34
  national guidelines for
    treatment 253
  operational criteria 3
  severe, chronic, and
    complex depression
    see DITCC
  unconscious generation of
    interpersonal stress 9
  unconscious projective and
    introjective
    processes 9–10

depression, chronic and
    complex 277–79
  distrust issues 278, 283–84
  emotional manifestations 281
  failure of mentalizing 279–83
  need for DIT adaptation 277
  need for therapeutic
    alliance 277
  pilot study 277
  relationship-interfering
    behaviours 279–80
  social isolation 278
derealization 44
descriptors, idiosyncratic 122–23
developmental theory 249
diagnosis, necessary
  antecedent 5–6
diagnostic categories 4, 6
  psychiatric vs psychodynamic
    diagnostic approach 4
diagnostic syndromes 5
Diamond, D 307
directive interventions 178–81
disavowal 44
discourse, monitoring multiple
    levels 160
displacement 44
displacement (of hostility) 217
dissociation 44
distrust
  depression, chronic and
    complex 278, 283–84
  see also epistemic trust
DIT
  see also DIT for complex care
    (DITCC); DIT-FSD; i-DIT
  accreditation, session
    recordings 237–38
  aims 59–60
    challenge to patient 15–18
    core features and
      strategies 59–73

motivation for, vs defensive
  state 16
and rationale 1–3
starting point 8–9
assessment for suitability 12–20
  response to exploratory
    approach 12–14
blended and i-DIT 327–28
competence rating scale
  Appendix 361
for complex care *see* DIT for
  complex care (DITCC);
  DIT-FSD
components 118
conflictual unconscious script/
  IPAF *see* IPAF
consent, information on 98–100
context of wider personality 5
contraindication 15, 246
defences conceptualization
  45–46
developmental theory and 249
directive techniques 180–81
and DITCC, commonalities and
  differences 283–84
dynamic interpretations 50
evaluation 237–38
evidence base 257–62
  practice-based
    evidence 253–54
external resources 18–19
face-to-face/blended,
  structure 329–33
foci 14, 64–70, 145–49
  on affect 66–67
  on interpersonal and affective
    issues 10–11
  on patient's mind 8, 68–70
  step-by-step guide 118–21
formulation
  aide-mémoire 119*b*
  idiographic approach 245

INDEX

frequently asked questions 245–51
future 347–52
group format 261, 348
internet-delivered DIT formats (i-DIT) 327–28
see also blended and i-DIT interventions 171
learning new model 145
patient checklist, *Appendix* 359
patient complexity subscale *Appendix* 365
patient information leaflet 71–72, 353
psychodynamic formulation 109–10
Randomized Evaluation of DIT; REDIT 258–59, 261–62
recurring object relationship 120
  clinical implications 266–67
  counsellor training 260
  DITCC 261
  IAPT outcome data 261
  meta-analytic evidence base 254–57
  practice-based evidence for DIT 261–62
  Randomized Evaluation of DIT; REDIT 258–59, 261–62
  RCTs 253, 260
  treatment fidelity, adherence, and competence 262–63
  working mechanisms 268
risk and self-harm 100–1
scope 348–50
self–object–affect part 5–6
sharing 97
shorter form 348–49
summarized 245–46
supervision and training protocol *see* Appendix 5
supportive nature/components 246
technical psychoanalytic concepts 37–51
theoretical framework 25–37
  core assumptions 25, 51
  core features and strategies 59, 60*b*
  ego functioning and theories of attachment 30–33
  interpersonal psychoanalysis (Sullivan) 33–36
  mentalizing 6, 36–37
  object-relations theory 26–30
training 248, 262
  accreditation 351
  expectations 250
  future 350–51
Training and Supervision Model *Appendix* 367
trajectory of therapy 60–64
  initial phase 1–4 61*t*, 61–62
  middle phase 5–12 62*t*, 62–63
  ending phase 13–16 63*t*, 63–64
  5 simple strategic steps 64
  see also initial phase; middle phase; ending phase; mentalizing
transference
  bridge to change 195–97
  criteria for interpreting 189–94
  exploring the IPAF 183–86
  formulation 186–89
  interpretion, case example 126–27
  'working in' ability 46–48, 183–97
vs DITCC 278
vs interpersonal psychotherapy (IPT) 245
see also mentalizing; transference relationship

DIT for complex care (DITCC) 59, 277–302
  attitude to learning from experience 283–84
  development 7
  and DIT, commonalities and differences 283–84
  endings 292–93
  enhanced social understanding 287
  epistemic trust 285–86
  failure of mentalizing 279–83
  intended/benefitting patients 277–80
  long-standing relationship difficulties 278
  mentalizing relationship with therapist 297–300
    we-mode 298
  mentalizing techniques 294–300
    intervention trajectory 295–97
  model in detail 288–93
    case example 291–92
  pilot data 261
  in practice 284–300
  primary and secondary care services 277
  relationship-interfering behaviours (RIBs) 278, 279–80, 291
  research, pilot data 261
  self-understanding 287
  structure 287–88
    insight phase 288
    set-up and engagement phase 288
    work-through and ending phase 288
  techniques 293–300
  transference
    interpretation 285–86
    negative or very unstable 278
    potential for distrust 286–87
  treatment 7
  two components 283–84
  vs DIT 278, 301
  see also DIT-FSD
DIT-FSD 313–22
  background and basic principles 313
  initial phase: engagement and case formulation 313–16
  middle phase: mentalizing and working through 316–22
  ending phase: empowerment and improvement 322
  see also functional somatic disorders (FSDs)
dreams 248–49
Driessen, E 254–56
drive theory, replacement by object-relations theory 28
DSM-III and ICD-11, reification 3–4
dynamic interpersonal therapy see DIT
dynamic interpersonal therapy for complex care see DIT for complex care (DITCC)
dynamic interpretations 49–51
dynamic unconscious, repression/reversal 41–42

early/repressed experiences, transference 46–47
eating disorders 45
ego functioning, interpersonal vulnerability 50
ego, and superego 48–49
egocentric perception 173–74
'elephant in the room' 296
embodied mentalizing 309–12, 317t
  RADLE mnemonic 317

emergence, vs structure 160–62
emotions
    amplifying 319
    differentiating 319–20
    embodied mentalizing, RADLE mnemonic 317
    highlighting emotional cost 321–22
    linking to presenting symptoms 320
    recognizing 318–19
    somatic markers 317*t*
empathy 35, 159
enactments 219, 221
ending phase of DIT 63*t*, 63–64, 199–218
    'acting out' 216
    difficulties 241–42
    evaluation 241–42
    goodbye letter 207–15, 241–42
        examples 211–15
        guidelines 210*b*
    interpreting the unconscious meaning 203–5
    mourning 200
    paranoid and manic phantasies 204
    patient's reactions 199–201
    premature/prolonged endings 205–6
    preparation for 201–3, 203*b*
    significant refinement of IPAF 152
    strategies 202*b*
    therapeutic stance 217–18
    therapist's perspective 206–7
    working with resistance 216–17
    see also initial phase of DIT; middle phase of DIT
Engel, G L 9–10
envy, reaction formation 45

epistemic trust 264–65, 266–67, 285–86, 298, 303–5, 312, 313–14, 315, 335
Etchegoyen, R H 37–38
Eubanks, C 266–67
event representations 31
evidence base for DIT 257–62
    practice-based evidence 253–54
expressive/exploratory techniques 162–71

Fairbairn, W R D 27, 28–29, 31
family history 85–86
Fehlbaum, L V 6
Feldman, C L 6, 261
Folkes-Skinner, J 261, 271, 347–48
formulating a transference interpretation 186–89
    case example 191–94
formulation *see* DIT, formulation; IPAF, formulation
frequently asked questions 245–51
Freud, A 30, 31, 48–49, 96
    assumption that psychic structure evolves 29–30
Freud, S 4, 29–30, 33–34, 40–42, 125, 347
Friedman, L 28–29
functional somatic disorders (FSDs) 303, 304, 306*f*
    attachment issues and IPAF 307–9
    attachment strategies
        hyperactivation 308
        primary/secondary 308
    biological vs psychological factors 304–5
    contemporary psychodynamic approach 306*f*, 306–12
    DIT approach to understanding 304–12

functional somatic disorders (FSDs) (*cont.*)
   emotions, bodily sensations and emotions 309–11
   epistemic mistrust 312
   establishing a therapeutic alliance 303–4
   formulating IPAF 309
   invalidating responses 307–8
   medical screening 305–6
   multicomponent, group-based DIT programme 304
   neurobiological circuits and brief psychodynamic treatment 304
   persistent somatic symptoms 307–8
   role of mentalizing 309–12
   somatic markers of inner mental states 318*t*
   specific adaptations to DIT model 303–4
   see also DIT-FSD

gambling/addictive behaviours 45
Gaskell, C 257
Gergely, G 36–37
Gill, M M 27–28, 54
goals for therapy 97–98
Goldfried, M R 266–67
goodbye letters 207–15
   CAT 207–15
   DIT-FSD 292, 322
   DITCC 290, 292
   examples 211–15
   guidelines 210*b*, 241
   i-DIT 333, 343
   purpose 64, 202, 241
Greenson, R R 37–38, 151–52, 159, 162, 234–35
group dynamic interpersonal therapy 261, 348
Gustafson, J P 347, 351

Haller, C 303
Hamill, M 207–8
Havsteen-Franklin, D 347–48
Heimann, P 46–47, 48
helplessness 282–83
here-and-now focus 66–68
Hilsenroth, C 267
history-taking vs history-making 82–84
hopelessnes, suicide risk 282–83
Horowitz, L M 91–92, 372
hostility, displacement 217
humanity, 'classic' and 'romantic' visions 29
hyper-embodiment 11
hyperactivating attachment strategies 45–46

i-DIT
   blended and i-DIT 329–33
   self-help 327–28
   types of 344
i-DIT, face-to-face/blended
   assessment of suitability 334–37
   balancing content focus and process focus 341–42
   ending phase 342–43
   goodbye letter 343
   IPAF 340–41
   motivation 337–38
   resistance to online work 338–40
   specific competences needed 333–43
   structure 329–33
id, ego, and superego 48–49
Improving Access to Psychological Therapies (IAPT) 102–3, 371–72
   DIT within 104

outcome data 261
outcome monitoring 104, 257, 258–59
infant, affect regulation 36–37
Ingrassia, A 207–8
initial phase of DIT
  aims and strategies 78–81
  engagement 75–77
  attachment strategy employed by patient 94–95
  'cautionary tales' 78–81, 242
  case examples 80–81
  cultural context 95–96
  difficulties 238–40
  family history 85–86
  history-taking vs history-making 82–84
  internal world of object relationships 87–90
  interpersonal context
    external reality 91
    on key attachment patterns 89–91, 90f
  interpersonal landscape map 87f, 87–96
  managing frame/setting 101–2
  medical history 86–87
  outcome monitoring 102–5
  presenting problem 84–85, 85b
  range of information 81
  relationship questionnaire 91–95, 92t
  risk and self-harm 100–1
  sharing a formulation 97
  video/audio recording 102–5
insecurity 35, 46, 158–59
intellectualization 44–45, 231
internal working models (IWMs) 30–33
  protective value 32
  transgenerational nature 31–32

internet-delivered DIT formats *see* i-DIT
interpersonal landscape 87–96
interpersonal learning, facilitation 36
interpersonal narratives (INs) 110, 143–45, 146, 189–90, 190b, 238, 288, 315, 327–28, 331–32, 337–38, 373
  abstracting interpersonal-affective patterns from 144f
  avoiding 143
  deconstruction 127
  elaboration, making IPAF apparent 143–45
  psychic equivalence 173–74
  see also relationships
interpersonal psychoanalysis (Sullivan) 33–36
interpersonal psychotherapy (IPT) 2, 64–65, 245
  object relationships 2
interpersonal-affective focus (IPAF) *see* IPAF
interpersonal-affective patterns 144f
interpretation 166–68
  dynamic 49–51
  helpful questions 168b
  unconscious meaning 203–5
interventions
  mentalizing 172–78
  remission rates 258
  steps 176b
IPAF 7–8, 41, 64–66
  agreed, not forgetting 143
  as an intellectual defence against feeling 230
  attachment strategy employed by patient 94–95
  cautious sharing with patient 129–37

IPAF (cont.)
  childhood experiences 42
  collaboration with patient 130
  conflictual unconscious script 8
  dimensions 111f, 112
  dynamic aspect 49
  focus on affect 66–67
  focus on current
    difficulties 67–68
  focus on patient's mind 68–70
  focus on therapeutic
    relationship 68
  focus of therapy 59–60
  formulation
    construction guide 118–21
    delivery 'in one go' 130
    trial interpretation, working
      towards sharing 121–22
  here-and-now focus 66–68
  identification 51
  linked areas of vulnerability 180
  negotiation, two key questions 89
  over-saturation of formulation 130
  overview 110–12
  patient's disagreement with 131
    case example 131–37
  patient's experience of 113–17
    case example 115–17, 117f
  patient's language and
    metaphors 122–25
    case example 123–25
  presentation 130
  psychodynamic
    formulation 109–10
  recurring object relationship 120
  reverse 233–34
  selecting a focus 128–29
    criteria 129f
  self and object descriptors,
    formulation of IPAF 112
  self-other poles 128, 147, 150
  sharing 121–22, 129–37
  significant refinement in ending
    phase 152
  tracking and activation 143–45
  transference
    interpretation 183–86
  transference/countertransference,
    informing
    formulation 125–27
  trial interpretation, working
    towards sharing 121–22
  unconscious aggression 50
  working with defences 150–53
  see also formulation
isolation 44–45

Johansson, O 334, 337
Joseph, B 227
Jurist, E L 309

Karyotaki, E 328–29
Kazdin, A E 253–54, 262–63
Kernberg, O 26, 28–29, 31, 33, 65, 111
Khalastchy, J 260, 348
Kiesler, D J 9, 34
Klein, J P 29
Kleinian School 27, 28–29
Koelen, J A 304
Kramer, S 26

Landström, C 347–48
Lane, R D 309
language and metaphors 122–25
  case example 123–25
Lear, J 125
Lee, A 10–11
Leichsenring, F 254–55, 267, 349
Leonidaki, V 268
Lindegaard, T 256–57, 328–29
listening
  analytic listening 159
  levels 161f

listening skills 70–71, 157–60
Loewald, H W 27–28
Lumley, M A 309
Lund, C 327–28

McEwen, B S 307
McFarquhar, T 9, 268
McLaughlin, J T 27–28
Mahler, M 30
Main, M 31
major therapies, compared 254–55
Malan, D H 347
manic defences 44
manic phantasies 204
Maunder, R G 307
medical history 86–87
mentalization-based treatment (MBT) 246–47
mentalizing 6, 36–37
  apparent dysfunctions in interpersonal cognition (mentalizing) 10
  attachment relationships 177
  constrained 174
  defined 36
  in DIT 247
  embodied 309–12, 317t
  enhancement, communication analysis 178
  failure 11–12, 172–74
    attachment theory 280–81
    chronic depression 279–83
  flexibility 36
  good, features of 173b
  hypermentalizing 282
  ineffective 280–81, 282–83
  interventions 172–78
    steps 176b
  pretend mode 281–82
  pseudomentalizing 174
  restricted (explains others) 177
  'rewinding' 176–77

second-order 297
teleological mode 281
therapeutic stance 177
treatment-resistant features of complex depression 280
mentalizing
  techniques 294–300
meta-analytic evidence base of psychological treatment 254–57
  brief psychotherapies 255–56
  cost-effectiveness 255–56
  moderation analyses 256
  pooled individual participant data 256
  systematic umbrella review 255
Michels, R 27–28
micro-slicing 338, 339
middle phase of DIT
  agreed IPAF 143–45
  aims and strategies 139–40, 142f
  difficulties 240
  priority of IPAF 145–46, 146b
  relational patterns, attempts at new behaviour 153–55
  relationship-interfering behaviours 154–55
  review of early goals 154
  sequence of sessions 140–42, 142f
  staying focused 145–49, 146b
    case example 147–49
    deviation 146–47
  strategies 142f
  strategies for exploring defences 152
  tracking IPAF 140–42, 143–45
  transference, attempts at new behaviour 153–55
  trial of different ways of responding 154

Mikulincer, M 6, 45–46, 308
Mitchell, S A 26, 28
Modell, A 27–28, 29, 56
mood changes 59, 61*t*, 102–3, 163
mood disorders 7–12, 248
　assumptions 25, 33
　attachment experiences 11
　DIT aims 59–60
　mentalization-based treatment (MBT) 246–47
　treatment 248
　see also depression and/or anxiety
motivation, assessment 16–17
Munholland, K A 31, 32

narcissism 5, 89–90, 103, 231–32, 285
　see also personality disorders
national guidelines, for treatment of depression and/or anxiety 253
National Institute for Health and Care Excellence (2022), data source 253
neurotic defences 44
neurotic phantasies 204–5
neutrality, with abstinence and anonymity 219–20

object relationship, recurring 120
object-related defences 150–51
object-relations theory 26–30
　drive theory replacement 28
　'hard' and 'soft' 28–29
　integration with structural theory 29
　shared assumptions 28
　transference 27–28
observing distance, therapeutic process 221
oedipal compromises 27–28, 46–47

oedipal phantasies 205
omnipotence 44
operational criteria, DSM-III and ICD-11 3–4
outcome monitoring 102–5

paranoid phantasies 204
patient
　defence against being 231
　ego strength 50
patient's current social world 284–85
patient's mind, focus on 68–70
patient's past 249–50
　relationship scenarios with propensity to evoke distress 8–9
patient's sense of agency 286–87
Perepletchikova, F 262–63
perfectionism 45
personality disorders 20, 33, 94–95, 126, 172, 177–78, 268, 280–81
　attachment styles 94–95
　borderline (BPD) 68–69, 247, 335–36
　Cluster C 268
　Kernberg 29
　severe depression 280–81
　see also DITCC; narcissism
personification 34
piercings, body modification 45
post-traumatic stress disorder, DIT approach 261
practice-based evidence 253–54
pretend mode, mentalizing 281–82
primitive defences 43
primitive withdrawal 44
projection 44
projective identification 44
psychiatric classification, operational criteria 3–4

psychic equivalence 173–74, 281
  and teleological modes, suicide
    risk 282–83
psychoanalytic technical
  concepts 37–51
psychoanalytic thought,
  formulation and 29
Psychodynamic Competences
  Framework 37
psychodynamic formulation 109–10
psychodynamic therapy,
  'evidence-based' 257
psychoeducation
  directive techniques 180–81
  vs interpretations 236–37
psychopathology, general or
  p factor 349
psychotherapy
  restricted mentalizing 173–74
  rupture and repair 266–67

questions 161–62, 168*b*

Rao, A S 261, 277, 303–4
rationalization 45
reaction formation 45
recurring interpersonal scenarios 88
reflective practice: monitoring
  countertransference 220–21
relational patterns, attempts at new
  behaviour 153–55
relationship history 91
relationship questionnaire 91–
  95, 92*t*
relationship-interfering behaviours
  (RIBs) 278, 279–80, 291
relationships
  building trust 284
  see also interpersonal narratives
    (INs); therapeutic
    relationship

repression 44
research
  China 260
  clinical competence and measures
    of outcome 266–67
  clinical implications 266–67
  credibility 253
  evidence base for DIT 257–62
    practice-based evidence
      outcomes 253–54, 261–62
  interpersonal relationships 267
  obstacles 262
  randomized controlled trials
    (RCTs) of DIT 253
  Randomized Evaluation of DIT
    (REDIT) 258–60, 268
  time limitation 59, 268
  treatment fidelity, adherence, and
    competence 262–67
  working mechanisms of
    DIT 267–68
resistance
  forms of 226–33
  working with 233–36
    ending phase 216–17
reversal 44
Richards, D 327–28
risk 100–1
  see also self-harm
role responsiveness 49
Ryan, A 347–48
Ryle, A 207
Ryle, C 207

Safran, J D 266–67
Sandler, J 31, 33, 100
Sbarra, D 307
Schafer, R 27–28
Schattner, E 309
schema-of-being-with-another 33
Schwaber, E 27–28

Second Edition, new material 20
secondary attachment
 strategies 308
secondary care patients *see* DIT for complex care (DITCC)
security 35
 earned security 159
 insecurity 35, 46, 158–59
Segal, H 220
Selders, M 261, 304
self and object descriptors, formulation of IPAF 112
self-absorption 285
self-descriptors 122–23
self-development paradox 30
self-esteem, vulnerability 285
self-harm 100–1
 body modification 45
 and risk-taking 45, 281
self-help, internet-delivered DIT formats 327–28
self-reported anxiety/depression, outcomes of DIT 257
self–object representations, sources of information 125
separation and loss 31
session recordings 237–38
Shaver, P R 6, 45–46, 308
Shaw, B 263
signifiers (of interpersonal dynamic) 124–25
silences 161–62
social referencing 30
somatic disorders *see* functional somatic disorders (FSDs)
somatic markers of inner mental states 318*t*
somatizing 45
somatoform disorder 261, 303
 DIT approach 261
Spearman, C 349

splitting 43
Sroufe, J A 31
statistical significance of studies 254–57
Steiner, J 220
Stern, D 28, 33
Stone, L 327–28
Strenger, C 29
stress-related disorders 306–12
structural theory, integration with object-relations theory 29
structure
 questions 161–62
 vs emergence 160–62
subjectivity
 individual, social origins 51
 pretend mode 174
 self–other 33
sublimation 45
substance abuse 45
suicide risk 282–83
 psychic equivalence and teleological modes 282–83
Sullivan, H S 26, 33–36, 76
 interpersonal psychoanalysis 33–36
supportive techniques 171–72
Svartberg, M 263

Tak, L M 307
Target, M 33, 173–74, 280–81
tattooing, body modification 45
Taylor, G J 309
techniques 157–82
teleological mode, restricted mentalizing 281
Thase, M E 327–28
therapeutic alliance, transference and 47–48
therapeutic frame
 in primary care setting 237
 defined 38–40

therapeutic relationship
  challenging the boundaries 230
  difficulties 219–43
  engaging the patient's interest 14
  experience with patient 19–20
  focus on 68
  forms of resistance 226–33
  goodbye letter 207–15
  idealizing therapist 231–32
  interpersonal and affective
    themes 14
  interpersonal scenario 127
  misunderstandings and
    misattunements 222–23
  observing distance 221
  patient's reflection 15
  personal questions about
    therapist 228–29
  requests for direction or
    advice 229–30
  requests for information
    227–28
  resistance
    to time-limited work 232–33
    working with 233–36, 235f
  sexualization 232
  testing by patient 219
  therapist effects 267
  unconscious conflict and
    defences 17–18
  see also therapeutic stance
therapeutic stance 70–72
  case example 223–26
  ending phase of DIT 217–18
  idealizing therapist 231–32
  mentalizing 177, 236–37
  misunderstandings 222–23
  when things go wrong 236–42
  summary 242
therapist, Training and Supervision
  Model Appendix 367

Therapist Competence Scale
  (TCS) 264, 265, 269
therapist effects
  clinical implications 266–67
  idealizing 231–32
  time-limited work 232–33
Town, J M 256
training see DIT training programme
transference
  adjustments 46–48
  bridge to change 195–97
    case example 195–97
  centrality 247–48
  and countertransference
    case example 126–27
    to inform the
      formulation 125–27
  criteria for interpreting 189–94
    case example 191–94
  definition and ubiquity 26, 40–
    41, 46–48
  development 38–39
  early, repressed
    experiences 46–47
  exploring the IPAF 183–86
  formulating a transference
    interpretation 186–89
  functions 125–26
  interpersonal-affective
    patterns 144f
  interpretion 40–41, 46–48
    case example 126–27
  key features of DIT
    transference 247–48
  manifestation 46–47
  negative 247–48
  or very unstable 278
  object-relations patterns 28
  patient's IWMs 46–47
  problematic interpersonal
    patterns 126

transference (*cont.*)
   strategies for exploring
      defences 152
   therapeutic alliance and 47–48
   therapist's understanding 186–89
   two-way unconscious
      communication 48
   unconscious communication 40–41
   understanding 35–36
   value 46–47
   'working in' ability 46–48,
      183–97
   see also countertransference; DIT
      transference; formulation
Truant, G S 16
trust *see* distrust; epistemic trust
trust/distrust issues
   building trusting
      relationships 284
   depression, chronic and
      complex 278, 283–84
Tudur Smith, C 256
'turning against the self' 44

unconscious, dynamic 41–42

unconscious communication
   40–42
   transference 40–41
unconscious phantasies 248–49
undoing 44

van der Vaart, R 327–28
Van Houdenhove, B 11, 307–8
Ventura Wurman, T 263, 264, 265,
   266n.2, 361, 365
verbal contract 99
video/audio recording 102–5
vulnerability 50

Wang, Y 260
Webb, C A 263
Whalley, H C 6
'when things go wrong' 236–42
Wienicke, F J 254–55, 256
Williams, T, *A Streetcar Named
   Desire* 281–82
Wilson, C 347–48
Winnicott, D W 27, 28–29, 39–40
working with resistance, ending
   phase 216–17

The manufacturer's authorised representative in the EU for product safety is Oxford University Press España S.A. of El Parque Empresarial San Fernando de Henares, Avenida de Castilla, 2 - 28830 Madrid (www.oup.es/en or product.safety@oup.com). OUP España S.A. also acts as importer into Spain of products made by the manufacturer.
Printed and bound by CPI Group (UK) Ltd, Croydon, CR0 4YY

02/04/2026

02083135-0007